T0228991

Feline Diabetes

Editor

JACQUIE S. RAND

VETERINARY CLINICS OF NORTH AMERICA: SMALL ANIMAL PRACTICE

www.vetsmall.theclinics.com

March 2013 • Volume 43 • Number 2

ELSEVIER

1600 John F. Kennedy Boulevard • Suite 1800 • Philadelphia, Pennsylvania, 19103-2899

http://www.theclinics.com

VETERINARY CLINICS OF NORTH AMERICA: SMALL ANIMAL PRACTICE Volume 43, Number 2
March 2013 ISSN 0195-5616, ISBN-13: 978-1-4557-7351-0

Editor: John Vassallo; j.vassallo@elsevier.com
Developmental Editor: Teia Stone

© 2013 Elsevier Inc. All rights reserved.

This journal and the individual contributions contained in it are protected under copyright by Elsevier, and the following terms and conditions apply to their use:

Photocopying

Single photocopies of single articles may be made for personal use as allowed by national copyright laws. Permission of the Publisher and payment of a fee is required for all other photocopying, including multiple or systematic copying, copying for advertising or promotional purposes, resale, and all forms of document delivery. Special rates are available for educational institutions that wish to make photocopies for non-profit educational classroom use. For information on how to seek permission visit www.elsevier.com/permissions or call: (+44) 1865 843830 (UK)/(+1) 215 239 3804 (USA).

Derivative Works

Subscribers may reproduce tables of contents or prepare lists of articles including abstracts for internal circulation within their institutions. Permission of the Publisher is required for resale or distribution outside the institution. Permission of the Publisher is required for all other derivative works, including compilations and translations (please consult www.elsevier.com/permissions).

Electronic Storage or Usage

Permission of the Publisher is required to store or use electronically any material contained in this journal, including any article or part of an article (please consult www.elsevier.com/permissions). Except as outlined above, no part of this publication may be reproduced, stored in a retrieval system or transmitted in any form or by any means, electronic, mechanical, photocopying, recording or otherwise, without prior written permission of the Publisher.

Notice

No responsibility is assumed by the Publisher for any injury and/or damage to persons or property as a matter of products liability, negligence or otherwise, or from any use or operation of any methods, products, instructions or ideas contained in the material herein. Because of rapid advances in the medical sciences, in particular, independent verification of diagnoses and drug dosages should be made.

Although all advertising material is expected to conform to ethical (medical) standards, inclusion in this publication does not constitute a guarantee or endorsement of the quality or value of such product or of the claims made of it by its manufacturer.

Veterinary Clinics of North America: Small Animal Practice (ISSN 0195-5616) is published bimonthly (For Post Office use only: volume 42 issue 1 of 6) by Elsevier Inc., 360 Park Avenue South, New York, NY 10010-1710. Months of issue are January, March, May, July, September, and November. Business and Editorial Offices: 1600 John F. Kennedy Blvd., Ste. 1800, Philadelphia, PA 19103-2899. Customer Service Office: 3251 Riverport Lane, Maryland Heights, MO 63043. Periodicals postage paid at New York, NY and additional mailing offices. Subscription prices are $294.00 per year (domestic individuals), $473.00 per year (domestic institutions), $143.00 per year (domestic students/residents), $390.00 per year (Canadian individuals), $580.00 per year (Canadian institutions), $433.00 per year (international individuals), $580.00 per year (international institutions), and $208.00 per year (international and Canadian students/residents). To receive student/resident rate, orders must be accompanied by name of affiliated institution, date of term, and the *signature* of program/residency coordinator on institution letterhead. Orders will be billed at individual rate until proof of status is received. Foreign air speed delivery is included in all *Clinics* subscription prices. All prices are subject to change without notice. **POSTMASTER:** Send address changes to *Veterinary Clinics of North America: Small Animal Practice*, Elsevier Health Sciences Division, Subscription Customer Service, 3251 Riverport Lane, Maryland Heights, MO 63043. Customer Service (orders, claims, online, change of address): Elsevier Periodicals Customer Service, Elsevier Health Sciences Division Subscription Customer Service 3251 Riverport Lane Maryland Heights, MO 63043. Tel: 1-800-654-2452 (U.S. and Canada); 314-447-8871 (outside U.S. and Canada). Fax: 314-447-8029. E-mail: journalscustomerservice-usa@elsevier.com (for print support); journalsonlinesupport-usa@elsevier.com (for online support).

Reprints. For copies of 100 or more of articles in this publication, please contact the Commercial Reprints Department, Elsevier Inc., 360 Park Avenue South, New York, NY 10010-1710. Tel.: 212-633-3812; Fax: 212-462-1935; E-mail: reprints@elsevier.com.

Veterinary Clinics of North America: Small Animal Practice is also published in Japanese by Inter Zoo Publishing Co., Ltd., Aoyama Crystal-Bldg 5F, 3-5-12 Kitaaoyama, Minato-ku, Tokyo 107-0061, Japan.

Veterinary Clinics of North America: Small Animal Practice is covered in *Current Contents/Agriculture, Biology and Environmental Sciences, Science Citation Index, ASCA, MEDLINE/PubMed (Index Medicus), Excerpta Medica,* and *BIOSIS.*

Printed and bound by CPI Group (UK) Ltd, Croydon, CR0 4YY

Transferred to digital print 2013

Contributors

EDITOR

JACQUIE S. RAND, BVSc, DVSc, MANZVS
Diplomate, American College of Veterinary Internal Medicine (Small Animal Internal Medicine); Professor of Companion Animal Health, Director, Centre for Companion Animal Health, School of Veterinary Science, The University of Queensland, Queensland, Australia

AUTHORS

CARLY ANNE BLOOM, DVM
Diplomate, American College of Veterinary Internal Medicine; Clinical Senior Lecturer, Small Animal Internal Medicine, Small Animal Clinic and Veterinary Teaching Hospital, School of Veterinary Science, The University of Queensland, St Lucia, Queensland, Australia

SARAH M.A. CANEY, BVSc, PhD
Diploma in Small Animal Medicine (Feline); MRCVS, Chief Executive, RCVS Specialist in Feline Medicine, Vet Professionals Limited, Midlothian Innovation Centre, Pentlandfield, Roslin, Midlothian, United Kingdom

DAVID B. CHURCH, BVSc, PhD, MACVSc, MRCVS
Vice-principal of Academic and Clinical Affairs, The Royal Veterinary College, University of London, North Mymms, Herts, United Kingdom

EDWARD C. FELDMAN, DVM
Diplomate, American College of Veterinary Internal Medicine; Professor of Small Animal Internal Medicine, Department of Medicine and Epidemiology, School of Veterinary Medicine, University of California-Davis, Davis, California

LINDA FLEEMAN, BVSc, PhD, MANZCVS
Director, Animal Diabetes Australia, Boronia Veterinary Clinic and Hospital, Boronia, Victoria, Australia

YAIZA FORCADA, DVM, MRCVS
Diplomate, European College of Veterinary Internal Medicine; Researcher in Pathogenesis of Feline Diabetes Mellitus, Department of Veterinary Clinical Sciences, The Royal Veterinary College, University of London, North Mymms, Herts, United Kingdom

SARA L. FORD, DVM
Diplomate, American College of Veterinary Internal Medicine (Internal Medicine); Chief of Internal Medicine, VCA Emergency Animal Hospital & Referral Center, San Diego, California

SUSAN GOTTLIEB, BVSc, MANZCVS, BSc(Vet), BAppSc
Veterinarian at The Cat Clinic, Currently enrolled MPhil at The University of Queensland, Brisbane, Queensland, Australia

HEATHER LYNCH, LVT
Technical Director, Tatum Point Animal Hospital, Phoenix, Arizona

STIJN J.M. NIESSEN, DVM, PhD, PGCVetEd, FHEA, MRCVS
Diplomate, European College of Veterinary Internal Medicine; Lecturer Internal Medicine, Department of Veterinary Clinical Sciences, The Royal Veterinary College, University of London, North Mymms, Herts, United Kingdom; Research Associate, Institute for Cellular Medicine, Medical School Newcastle, Newcastle-upon-Tyne, Tyne and Wear, United Kingdom

ISABELLE PADRUTT, DVM
Clinic for Small Animal Internal Medicine, Zurich, Switzerland

CARRIE A. PALM, DVM
Diplomate, American College of Veterinary Internal Medicine; Assistant Clinical Professor of Small Animal Internal Medicine, Department of Medicine and Epidemiology, School of Veterinary Medicine, University of California-Davis, Davis, California

JACQUIE S. RAND, BVSc, DVSc, MANZVS
Diplomate, American College of Veterinary Internal Medicine (Small Animal Internal Medicine); Professor of Companion Animal Health, Director, Centre for Companion Animal Health, School of Veterinary Science, The University of Queensland, Queensland, Australia

CLAUDIA E. REUSCH, DVM, Dr Med Vet
Diplomate, European College of Veterinary Internal Medicine (Companion Animals); Professor of Small Animal Internal Medicine, Clinic for Small Animal Internal Medicine, Zurich, Switzerland

KIRSTEN ROOMP, MSc, Dr rer nat
Luxembourg Centre for Systems Biomedicine, University of Luxembourg, Esch-Belval, Luxembourg

SEAN SURMAN, DVM, MS
Diplomate, American College of Veterinary Internal Medicine; Clinical Senior Lecturer, Small Animal Internal Medicine, Small Animal Clinic and Veterinary Teaching Hospital, School of Veterinary Science, The University of Queensland, St Lucia, Queensland, Australia

DEBRA L. ZORAN, DVM, PhD
Diplomate, American College of Veterinary Internal Medicine (Small Animal Internal Medicine); Associate Professor and Chief of Medicine, Department of Small Animal Clinical Sciences, College of Veterinary Medicine and Biomedical Sciences, Texas A&M University, Texas

Contents

poor glycemic control, hypertension, and microalbuminuria, as well as genetic factors. In both type 1 and 2 diabetics with nephropathy, structural changes occur in the kidneys before overt clinical disease. Studies suggest that some of the risk factors and structural renal changes of human diabetes also exist in diabetic dogs and cats. This article assembles existing information on the presence of risk factors, laboratory and histologic findings, and consequences of human diabetic nephropathy as applied to cats.

Jacquie S. Rand

Diabetic ketoacidosis and hyperosmolar hyperglycemic state are 2 potentially life-threatening presentations of feline diabetes mellitus. Presentations range from mildly anorexic cats with diabetic ketoacidosis to comatose cats with diabetic ketoacidosis or hyperosmolar hyperglycemic state. Such cases are the result of severe insulin deficiency and/or concurrent disease, resulting in nausea and vomiting, electrolyte and water losses, acidosis, and circulatory collapse. The condition requires careful attention to supportive care to correct fluid and electrolyte abnormalities, treatment of concurrent diseases, and reversal of the effects of insulin deficiency. However, early diagnosis of diabetes mellitus and institution of appropriate insulin therapy prevents these complications.

Sean Surman and Linda Fleeman

The use of continuous glucose monitoring systems in veterinary patients is summarized and discussed. The current clinical uses in veterinary medicine, including monitoring of hospitalized/sick diabetic patients, long-term monitoring of stable diabetic patients, anesthetized patients, and other patients with altered blood glucose homeostasis are presented. The most important advantage of these systems over intermittent blood glucose measurements is that they facilitate detection of brief periods of hypoglycemia and provide information overnight. The accuracy and advantages/disadvantages compared with traditional monitoring are addressed. The technology involved in the currently available monitoring systems is also discussed.

Carrie A. Palm and Edward C. Feldman

Diabetes mellitus is a common disease in cats. Similar to people, cats with diabetes mellitus often have type 2 disease. Oral hypoglycemic drugs can be a potential treatment option for affected cats, especially when cats or owners do not tolerate administration of injectable insulin. Several classes of oral hypoglycemic drugs have been evaluated in cats but these drugs have not been commonly used for treatment of diabetic cats. With the advent of newer oral hypoglycemic drugs, and a better understanding of diabetes mellitus in cats, further investigation may allow for better diabetic control for feline patients.

Incretins (gastric inhibitory polypeptide and glucagon-like peptide 1 [GLP-1]) are hormones released from the gastrointestinal tract during food intake that potentiate insulin secretion. Native GLP-1 is quickly degraded by the enzyme dipeptidylpeptidase-4 (DPP-4), which has led to the development of GLP-1 agonists with resistance to degradation and to inhibitors of DPP-4 activity as therapeutic agents in humans with type 2 diabetes. In healthy cats, GLP-1 agonists and DPP-4 inhibitors have produced a substantial increase in insulin secretion. Although results of clinical studies are not yet available, incretin-based therapy promises to become an important new research area in feline diabetes.

VETERINARY CLINICS OF NORTH AMERICA: SMALL ANIMAL PRACTICE

THE CLINICS ARE NOW AVAILABLE ONLINE!
Access your subscription at:
www.theclinics.com

Preface

Feline Diabetes

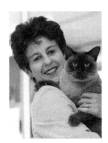

Jacquie S. Rand, BVSc, DVSc, MANZVS, DACVIM
Editor

This feline diabetes edition was inspired by the many feline patients, their owners, and their veterinarians around the globe who asked questions and challenged the dogma.

In the last 8 years there have been major changes in the way we manage our feline patients, which have resulted in vastly improved outcomes for newly diagnosed diabetic cats. With the advent of long-acting insulin and low-carbohydrate diets, we are achieving outcomes that were not attainable 10 years ago. The next revolution in managing diabetics, I believe, will involve home monitoring and tighter glycemic control.

Successful outcomes rely on committed owners working closely with veterinarians who are up to date with the latest research on the management of diabetes. This issue is a compilation of knowledge from some of the most experienced veterinarians in the world in the area of feline diabetes.

My hope is that this feline diabetes edition will support veterinarians in practice and assist them to help their feline diabetic patients better.

Many thanks to the contributing authors; without their expert knowledge, this edition would not be possible. Thanks also to John Vassallo, editor at Saunders/Elsevier, for his patience and assistance in completing this work.

This edition is dedicated to those who shaped my life:

To my husband Tom, my rock, my greatest supporter, and my sanctuary in stormy seas.

To my dad, who taught me that "if a job is worth doing, it is worth doing well," and that "a job is not done until it is finished."

To my mum, who was always a cheerful supporter in all the twists and turns in my life.

To my daughter, Lisette, who reminded me when it was time to play, and the importance of having a balanced life.

To the owners, their diabetic pets, veterinarians, and students, who inspired, taught, and challenged me.

Vet Clin Small Anim 43 (2013) xi–xii
http://dx.doi.org/10.1016/j.cvsm.2013.02.001
0195-5616/13/$ – see front matter © 2013 Published by Elsevier Inc.

vetsmall.theclinics.com

And, finally, to Merlin (pictured), our Burmese cat, with a very special personality, who was rescued from the municipal pound and who helped me understand better the effect of high-carbohydrate diets in cats. Merlin was insulin resistant all his adult life and was glucose intolerant and prediabetic for much of his senior years, but thanks to a low-carbohydrate diet and calorie counting, he never developed diabetes.

Thank you all and bless you.

Jacquie S. Rand, BVSc, DVSc, MANZVS, DACVIM
(Small Animal Internal Medicine)
Centre for Companion Animal Health
School of Veterinary Science
The University of Queensland
Queensland 4072, Australia

E-mail address:
j.rand@uq.edu.au

Pathogenesis of Feline Diabetes

Jacquie S. Rand, BVSc, DVSc, MANZVS, DACVIM

KEYWORDS

- Feline • Diabetes mellitus • Type 2 diabetes • Pathogenesis

KEY POINTS

- Diabetes is essentially a disease of insulin secretory failure caused by damage to pancreatic islet β cells.
- Diabetes in cats is most commonly type 2, which is caused by β-cell failure in the presence of insulin resistance caused by obesity.
- The mechanisms of β-cell failure are still debated, but intracellular amyloid oligomers are a likely contributor in early stages, and glucose toxicity contributes to further β-cell damage and maintenance of the diabetic state.
- Other causes of β-cell failure include widespread damage to the pancreas by pancreatitis, and diseases that increase insulin resistance such as acromegaly.
- Diabetes is a disease of insulin deficiency.
- Insulin requirement can be increased by obesity, acromegaly, inflammation, and concurrent endocrine disease.
- Insulin secretion can be decreased by damage to pancreatic β cells by inflammation, glucose toxicity, reactive oxygen species, toxic intracellular oligomers, or mechanisms as yet unknown.

INTRODUCTION

Diabetes mellitus (diabetes) is defined as persistent hyperglycemia caused by a relative or absolute insulin deficiency. Insulin is exclusively produced by the β cells of the islets of Langerhans in the pancreas, and insulin deficiency occurs when β cells are destroyed or their function is impaired. The mechanisms involved in causing loss of β-cell function are the basis for the classification of diabetes. The mechanisms underlying β-cell damage might also create therapeutic targets to prevent the onset of diabetes or specific treatment of the underlying disease process.

At present there is no consensus in the veterinary literature on what blood glucose concentration should be classed as diabetic. Typically diabetes is diagnosed when blood glucose concentration is above the renal threshold, causing obligatory water loss and hence the signs of polyuria and polydipsia. These signs are associated with

Centre for Companion Animal Health, School of Veterinary Science, The University of Queensland, Australia
E-mail address: j.rand@uq.edu.au

Vet Clin Small Anim 43 (2013) 221–231
http://dx.doi.org/10.1016/j.cvsm.2013.01.003
0195-5616/13/$ – see front matter Crown Copyright © 2013 Published by Elsevier Inc. All rights reserved.

vetsmall.theclinics.com

a blood glucose concentration of 14 to 16 mmol/L (234–288 mg/dL) or higher.[1] Various cutpoints have been used in the veterinary literature, and 10 mmol/L (180 mg/dL) was proposed by Crenshaw and Peterson.[2] In human patients, however, the cutoff blood glucose concentration for diabetes mellitus has been lowered consistently over time as more information has become available on the adverse effects of mild hyperglycemia, including microvascular damage and retinopathy. At present, 7.1 mmol/L or 126 mg/dL is used.[3] Cats notably have fasting glucose concentrations similar to those of humans.[4] Recent research in client-owned cats suggest that the cutpoint for normal fasting glucose concentration is 6.3 mmol/L in healthy, nonobese cats 8 years of age or older, and cats with persistent glucose concentrations above this value but below diabetic concentrations should be considered as having impaired fasting glucose.[5] Humans with impaired fasting glucose or impaired glucose tolerance based on increased 2-hour glucose concentrations in a glucose tolerance test are considered prediabetic and at greatly increased risk of developing diabetes. A recent study of diabetic cats in remission found that fasting glucose concentrations greater than 6.5 mmol/L (117 mg/dL) or glucose concentration greater than 6.5 mmol/L (117 mg/dL) at 4 hours after a glucose challenge (1 g/kg) were predictive of relapse, suggesting that cats with glucose concentrations greater than 6.5 mmol/L should also be considered prediabetic.[5] In humans, approximately 50% of patients with diabetes are undiagnosed, and there are 2 to 4 times more patients considered prediabetic than diabetic.[3] It is likely that there are also many undiagnosed diabetic and prediabetic cats.

In humans, diabetes is classified based on the pathogenesis of β-cell failure as type 1, type 2, gestational diabetes, and other specific types of diabetes.[6] Type 1 diabetes is caused by autoimmune damage to pancreatic β cells. Type 2 diabetes is characterized by insulin resistance with concomitant β-cell failure, which in humans is often relative rather than absolute failure of insulin secretion. Type 2 diabetes occurs when β cells fail to secrete adequate insulin, although there is no consensus about the leading mechanism(s) of β-cell damage. Typically type 2 diabetes occurs when insulin requirements are increased by a chronic fuel surfeit and insulin resistance.[7] Insulin sensitivity/resistance has a genetic predisposition,[8] but the most common acquired insulin resistance in type 2 diabetes is obesity associated. In type 2 diabetes insulin secretion is defective, and is insufficient to compensate for the insulin resistance. Gestational diabetes is defined as diabetes that is first diagnosed during pregnancy.[9] If diabetes persists after the end of pregnancy, it is reclassified as one of the other types. The classification "other specific types of diabetes" includes all the other causes of diabetes.[6] Broadly these include diseases that damage the whole pancreas (such as pancreatitis, pancreatic carcinoma, and pancreatectomy), toxic causes of β-cell damage (such as by the antineoplastic drug streptozotocin or rare drug reactions such as to the thiazide diuretics, glucocorticoids, and thyroid hormone), genetic causes of diabetes (resulting in β-cell failure or insulin resistance, such as various rare single-gene causes of diabetes and leprechaunism), and diabetes types associated with other endocrine diseases (such as hyperadrenocorticism, acromegaly, and glucagonoma).

In cats, diabetes that is analogous or similar to several human diabetes types has been recognized. Most commonly, feline diabetes is of a type similar to type 2 diabetes.[10] Cats also exhibit several types of diabetes that under the human classification system would be classified as other specific types, including diabetes associated with acromegaly,[11] hyperadrenocorticism, and pancreatic carcinoma.[12] Although many diabetic cats have histologic evidence of pancreatitis, in some cats it is not clear whether the diabetes is the cause or consequence of chronic pancreatitis.[12,13] Some diabetic cats, however, do have classic signs and biochemical evidence of acute pancreatitis at the time of onset of diabetes, and may later achieve remission at a time when clinical and biochemical signs of pancreatitis have resolved. Clinical and histologic findings consistent with type 1 diabetes was reported in a 5-month-old kitten,[14] and recent research has demonstrated T-cell lymphocytes within pancreatic islets of diabetic cats, suggesting that autoimmune damage and, therefore, type 1 diabetes might occur in cats,[13] although it appears to be very rare.

PATHOGENESIS OF TYPE 2 DIABETES IN CATS

Human type 2 diabetes has a complex etiology and is caused by a combination of genetic factors and environmental interactions, and there is an increased risk with aging. There is strong evidence that the same factors are also important in cats.

The susceptibility to type 2 diabetes in human beings, monkeys, and rodents is inherited, and there are preliminary data supporting a genetic influence in cats.[12] Diabetes is most common in domestic long-haired and short-haired cats. Burmese cats are overrepresented, and many other pure breeds are underrepresented, in comparison with the incidence in domestic cats. The Burmese breed is overrepresented in Australia, New Zealand,[15,16] and the United Kingdom.[17] The frequency of diabetes in the Burmese breed is approximately 4 times the rate in domestic cats in Australia, with 1 in 50 Burmese affected compared with less than 1 in 200 domestic cats.[18] In some Burmese families, more than 10% of the offspring are affected.[18] The genetic factors predisposing cats to diabetes are unknown.

In human patients, a family history of type 2 diabetes is an important risk factor, increasing the risk by 3.5 and 6 times if one or both parents are diabetic, respectively.[19] There is a high concordance rate of diabetes in identical twins, and to a lesser degree also in nonidentical twins. In one study of identical twins the concordance rate was 58%, in contrast to an expected prevalence of 10%.[20] This high concordance rate is highly suggestive of a genetic determination. However, the fact that concordance rates do not reach 100% in identical twins, which share 100% of their genes, means that genetic factors are not solely responsible for the development of diabetes.

Although the genetics of type 2 diabetes are far from being well established, there are interesting trends emerging. It has been discovered that most of the genetic markers associated with increased risk for the metabolic syndrome, a prediabetic syndrome in humans, are located within genes known to be associated with lipid metabolism.[8] Studies in humans examining genetic contributors to obesity, the major preventable risk factor for type 2 diabetes, have found more than 30 associated genes, with many of these involved in neural function.[21] This finding supports the hypothesis that hypothalamic or other neural function underlies the development of obesity.[22] Other genes associated with type 2 diabetes code for proteins that are involved in insulin sensitivity, insulin signaling, and the regulation of gene transcription.[21]

In a recent study in Burmese cats, lean Burmese demonstrated gene expression patterns similar to those of as age-matched and gender-matched obese domestic cats for the majority of the genes examined, and the pattern of gene expression suggested possible aberrations in lipogenesis.[23] Moreover, lean Burmese displayed an approximately 3- to 4-fold increase in the percentage of very-low-density cholesterol fraction, which was double that of obese domestic cats, indicating an increased degree of lipid dysregulation, especially in relation to triglycerides. The findings of this study suggest that Burmese cats have a genetic propensity for dysregulation in lipid metabolism, which may predispose them to diabetes in their senior years.[23]

The key to understanding the pathogenesis of type 2 diabetes is to recognize that in normal individuals β cells are responsive to the need for insulin secretion, and will undergo hypertrophy and hyperplasia to meet increased insulin needs.[24] Insulin needs change largely as a result of changes in insulin sensitivity. Insulin sensitivity is defined as the effectiveness of a given concentration of insulin to decrease blood glucose. If insulin sensitivity is decreased (ie, if insulin resistance occurs), more insulin is needed to maintain glucose concentrations below the set point for insulin secretion. Type 2 diabetes occurs when insulin sensitivity is decreased and compensatory insulin secretion fails in association with β-cell failure.

Decreased Insulin Sensitivity

Insulin sensitivity varies widely even in normal cats, but is lower in males and is decreased in obesity.[25] In human beings, insulin sensitivity is also decreased in various disease states including inflammatory disease,[26] polycystic ovary syndrome,[27] hyperadrenocorticism,[28] and pheochromocytoma,[29,30] in response to drugs such as glucocorticoids and atypical antipsychotic agents,[31,32] and during pregnancy.[9] In both cats and humans, obesity is the leading acquired cause of insulin resistance. For example, weight gain of 44% over 10 months in cats resulted in a 50% decrease in insulin sensitivity.[25] Obesity causes insulin resistance through a variety of mechanisms, including changes in adipose-secreted hormones, and through systemic inflammatory mediators.[33,34] Acromegaly appears to be an underdiagnosed cause of insulin resistance in diabetic cats[11] (see the article elsewhere in this issue on hypersomatotropism, acromegaly, and hyperadrenocorticism and feline diabetes mellitus.), whereas hyperadrenocorticism is a rare cause of feline diabetes[35] (see article by Niessen SJM and collegues elsewhere in this issue).

Hormones secreted by adipose tissue (adipokines) were first discovered around 20 years ago, and since then more than 100 such hormones have been discovered. One adipokine of particular importance to diabetes is adiponectin, a hormone that has effects on the liver, skeletal muscle, the pancreatic islets, and adipose tissue itself.[36] Unlike other adipokines, adiponectin concentrations are decreased with increasing obesity. Because adiponectin increases insulin sensitivity, the decreased concentrations that occur with obesity are associated with insulin resistance. Adiponectin is present in circulation as multimers composed of varying numbers of trimers.[37] Low molecular weight trimers and hexamers (collectively called low molecular weight adiponectin) have less biological activity on glucose homeostasis than high molecular weight multimers composed of 12, 18, or more adiponectin monomers.[38] In cats, adiponectin has been shown to be associated with diet[39] and obesity,[40] but studies linking it with insulin sensitivity and diabetes are currently lacking. Leptin has also been examined in cats. Leptin concentrations are increased in obesity,[40–42] and are independently associated with decreased insulin sensitivity,[41] and therefore may be associated with the pathogenesis of diabetes in cats.

Other adipokines are secreted by adipose tissue in increasing concentrations in the presence of obesity.[33] Many of these are inflammatory mediators, including interleukins and tumor necrosis factor.[34,43] These hormones decrease the intracellular effects of insulin by increasing phosphorylation of insulin receptor substrate, which mediates the effects of insulin after it binds to insulin receptors in muscle and adipose tissue.[43] By decreasing the effects of insulin, these proinflammatory adipokines are involved in decreasing insulin sensitivity.

Decreased Insulin Secretion

Insulin secretion is increased in response to decreased insulin sensitivity.[24] In normal individuals, insulin secretion increases as insulin sensitivity decreases, and the product of insulin secretion and insulin sensitivity (ie, insulin secretion multiplied by insulin sensitivity) stays constant.[44] However, compensation fails once β cells are unable to further increase insulin production, or when more insulin-producing β cells cannot be produced by compensatory hypertrophy. In the past, β-cell "exhaustion" secondary to chronic hyperfunction has been invoked as a simplistic explanation of β-cell failure in insulin-resistant individuals. However, many individual insulin-resistant cats[10] and humans[45,46] compensate adequately for insulin resistance and do not progress to diabetes mellitus. Similarly, type 2 diabetes does not appear to occur at all in other species such as dogs, even though they do exhibit similar degrees of insulin resistance.[47] The concept of β-cell exhaustion lacks a mechanistic basis and fails to explain species differences in susceptibility to type 2 diabetes, which occurs in humans,[6] cats,[10] some nonhuman primates,[48] and laboratory rodents,[49] but not in dogs[10] or other species, regardless of the presence of obesity. Other endocrine cells do not exhibit exhaustion (eg, chronic stress does not lead to hypoadrenocorticism and chronic dehydration does not cause diabetes insipidus), so it seems improbable that an increased requirement for insulin secretion per se leads to β-cell failure.

Recent work in gestational diabetes in human beings has advanced the understanding of the development of diabetes mellitus in insulin-resistant states.[9] Pregnant women are insulin resistant, and some women develop diabetes during pregnancy but recover after giving birth.[50] These women are at increased risk for developing diabetes subsequently, and the relative prevalence of each of the categories of diabetes that these women subsequently develop is very similar to that in the wider population.[9] This fact suggests that insulin resistance itself does not cause diabetes, but rather that it highlights individuals with early stages of β-cell failure by increasing the demand for insulin. This increased demand cannot be met by the failing β cells. It seems likely that obesity and other insulin-resistant states act similarly to increase the need for insulin secretion by β cells, which cannot be met in individuals whose β cells are damaged by some other disease process. In fact, obesity increases the demand on β cells to produce insulin while processes associated with obesity simultaneously appear to damage β cells, reducing secretory capacity.

Theories about the cause of this failure of compensation have included damage to pancreatic islets by amyloid deposition and a variation of the amyloid hypothesis called the toxic oligomer hypothesis; toxicity by glucose, lipids, or both; reactive oxygen species; and inflammatory cytokines.

Amyloid is an accumulation of protein strands that have refolded from their normal, functional shape to form abnormal, nonfunctional, β-pleated sheets.[51] Protein in β-pleated sheet conformation is resistant to degradation by proteases, and tends to recruit more protein to transform into the altered conformation, so that more and more amyloid material accumulates.[51] Within pancreatic islets, the abnormal protein that forms amyloid has been identified as amylin (also called islet amyloid polypeptide), a hormone that is cosecreted with insulin and is secreted in disproportionately larger quantities in individuals with insulin resistance, which increases the amount of amylin available to contribute to amyloid accumulation within pancreatic islets.[51] Amyloid is almost universally present in individuals with type 2 diabetes (both humans and cats[51,52]). In an experimental model of induced diabetes in cats, islet amyloid was not evident before the induction of diabetes, but was present in all 4 glipizide-treated and in 1 of 4 insulin-treated cats 18 months after diabetes was induced by 50% pancreatectomy and 4 months of dexamethasone and growth hormone treatment.[53] Islet amyloid was an appealing potential cause of β-cell failure, especially because it explains the species differences in susceptibility to type 2 diabetes. The amino acid sequence of amylin in dogs is different from that in humans and cats, and does not form β-pleated sheets in dogs. However, the amyloid theory has largely been abandoned as a viable hypothesis for several reasons. First, the amyloid hypothesis fails the test of dose-response; that is, the severity or likelihood of diabetes and the degree of impairment of insulin secretion are not related to the amount of amyloid present in islets. Second, many normal individuals have amyloid within the islets but have normal insulin secretion. Finally, the amyloid hypothesis seems implausible because all cells within pancreatic islets (α, β, and δ cells) are exposed to amyloid but only β-cell function is impaired, whereas glucagon production by α cells is increased in type 2 diabetes.[54,55]

The toxic oligomer hypothesis is similar to the amyloid hypothesis in that it is also based on toxicity of polymerized, misfolded amylin, but differs from the amyloid hypothesis because toxicity is attributed to intracellular amyloid fibril rather than the inert extracellular form.[56,57] Unlike amyloid, which is visible with light microscopy, intracellular amyloid fibrils are not visible at the microscopic level but trigger β-cell death through the misfolded protein response, which triggers programmed cell death (apoptosis) when misfolded protein is detected within the endoplasmic reticulum.[57,58] The toxic oligomer hypothesis helps explain why β cells are affected by amyloid toxicity whereas other islet cells are not, because only β cells produce amyloid, and so are the only cells that are exposed to the more toxic nanofibrils that form intracellularly.[58] It also accounts for why cats and humans, but not dogs, are susceptible to type 2 diabetes. However, more work is needed to clarify the role of amylin oligomers in the pathogenesis of type 2 diabetes, because there are still limitations with this hypothesis, including clarification of the oligomers involved and the importance of the role of toxic oligomers.[59] One important limitation is that amylin and insulin are cosecreted, so that individuals with insulin resistance and compensatory hyperinsulinemia also have high amylin secretion and should form toxic amylin oligomers. However, this does not occur for many individuals. Modifications of the theory are still needed to clarify the conditions under which amylin forms toxic intracellular oligomers.[59]

Glucose toxicity was initially proposed to occur at very high glucose concentrations (>15 mmol/L, 540 mg/dL) and to act as a secondary mechanism that would accelerate β-cell failure in individuals with some other cause of inadequate insulin secretion.[60] However, subsequent studies in rats found that glucose toxicity can cause impaired β-cell function at glucose concentrations that are only 1 mmol/L (18 mg/dL) higher than normal, suggesting that it acts much earlier in the pathogenesis of diabetes than had previously been thought. Chronic hyperglycemia and hyperlipidemia contribute to changes in the microenvironment in the endoplasmic reticulum, where proteins are assembled, modified, and folded. These changes in the endoplasmic reticulum can trigger β-cell death through the unfolded protein response, a mechanism that monitors the volume of proteins that have not folded and assembled properly and which can trigger apoptosis if the number of such proteins is too high. This mechanism is an important contributor to β-cell death in diabetes.[61] Cats are susceptible to glucose toxicity at high glucose concentrations,[62] and good control of blood glucose concentrations in diabetic cats can lead to remission of diabetes,[63] so glucose toxicity very likely plays an important role in the development or maintenance of inadequate insulin secretion in type 2 diabetes in cats. However, the initial development of abnormally high blood glucose concentrations implies that insulin secretion is already impaired before glucose toxicity can exist, meaning that glucose toxicity is an unlikely primary mechanism in the development of type 2 diabetes.

Damage to β cells by reactive oxygen species is proposed as a primary mechanism causing initiation of β-cell damage, thus triggering the development of impaired insulin secretion, and also as a mechanism to promote or maintain further β-cell death in individuals with existing diabetes.[64] Reactive oxygen species are generated when there is excess fuel (such as glucose or fatty acids) in the cell.[64,65] β Cells are particularly prone to this because intracellular glucose concentrations reflect plasma glucose concentrations, allowing β cells to sense and respond to changes in plasma glucose.[64] Oxidation of intracellular glucose and fatty acids causes increased electrochemical gradients across the mitochondrial membrane, which can damage the cell by causing increased production of reactive oxygen species. Affected cells respond by producing uncoupling protein 2, which safely dissipates the increased electrochemical gradient, but at the expense of production of adenosine triphosphate (ATP). Because ATP production within β cells is the trigger for insulin secretion, production of uncoupling protein 2 has the effect of keeping the β cells alive, but still has the effect of decreasing insulin production.[65] However, this theory by itself does not explain why cats and humans, but not dogs, develop type 2 diabetes.

Inflammation triggered by autoimmunity has long been known to have a role in type 1 diabetes, but there is also evidence of inflammation in type 2 diabetes.[66] Pancreatic islets in humans with type 2 diabetes exhibit inflammatory cell infiltration, increased cytokine expression, and fibrosis, the hallmark of chronic inflammation.[66] Inflammation is triggered within pancreatic islets as well as systemically by adipose tissue. Adipose tissue (adipocytes themselves and macrophages that reside alongside adipocytes) can secrete many cytokines, and obesity is associated with systemic changes in inflammatory proteins including cytokines such as tumor necrosis factor and interleukins,[67] and acute phase proteins such as C-reactive protein, haptoglobin, and fibrinogen.[66] In addition, β cells themselves secrete cytokines, especially interleukin-1, which initiate an inflammatory cascade in response to nutrient overload.[66] Proinflammatory cytokines, whether secreted remotely or locally by β cells, affect β-cell function and can trigger apoptosis. Recent trials in humans suggest that this mechanism can be targeted to protect against the development of type 2 diabetes.[68] Studies of this group of mechanisms in cats have not been done.

In summary, none of the proposed mechanisms of β-cell failure, except amyloid oligomers, explains the difference in species susceptibility to type 2 diabetes, and this theory needs further refinement to explain individual differences in susceptibility of insulin-resistant individuals to type 2 diabetes.

PATHOGENESIS OF FELINE ACROMEGALY (HYPERSOMATOTROPISM)

Although obesity is the most common cause of insulin resistance that leads to increased insulin requirements and diabetes mellitus, other causes have been documented. One such is acromegaly, which is the result of increased secretion of growth hormone by a pituitary tumor.[11] Diabetes caused by acromegaly typically involves cats with extreme insulin resistance and, hence very high insulin dose requirements.[69] However, with increased surveillance for acromegaly, feline diabetic patients are being diagnosed that are not clinically insulin resistant based on insulin dose, and occasionally achieve remission without treatment for acromegaly (Stjin Niessen, personal communication, 2012). What is not currently understood is whether or how acromegaly (and other endocrine diseases that cause insulin resistance and are associated with other specific types of diabetes) contributes to β-cell failure. Acromegalic cats have evidence of β-cell hyperplasia and following successful tumor removal, some cats exhibit transient signs of hypoglycemia, which can be severe and life threatening (Hans Kooistra, personal communication, 2012). This subject is covered in more detail in the article elsewhere in this issue on hypersomatotropism, acromegaly, hyperadrenocorticism, and feline diabetes mellitus.

PATHOGENESIS OF PANCREATITIS-ASSOCIATED DIABETES

Pancreatitis causes diabetes by causing widespread inflammatory damage and fibrosis throughout the exocrine pancreas, which incidentally also destroys the endocrine pancreas.[10] The difficulty of reliably diagnosing pancreatitis in cats is exacerbated by the limited research on this clinical entity,[70] but there are several features expected in cats with pancreatitis-associated diabetes. Pancreatitis in cats is strongly associated with inflammatory bowel disease and cholangiohepatitis.[71] These disorders are chronic inflammatory diseases that are expected to cause waxing and waning insulin resistance as well as very variable insulin requirements, intermittent loss of appetite and ketosis, and weight loss. The outcome is diabetic cats that are difficult to regulate well because of changing insulin requirements and periodic appearance of signs such as inappetence associated with the underlying disease (see the article elsewhere in this issue on pancreatitis and diabetes).

SUMMARY

Diabetes is essentially a failure of insulin secretion caused by damage to pancreatic islet β cells. Diabetes in cats is most commonly type 2, which is caused by β-cell failure in the presence of insulin resistance resulting from obesity. The mechanisms of β-cell failure are still debated, but intracellular amyloid oligomers are a likely contributor in the early stages, and glucose toxicity contributes to further β-cell damage and maintenance of the diabetic state. Other causes of β-cell failure include widespread damage to the pancreas by pancreatitis, and diseases of increased insulin resistance such as acromegaly.

ACKNOWLEDGMENTS

Manuscript preparation and editorial assistance was provided by Kurt Verkest of VetWrite (vetwrite@gmail.com).

REFERENCES

1. Rand JS. Feline diabetes mellitus. In: Mooney CT, Peterson ME, editors. BSAVA Manual of Canine and Feline Endocrinology. 4th edition. UK: British Small Animal Vet. Assoc; 2012. p. 133–47.
2. Crenshaw K, Peterson M. Pretreatment clinical and laboratory evaluation of cats with diabetes mellitus: 104 cases (1992-1994). J Am Vet Med Assoc 1996;209(5): 943.
3. American Diabetes Association. Diagnosis and classification of diabetes mellitus. Diabetes Care 2010;33(Suppl 1):S62–9.
4. Reeve-Johnson M, Rand J, Anderson S, et al. Determination of reference values for casual blood glucose concentration in clinically-healthy, aged cats measured with a portable glucose meter from an ear or paw sample [abstract]. J Vet Int Med May 1, 2012;26(3):755.
5. Gottlieb S, Rand J, Marshall R. Diabetic cats in remission have mildly impaired glucose tolerance [abstract]. Paper presented at: Australian College of Veterinary Scientists Science Week June, 2012. Gold Coast, Australia.
6. Expert Committee on the Diagnosis and Classification of Diabetes Mellitus. Report of the Expert Committee on the Diagnosis and Classification of Diabetes Mellitus. Diabetes Care 1997;20(7):1183–97.
7. Nolan CJ, Damm P, Prentki M. Type 2 diabetes across generations: from pathophysiology to prevention and management. Lancet 2011;378(9786):169–81.
8. Povel C, Boer J, Reiling E, et al. Genetic variants and the metabolic syndrome: a systematic review. Obes Rev 2011;12(11):952–67.

9. Buchanan TA, Xiang A, Kjos SL, et al. What is gestational diabetes? Diabetes Care 2007;30(Suppl 2):S105–11.

10. Rand JS, Fleeman LM, Farrow HA, et al. Canine and feline diabetes mellitus: nature or nurture? J Nutr 2004;134(Suppl 8):2072S–80S.

11. Niessen SJM, Petrie G, Gaudiano F, et al. Feline acromegaly: an underdiagnosed endocrinopathy? J Vet Intern Med 2007;21(5):899–905.

12. Goossens MM, Nelson RW, Feldman EC, et al. Response to insulin treatment and survival in 104 cats with diabetes mellitus (1985-1995). J Vet Intern Med 1998; 12(1):1–6.

13. Zini E, Lunardi F, Zanetti R, et al. Histological investigation of endocrine and exocrine pancreas in cats with diabetes mellitus [abstract]. The European College of Veterinary Internal Medicine, Companion Animals Congress. Maastricht, September, 2012: EN-0-2.

14. Woods J, Panciera D, Snyder P, et al. Diabetes mellitus in a kitten. J AM Anim Hosp Assoc 1994;30:177–80.

15. Wade C, Gething M, Rand J. Evidence of a genetic basis for diabetes mellitus in Burmese cats. J Vet Intern Med 1999;13(3):269.

16. Rand J, Bobbermien L, Hendrikz J, et al. Over representation of Burmese cats with diabetes mellitus. Aust Vet J 1997;75(6):402–4.

17. McCann TM, Simpson KE, Shaw DJ, et al. Feline diabetes mellitus in the UK: the prevalence within an insured cat population and a questionnaire-based putative risk factor analysis. J Feline Med Surg 2007;9(4):289–99.

18. Lederer R, Rand J, Jonsson N, et al. Frequency of feline diabetes mellitus and breed predisposition in domestic cats in Australia. Vet J 2009;179(2):254–8.

19. Meigs JB, Cupples LA, Wilson P. Parental transmission of type 2 diabetes: the Framingham Offspring Study. Diabetes 2000;49(12):2201–7.

20. Newman B, Selby J, King MC, et al. Concordance for type 2 (non-insulin-dependent) diabetes mellitus in male twins. Diabetologia 1987;30(10):763–8.

21. Feero WG, Guttmacher AE, McCarthy MI. Genomics, type 2 diabetes, and obesity. N Engl J Med 2010;363(24):2339–50.

22. Hochberg I, Hochberg Z. Expanding the definition of hypothalamic obesity. Obes Rev 2010;11(10):709–21.

23. Lee P, Mori A, Coradini M, et al. Potential predictive biomarkers of obesity in Burmese cats. Vet J 2012. [Epub ahead of print].

24. Ahrén B, Pacini G. Islet adaptation to insulin resistance: mechanisms and implications for intervention. Diabetes Obes Metab 2005;7(1):2–8.

25. Appleton DJ, Rand JS, Sunvold GD. Insulin sensitivity decreases with obesity, and lean cats with low insulin sensitivity are at greatest risk of glucose intolerance with weight gain. J Feline Med Surg 2001;3(4):211–28.

26. Browning LM. n-3 Polyunsaturated fatty acids, inflammation and obesity-related disease. Proc Nutr Soc 2003;62(2):447–53.

27. Legro RS, Finegood D, Dunaif A. A fasting glucose to insulin ratio is a useful measure of insulin sensitivity in women with polycystic ovary syndrome. J Clin Endocrinol Metab 1998;83(8):2694–8.

28. Biering H, Knappe G, Gerl H, et al. [Prevalence of diabetes in acromegaly and Cushing syndrome]. Acta Med Austriaca 2000;27(1):27–31 [in German].

29. Blüher M, Windgassen M, Paschke R. Improvement of insulin sensitivity after adrenalectomy in patients with pheochromocytoma. Diabetes Care 2000;23(10):1591.

30. Stenstrom G, Sjostrom L, Smith U. Diabetes mellitus in phaeochromocytoma. Fasting blood glucose levels before and after surgery in 60 patients with phaeochromocytoma. Acta Endocrinol (Copenh) 1984;106(4):511–5.

31. Elias AN, Hofflich H. Abnormalities in glucose metabolism in patients with schizophrenia treated with atypical antipsychotic medications. Am J Med 2008;121(2): 98–104 [see comment].
32. Qi D, Pulinilkunnil T, An D, et al. Single-dose dexamethasone induces whole-body insulin resistance and alters both cardiac fatty acid and carbohydrate metabolism. Diabetes 2004;53(7):1790–7.
33. Hutley L, Prins JB. Fat as an endocrine organ: relationship to the metabolic syndrome. Am J Med Sci 2005;330(6):280–9.
34. Dandona P, Aljada A, Bandyopadhyay A. Inflammation: the link between insulin resistance, obesity and diabetes. Trends Immunol 2004;25(1):4–7.
35. Neiger R, Witt AL, Noble A, et al. Trilostane therapy for treatment of pituitary-dependent hyperadrenocorticism in 5 cats. J Vet Intern Med 2004;18(2):160–4.
36. Li S, Shin HJ, Ding EL, et al. Adiponectin levels and risk of type 2 diabetes: a systematic review and meta-analysis. JAMA 2009;302(2):179–88.
37. Richards AA, Stephens T, Charlton HK, et al. Adiponectin multimerization is dependent on conserved lysines in the collagenous domain: evidence for regulation of multimerization by alterations in posttranslational modifications. Mol Endocrinol 2006;20(7):1673–87.
38. Lara-Castro C, Luo N, Wallace P, et al. Adiponectin multimeric complexes and the metabolic syndrome trait cluster. Diabetes 2006;55(1):249–59.
39. Tan HY, Rand JS, Morton JM, et al. Adiponectin profiles are affected by chronic and acute changes in carbohydrate intake in healthy cats. Gen Comp Endocrinol 2011;172(3):468–74.
40. Hoenig M, Thomaseth K, Waldron M, et al. Insulin sensitivity, fat distribution, and adipocytokine response to different diets in lean and obese cats before and after weight loss. Am J Physiol Regul Integr Comp Physiol 2007;292(1):R227–34.
41. Appleton DJ, Rand JS, Sunvold GD. Plasma leptin concentrations are independently associated with insulin sensitivity in lean and overweight cats. J Feline Med Surg 2002;4:83–93.
42. Appleton DJ, Rand JS, Sunvold GD. Plasma leptin concentrations in cats: reference range, effects of weight gain and relationship with adiposity a measured by dual energy X-ray absorptiometry. J Feline Med Surg 2000;2:191–9.
43. Tilg H, Moschen AR. Inflammatory mechanisms in the regulation of insulin resistance. Mol Med 2008;14(3–4):222.
44. Ahren B, Pacini G. Importance of quantifying insulin secretion in relation to insulin sensitivity to accurately assess beta cell function in clinical studies. Eur J Endocrinol 2004;150(2):97–104.
45. Kelishadi R, Cook SR, Motlagh ME, et al. Metabolically obese normal weight and phenotypically obese metabolically normal youths: the CASPIAN Study. J Am Diet Assoc 2008;108(1):82–90.
46. Leahy JL. Pathogenesis of type 2 diabetes mellitus. Arch Med Res 2005;36(3): 197–209.
47. Verkest KR, Fleeman LM, Rand JS, et al. Evaluation of beta-cell sensitivity to glucose and first-phase insulin secretion in obese dogs. Am J Vet Res 2011; 72(3):357–66.
48. Wagner JD, Kavanagh K, Ward GM, et al. Old world nonhuman primate models of type 2 diabetes mellitus. ILAR J 2006;47(3):259.
49. Rees DA, Alcolado JC. Animal models of diabetes mellitus. Diabet Med 2005; 22(4):359–70.
50. Kjos SL, Buchanan TA. Gestational diabetes mellitus. N Engl J Med 1999; 341(23):1749–56.

51. Johnson KH, O'Brien TD, Betsholtz C, et al. Islet amyloid polypeptide: mechanisms of amyloidogenesis in the pancreatic islets and potential roles in diabetes mellitus. Lab Invest 1992;66(5):522–35.
52. Yano BL, Hayden DW, Johnson KH. Feline insular amyloid: association with diabetes mellitus. Vet Pathol 1981;18:621–7.
53. Hoenig M, Hall G, Ferguson D, et al. A feline model of experimentally induced islet amyloidosis. Am J Pathol 2000;157(6):2143.
54. Clark A, Wells C, Buley I, et al. Islet amyloid, increased A-cells, reduced B-cells and exocrine fibrosis: quantitative changes in the pancreas in type 2 diabetes. Diabetes Res 1988;9(4):151.
55. Guardado-Mendoza R, Davalli AM, Chavez AO, et al. Pancreatic islet amyloidosis, β-cell apoptosis, and α-cell proliferation are determinants of islet remodeling in type-2 diabetic baboons. Proc Natl Acad Sci U S A 2009;106(33):13992–7.
56. Khemtemourian L, Antoinette Killian J, Hoppener JW, et al. Recent insights in islet amyloid polypeptide-induced membrane disruption and its role in β-cell death in type 2 diabetes mellitus. Exp Diabetes Res 2008;2008:421287.
57. Haataja L, Gurlo T, Huang CJ, et al. Islet amyloid in type 2 diabetes, and the toxic oligomer hypothesis. Endocr Rev 2008;29(3):303–16.
58. Scheuner D, Kaufman RJ. The unfolded protein response: a pathway that links insulin demand with beta-cell failure and diabetes. Endocr Rev 2008;29(3):317–33.
59. Zraika S, Hull R, Verchere C, et al. Toxic oligomers and islet beta cell death: guilty by association or convicted by circumstantial evidence? Diabetologia 2010;53(6):1046–56.
60. Poitout V. Glucolipotoxicity of the pancreatic beta-cell: myth or reality? Biochem Soc Trans 2008;36(Pt 5):901–4.
61. Back SH, Kaufman RJ. Endoplasmic reticulum stress and type 2 diabetes. Annu Rev Biochem 2012;81(1):767–93.
62. Zini E, Osto M, Franchini M, et al. Hyperglycaemia but not hyperlipidaemia causes beta cell dysfunction and beta cell loss in the domestic cat. Diabetologia 2009;52(2):336–46.
63. Tschuor F, Zini E, Schellenberg S, et al. Remission of diabetes mellitus in cats cannot be predicted by the arginine stimulation test. J Vet Intern Med 2011;25(1):83–9.
64. Nolan CJ, Prentki M. The islet beta-cell: fuel responsive and vulnerable. Trends Endocrinol Metab 2008;19(8):285–91.
65. Prentki M, Nolan CJ. Islet beta cell failure in type 2 diabetes. J Clin Invest 2006;116(7):1802–12.
66. Donath MY, Shoelson SE. Type 2 diabetes as an inflammatory disease. Nat Rev Immunol 2011;11(2):98–107.
67. Donath MY, Storling J, Berchtold LA, et al. Cytokines and {beta}-cell biology: from concept to clinical translation. Endocr Rev 2008;29(3):334–50.
68. Dinarello CA, Donath MY, Mandrup-Poulsen T. Role of IL-1[beta] in type 2 diabetes. Curr Opin Endocrinol Diabetes Obes 2010;17(4):314–21, 310.1097/MED.1090b1013e32833bf32836dc.
69. Peterson ME, Taylor RS, Greco DS, et al. Acromegaly in 14 cats. J Vet Intern Med 1990;4(4):192–201.
70. Zoran DL. Pancreatitis in cats: diagnosis and management of a challenging disease. J Am Anim Hosp Assoc 2006;42(1):1–9.
71. Xenoulis PG, Steiner JM. Current concepts in feline pancreatitis. Top Companion Anim Med 2008;23(4):185–92.

The Role of Diet in the Prevention and Management of Feline Diabetes

Debra L. Zoran, DVM, PhD[a],*,
Jacquie S. Rand, BVSc, DVSc, MANZVS, DACVIM[b]

KEYWORDS

- Feline • Diabetes mellitus • Diet • Protein • Obesity • Carbohydrates • Glucose

KEY POINTS

- To maximize the probability of remission, a low-carbohydrate diet should be introduced soon after diagnosis of diabetes when the cat is eating well.
- Because diabetic remission is an important goal, frequent monitoring (both of body weight and glycemic control) and access to controlled amounts of low-carbohydrate/high-protein food is the best strategy.
- Low-carbohydrate diets should be continued after remission to minimize postprandial glycemia, and the demand on beta cells to secrete insulin.
- For cats already on insulin therapy, when changing from a high-carbohydrate to a low-carbohydrate diet, the insulin dose initially should be reduced by 30% to 50% to avoid hypoglycemia.
- Combined with high protein to facilitate weight loss and maintenance of muscle mass, low-carbohydrate diets should be used in obese cats that have the potential to achieve remission.

BACKGROUND

Feline diets and their role in the prevention or treatment of diabetes have been the source of considerable discussion over the past 10 years, primarily because of the ongoing controversy as to whether the cat, an obligate carnivore, is best fed a diet more closely patterned after its ancestors, or whether diets created to meet their essential needs, but containing lower amounts of protein and higher amounts of carbohydrates, are a more economical, user friendly, and acceptable alternative.

Disclosure: Consultant for Nestle Purina PetCare.
[a] Department of Small Animal Clinical Sciences, College of Veterinary Medicine and Biomedical Sciences, Texas A&M University, Mail Stop (MS) 4474, College Station, TX 77843-4474, USA;
[b] Centre for Companion Animal Health, School of Veterinary Science, The University of Queensland, Queensland 4072, Australia
* Corresponding author.
E-mail address: dzoran@cvm.tamu.edu

Vet Clin Small Anim 43 (2013) 233–243
http://dx.doi.org/10.1016/j.cvsm.2012.11.004
0195-5616/13/$ – see front matter © 2013 Elsevier Inc. All rights reserved.

The arguments for the alternative approach range from cats are living longer, to it is what consumers want, to there is no evidence that these diets are the cause of some of the most currently problematic feline diseases (such as obesity and diabetes). If one examines carefully the current state of feline health, however, we can clearly see we have traded one set of issues (a shortened life span due to fatal infectious diseases, parasites, dog attacks, and car accidents) for another set of equally big problems, with obesity topping the list and diabetes incidence increasing more than 100-fold. To be fair, it would be completely irrational to blame all of the ills of our indoor-living cats on their diets; however, to completely ignore diet as a risk factor when it is legitimate to do so, is also equally dangerous. So, the focus of the first part of this article is to review the currently available evidence and focus on how diet may play a role in lowering (or increasing) the risk of diabetes.

As in many feline diseases, dietary therapy is a very important aspect of successful management of the diabetic cat; however, dietary therapy of diabetes in the cat is not aimed solely at feeding a particular diet consistently, both in timing and energy. In contrast to dogs, because cats with diabetes most commonly have type 2 diabetes, the goal of therapy is to achieve diabetic remission, not just to manage the disease for the duration of the cat's life. Diet is a very important part of this process to minimize the demand on beta cells to produce insulin. In addition, dietary therapy of diabetes must also help normalize body weight and muscle mass (ie, resolve obesity or promote regain of lost muscle), reduce postprandial hyperglycemia, and minimize fluctuations in blood glucose. There is strong clinical and research evidence that a diet containing protein as the main ingredient (>40% metabolizable energy [ME], >10 g/100 kcal) and very low concentrations of carbohydrate (eg, carbohydrates <15% ME, <25% dry matter [DM], or <3 g/100 kcal) is most effective in achieving these goals in cats.[1–3] In addition, because many feline diabetics have poor muscle condition scores, high-protein diets are essential to replacement of that lost muscle, are needed for prevention of hepatic lipidosis during weight loss, and are essential to increasing metabolism to help promote fat burning and normal insulin function.[4–7] The second half of this article reviews the role of diet in treatment of diabetes. To the extent that it exists, evidence from published studies are cited; however, in areas where research evidence is lacking, clinical experience and physiologic principles are used as important sources of guidance.

THE ROLE OF DIET IN REDUCING THE RISK OF DIABETES IN CATS

Diabetes is a complex endocrine disease that results from a convergence of a multiple risk factors, including genetic risk.[8] As such, a single factor, such as the diet, is not in and of itself, a causative factor for the disease. However, there are several features of the current most popular feline diets (eg, extruded dry, high-carbohydrate diets, high-energy density) that may increase risk or promote conditions that increase risk, and for that reason it is important to carefully consider diet when examining the situation concerning feline health: feline diabetes is clearly more common that it was 15 years ago when it did not even make the top 25 list of most important feline diseases.[9] In the ensuing 15 years, several epidemiologic studies have evaluated the prevalence of diabetes, and examined diet as a risk factor for development of diabetes mellitus in cats. No studies of first opinion practices in the United States have been completed in the past few years, but an estimated prevalence of diabetes at 1.2% of feline patients seen at US veterinary teaching hospitals was reported in 2007.[10] Moreover, in all studies, 2 common themes persist: increased age and body weight consistently appear as risk factors for feline diabetes.[9–12] Thus, because obesity is one of the most important risk factors for development of diabetes in cats, it can be stated that improper nutrition plays a critical role in diabetes risk.[13,14] A large majority of cats (70% by one recent estimate) are either overweight (15%–20% over ideal body weight [BW]) or obese (>20% over ideal BW).[15,16] Thus, prevention of obesity in young cats and achieving weight loss in obese older cats are key strategic components of dietary therapy aimed at reducing this risk factor for diabetes. There are multiple components to prevention of obesity in cats, but from the perspective of diet, one factor is key: providing excess energy through free choice or ad libitum feeding of neutered, inactive, indoor cats is to be strongly discouraged.[11,13,17,18] In addition to counseling owners about the importance of feeding cats a measured amount of food matched to their energy needs, it is also crucial to advise owners on how to help maintain dietary flexibility in cats. Cats will become habituated to a single food (eg, flavor, texture, odor) if they are fed only one food, and this will create great challenges if a diet change or adjustment is required. Thus, it is important to introduce cats to both canned and dry foods, and continue feeding a mixture of these foods throughout life to help maintain dietary flexibility.

To induce safe, permanent weight loss in cats, a dietary strategy must be embraced that includes the following: (1) feeding a diet high in protein (>40% ME, >45% DM, or >10 g/100 kcal) to prevent loss of muscle mass that can occur with severe energy restriction; (2) feeding a diet that is reduced in energy, and restricted in both fat and carbohydrate, to stimulate fat mobilization (and so that effective energy restriction can be achieved); and, finally, (3) monitoring and adjusting energy intake to achieve effective fat loss. Lean muscle tissue is an essential element of basal metabolism and is necessary for normal insulin function as well. Many weight loss diets are low energy, but not high enough in protein to preserve lean muscle tissue. In studies of cats comparing high-protein or moderate-protein diets during weight loss, cats on high-protein diets had greater success in achieving weight loss, lost fat mass while preserving lean tissue, and had a greater tendency to maintain stable weight after weight loss.[19] A number of diets may be acceptable for preservation of lean muscle tissue, but the goal should be to have fat less than 4 g/100 kcal, carbohydrates less than 3 g/100 kcal, and protein content greater than 10 g/100 kcal. Diets with this profile are easily obtained using canned food diets, and many options exist. In addition, the added water in canned foods increases hydration and food volume, which increases satiety, and both issues are important husbandry concerns in cats.[20] Conversely, extruded dry foods require some carbohydrate in processing for the creation of the shape and texture, and the removal of carbohydrate requires the addition of fat to the diet for processing. Thus, high-protein dry foods are often high fat (and thus high energy), making it very difficult to feed an appropriate amount of the food during weight loss when the need for energy restriction may be extreme. Alternatively, if fat is restricted, the carbohydrate content is typically high, because the manufacturing process limits the amount of protein that can be added to dry food; however, the high carbohydrate content exacerbates postprandial glycemic response, which in some obese cats, results in peak postprandial glucose concentrations in the diabetic range.[21] Addition of fiber may help to attenuate the postprandial glycemic response, but there are no well-designed studies yet in cats that address this.

The other essential aspect of achieving weight loss is to control energy intake. In obese cats, meal feeding will be necessary to meet the specific number of calories required to achieve weight goals. Maintenance energy needs for indoor neutered cats that are of ideal body weight are estimated to be approximately 40 kcal/kg/d (or for the average 4–5-kg cat, an intake of 160–200 kcal/d); however, to achieve weight loss, the energy intake must be restricted much further, with a reduction in energy from this maintenance rate by 10% to 40%, or to 20 to 30 kcal/kg, which may mean intakes of 120 to 140 kcal/d for some cats. It is possible to achieve this level of energy restriction and maintain high levels of protein with canned foods. It is very difficult to achieve this level of restriction with a high-protein dry food unless some of the energy has been replaced with fiber. If the cat has been eating free-choice food, the first step is to establish a meal-feeding regimen so that energy intake can be controlled. In a recent comparison between a high-fiber food and a canned food with equal ingredients, cats fed the canned diets begged less and showed more signs of satiety than those on the dry high-fiber diets.[20] Thus, because energy intake can be controlled, it is easier to feed a diet with a high-protein/low-carbohydrate nutrient profile. In addition, the added water increases both moisture and volume to the meal; canned foods are a highly desirable option for cats needing to lose weight.

Although there is clear evidence that the incidence of diabetes has increased with the increasing incidence of obesity, it is clearly not a one-to-one ratio, or diabetes would have become a disease of epidemic proportions in recent years. Further, multiple studies show that no single dietary factor is responsible for development of obesity. In fact, the dietary factor most important in development of obesity is diets high in fat, rather than carbohydrate-dense diets (which are sometimes very low in fat).[22] Other important risk factors are neutering, overfeeding (particularly free-choice feeding), and indoor/inactive lifestyle.[11,17,22] For more information on strategies for obesity management, the reader is urged to consult one of several recent reviews for more information on this topic.[18,23]

What are the other dietary factors that might play a role in reduction of risk of diabetes in cats? There are a number of ways that the diet composition itself would possibly be important, and of all of the nutrients, dietary carbohydrates have generated the most attention. In a study among feline patients in the United Kingdom, consumption of a mix of wet and dry foods was associated with a lower risk for diabetes, compared with only dry (high-carbohydrate) diets, or only wet (lower-carbohydrate) diets.[12] Cats fed wet diets were 3 times more likely to develop diabetes than cats fed mixed diets; cats fed dry diets had 2 times the risk. Slingerland and colleagues[24] reported that there was no difference in diabetic risk of healthy cats with consumption of dry or wet foods, but most cat owners fed a mixture of wet and dry foods and the number of cats in the study solely fed dry food was too low to detect a difference if one was present, given the incidence of diabetes in the cat population. Indoor housing and inactivity were associated with an increased risk for diabetes in their study. Thus, in only one epidemiologic study, the type of food (dry vs canned) was a determinant of increased risk for development of diabetes and obesity. Living indoors, physical inactivity, and increasing age were found to be the most important risks for development of diabetes in cats. To better elucidate the contribution of diet to the development of diabetes, well-designed studies are required that have the power to detect differences if they are present.

Recently, there have been a number of published studies comparing the effects of diets differing in dietary carbohydrate, fat, and protein on glucose metabolism in healthy lean and obese cats.[7,20,21,25–30] These studies had different points of focus, test protocols, and all were short-term studies in which the level of dietary carbohydrate varied widely: from 0 to 16 g/100 kcal ME (>50% carbohydrate [CHO]). In addition, the level of protein varied inversely to carbohydrate, and ranged from 6.0 to 13.5 g protein/100 kcal ME; thus, the results of these studies were at least partly confounded by alterations in protein concentrations. To date, there is only one study that attempted to address the effect of levels of carbohydrate in the diet on protein intake and use, and in that article, the investigators found that a ceiling effect of high carbohydrate concentrations on protein intake occurred in cats on diets with a greater than 40% DM carbohydrate.[31] This simply illustrates the difficulty of attempting to study the effects of a single nutrient, because in the body, the interactions of these nutrients are vital and confounding. Finally, the duration of fasting before the initial sample collection and the duration of postprandial collections varied greatly between studies, and, consequently, the results obtained are highly variable, making comparisons difficult, if not inaccurate. For example, it has been documented that it can take 8 or more hours to reach a postprandial peak in blood glucose and 12 to 24 hours for the blood glucose to return to fasting levels in cats fed a single meal.[21,28–30,32] Although there have been 10 studies evaluating carbohydrate effects on blood glucose, only 5 used a 24-hour fast. If only those 5 studies with appropriate 24-hour fasting times are considered, a total of 17 different diets ranging in carbohydrate from 3.2 (<25%) to 14.5 g/100 kcal ME (>50%) were examined.[21,25,30,32–35] For 5 diets with carbohydrate levels of 6.65 g/ kcal or greater,[21,27,30,32] peak postprandial glucose concentrations in many cats, and mean 24-hour glucose concentrations in some cats were above the upper limit of the reference interval established for healthy fasted cats of less than 6.0 to 6.5 mmol/L (108–117 mg/dL).[21,32,33,36] Four of these diets resulted in peak glucose concentrations greater than 8 mmol/L in some cats, which is above the level defined by the International Diabetes Federation as representing postprandial hyperglycemia (7.8 mmol/L) in humans.[21,27,32,37] In one study, when cats fed 12.1 g carbohydrate/100 kcal ME were compared with cats fed diets containing 3.2 (<25% DM) or 8.3 g carbohydrate/100 kcal ME (35% DM), the mean blood glucose was significantly higher, and it remained elevated through the end of the 19-hour period of evaluation.[30] Perhaps the most important finding was that the magnitude[21] and duration[33] of postprandial hyperglycemia observed was exacerbated by weight gain, and in overweight cats, mean postprandial glucose concentration over the entire 24-hour period was between 8 and 9 mmol/L (144–162 mg/dL).[21] Notably, the diet with 14.5 g/100 g/kcal resulted in peak glucose concentrations as high as 10.8 mmol/L (194 mg/dL) in lean cats, and 13.4 mmol/L (241 mg/dL) after moderate weight gain (mean body condition score 6.3), which is considered in the diabetic range for cats.[21] This finding is particularly alarming, considering that in the United States, feline obesity is approaching 70% of all cats presented to veterinarians.[15] Thus, if a large number of these cats have serum blood glucose above what is currently accepted as the glucose reference range for many hours out of the day, what are the long-term implications for beta cell function?

Minimizing the increase in glucose concentration following a meal, and the subsequent demand on beta cells to secrete insulin, is a primary goal for management of prediabetic and diabetic human patients,[38,39] and logically should also apply to feline patients, and especially obese cats. In human studies, it has been shown to be more important (but also more difficult) to normalize postprandial hyperglycemia, as compared with fasting glucose concentrations.[38,39] Although the International Diabetes Federation defines postprandial hyperglycemia in humans as a plasma glucose concentration higher than 7.8 mmol/L (140 mg/dL),[37] currently, there are no similar recommendations for cats; however, knowing that persistent postprandial hyperglycemia is likely to place a burden on beta cells over months or years, reducing carbohydrate content may be an important step in prevention of diabetes in cats. This is likely most relevant to cats at increased risk of diabetes, such as older cats that are obese, Burmese breed of Australasian or European origin, and/or having repeated corticosteroid administration.

In humans, dogs, and cats, the carbohydrate load of the diet is the primary determinant of postprandial glucose and insulin concentrations.[26,32,40] Although protein also stimulates insulin secretion, and protein content is usually increased in low-carbohydrate diets, in cats, as in other species, it is the carbohydrate content, rather than the protein content, that determines postprandial glucose concentrations.[32] For example, in healthy cats, a high-protein meal (46% ME protein; 26% fat; 27% carbohydrate) and a high-fat meal (26% protein; 47% fat; 26% carbohydrate) gave similar postprandial glucose concentrations, whereas a high-carbohydrate meal (25% protein; 26% fat; 47% carbohydrate) produced approximately 20% to 25% significantly higher postprandial glucose concentrations.[32] Thus, when attempting to lower postprandial glucose concentrations using diet, lowering dietary carbohydrate is the only effective approach.

Although the dietary carbohydrate concentration is a point of focus for its effects on postprandial peak blood glucose and insulin concentrations, perhaps more important in its long-term impact is the duration of the postprandial period that occurs in cats fed high-carbohydrate meals. Previous studies in cats fed diets ranging from 30% to 50% ME carbohydrate, resulted in increases in postprandial glucose and insulin concentrations for an average of 12 to 19 hours in lean cats, with some cats of more than 24 hours, and for at least 18 hours in obese cats.[14,21,30,41] This is in contrast to approximately 6 hours in lean dogs fed a similar meal.[40] The effect of a prolonged elevation of glucose and insulin in the postprandial period over years has not been studied in cats, but in other species, glucose toxicity, hyperamylinemia, and beta cell apoptosis are consequences that may also be predicted in susceptible cats.

In cats allowed continuous access to food, the effect on blood glucose is more complicated because the intake load per meal is often reduced and more variable. One study used constant glucose monitoring and showed that blood glucose in most cats is fairly stable over the course of the day in cats fed a moderate-carbohydrate (6 g/100 kcal ME) diet ad libitum.[36] Another study monitored blood glucose every 3 hours over a 24-hour period in cats fed with either a higher (9.8 g/100 kcal ME) or a lower (2.5 g/100 kcal ME) carbohydrate diet, and showed no difference in total glucose area under the curve.[27] However, there is strong evidence that cats allowed free access to food are more likely to become obese, so the risk for development of glucose intolerance and persistent postprandial hyperglycemia are increased with the development of obesity.

To date, there are no publications reporting controlled, lifelong, or even multiyear studies comparing the long-term effects of high-carbohydrate with low-carbohydrate intake in cats. However, considering that multiple lines of evidence show that cats have a prolonged postprandial increase in blood glucose concentration following ingestion of moderate or high carbohydrate diets, and that this effect may be greatly magnified for both duration and peak concentration in obese cats, there appears to be ample evidence that a return to a higher protein/lower carbohydrate diet more typical of the domestic cat's ancestors is needed.

THE ROLE OF DIETARY THERAPY IN MANAGEMENT OF DIABETES IN CATS

The goal of treatment of cats with newly diagnosed diabetes mellitus has changed from controlling clinical signs to achieving diabetic remission. Cats in diabetic remission are normoglycemic without the need for insulin. Achieving diabetic remission has substantial benefits for the quality of life of diabetic cats, along with many lifestyle benefits for their owners. Therefore, the treatment protocol selected should aim to maximize the probability of achieving remission. There are several important factors in achieving remission, and they include the following: early institution of a treatment protocol aimed at achieving excellent glycemic control,[42] use of long-acting insulin (glargine or detemir) twice daily,[42–44] and use of a low-carbohydrate diet.[1–3] When good glycemic control is achieved early in newly diagnosed diabetic cats, high remission rates (>80%) are obtained.[42,44] The interested reader is referred to other sections in this issue or more information on the best approaches to attain this goal.

There are several goals in dietary therapy of feline diabetics, and they include, firstly and most importantly, to use diet to assist in reducing postprandial blood glucose concentrations to facilitate reversal of beta cell toxicity and recovery of insulin secretory capacity. This is particularly important if remission is a goal. A second dietary goal is to reduce fluctuation of blood glucose concentrations after eating and the potential for marked hyperglycemia or clinical hypoglycemia. This is more of a consideration when using long-acting, "peakless" insulin, such as detemir or glargine. Third, to normalize BW, which for many diabetic cats means weight loss, but also can mean regaining muscle mass. To meet or achieve these goals, the diet should be a high-protein (>40% ME, >10 g/100 kcal), low-carbohydrate (<12 ME, <3 g/100 kcal), and moderate-fat to low-fat (if dry) diet, so that energy control can be achieved. If the cat will eat canned/wet food, the energy content is easier to control because of the water in the food.

To increase the probability of diabetic remission in newly diagnosed diabetic cats, the goal of therapy is to achieve blood glucose concentrations as close to the normal range as possible while avoiding life-threatening hypoglycemia.[42] Achieving normal or near-normal blood glucose concentrations facilitates recovery of beta cells from glucose toxicity. Several studies have shown the benefits of using low-carbohydrate diets in diabetic cats.[1–3] However, the study by Benett and coworkers was the best designed and compared the glycemic control of a moderate-carbohydrate/high-fiber diet (26% CHO ME) with a low-carbohydrate/low-fiber diet (12% CHO ME) over 16 weeks in newly diagnosed (n = 19) and previously diagnosed (n = 43) diabetic cats.[2] Sixty-eight percent of cats fed the low-carbohydrate diet achieved diabetic remission compared with the higher carbohydrate group (only 41% achieved remission). At the end of the study, of the cats that still required insulin, 40% on the low-carbohydrate diet were considered well regulated, whereas only 26% on the higher carbohydrate diet were considered to be well regulated and stable. The authors concluded that diabetic cats were significantly more likely to revert to a non-insulin dependent state when fed the canned low carbohydrate food. In the other studies, feeding a low carbohydrate diet to diabetic cats improved diabetic regulation (compared with use of a moderate carbohydrate diet), and lowered the insulin dose and increased diabetic remission by 50%, but both studies lacked adequate controls for comparison to moderate carbohydrate diets.[1,3]

In addition to the amount of carbohydrate, the type of carbohydrate in the diet also appears to be important. Thus, for cats that will consume only dry-food diets and will have some carbohydrate in their food, the source of carbohydrate should be a complex carbohydrate with a low glycemic index (eg, whole grains such as barley). In a limited number of studies, postprandial glucose and insulin response after consumption of diets with different carbohydrate sources have been compared in healthy cats. Rice, barley, corn, and wheat had relatively higher responses than sorghum, lentil, and cassava flour (tapioca).[25,33,45,46] To date, most studies comparing differing levels of carbohydrate in diabetic and healthy cats have used diets with carbohydrate sources, such as corn, soy, sorghum, and wheat: all grains that result in a significant postprandial increase in glucose and insulin concentrations. Novel carbohydrate sources, such as lentil and cassava flour, were associated with no postprandial increase in glucose and minimal insulin responses after being fed as a single meal of approximately 68 kcal/kg.[25] Currently, a postprandial glycemia index has not been developed in veterinary medicine equivalent to the glycemic index in human medicine, so a comparison of the glucose response of a meal with a particular grain to that of a very highly digestible/high glycemic index carbohydrate (such as white bread) is not validated. Total carbohydrate load includes both the carbohydrate content and the glycemic response of that carbohydrate source, and is believed to be more important than just the carbohydrate content alone. Commercial diets with novel carbohydrate sources have been developed for cats, but currently there are no data on their effect on glycemic response.

Cats in diabetic remission continue to have impaired glucose tolerance and some have impaired fasting glucose concentrations despite having normal blood glucose levels, and thus, should be considered prediabetic and at risk of redeveloping overt diabetes.[47] In 3 recent studies, at least 25% of cats in diabetic remission reverted to overt diabetes and again required exogenous insulin to control their clinical signs.[43,48] Thus, cats in diabetic remission will continue to benefit from feeding of a low-carbohydrate/high-protein diet indefinitely.

Although it is important to implement a low-carbohydrate diet in the management of cats with diabetes as soon as possible, there are circumstances where this should be delayed or may be inappropriate. In sick, inappetant diabetic cats, the first priority is to offer food the cat will eat. Because of the risk of food aversion developing in cats, dietary changes should be implemented when the cat is eating readily and made slowly over 7 to 10 days, gradually replacing the original diet. In long-term diabetic cats (diagnosed >2–3 years previously), or those with concurrent disease, such as untreated acromegaly or irreversible end-stage pancreatitis, in which the probability of remission is low, in these cats, the goal of therapy should be to control clinical signs by minimizing hyperglycemia, avoid life-threatening hypoglycemia, and use appropriate dietary management of other health issues as indicated. For example, in cats with stage 3 chronic kidney disease requiring phosphorus restriction and a reduction in dietary protein, high-protein/low-carbohydrate diabetic diets may not be appropriate. In cats with earlier stages of chronic kidney disease, phosphorus should be restricted, if possible using other methods than changing to a protein-restricted diet (higher in carbohydrate), because this will likely reduce the probability of remission, and chronic hyperglycemia likely has adverse effects on the kidney, as it does in other species. Of note, grocery-line diets with very low carbohydrate are often predominantly fish or meat, and have substantially higher phosphate levels than the some of the veterinary prescription diets designed for diabetes.

Finally, although cats prefer to eat small, frequent meals (nibble or graze), it is helpful if diabetic cats are fed a measured amount of food at the time of the insulin injection so the owner can observe if the cat is eating appropriately at least twice daily. At this stage, there are no published data on the effect of once-daily, twice-daily, or multiple meals on postprandial glucose concentrations in cats to make firm recommendations on the best feeding pattern for diabetic cats. If the cat is prone to hypoglycemia or prefers small frequent meals, it is completely reasonable to divide the daily energy requirement into 4 separate feedings. This can be easily achieved by using timed feeders, so the cat has the opportunity to eat multiple times per day while controlling intake, but at the same time providing an energy source mid-day should the cat need or prefer it.

SUMMARY

To maximize the probability of remission, a low-carbohydrate diet should be introduced soon after diagnosis of diabetes when the cat is eating well. Low-carbohydrate diets should be continued after remission to minimize postprandial glycemia, and the demand on beta cells to secrete insulin. For cats already on insulin therapy, when changing from a high-carbohydrate to a low-carbohydrate diet, the insulin dose initially should be reduced by 30% to 50% to avoid hypoglycemia. Combined with high protein to facilitate weight loss and maintenance of muscle mass, low-carbohydrate diets should be used in obese cats that have the potential to achieve remission. Diabetic cats with advanced chronic kidney disease resulting in inappetance will need a protein-restricted diet (therefore, higher carbohydrate). In earlier stages of renal disease, to maximize the probability of remission, phosphorus should be managed using methods other than restricting protein. Cats should be fed the diet that is most appropriate for any medical problem requiring dietary intervention if they have a very low probability of remission; that is, cats diabetic for longer than 2 years despite excellent glycemic control, and cats with untreatable concurrent disease causing loss of beta cells (pancreatic neoplasia, or advanced chronic pancreatitis evidenced by concurrent loss of exocrine function). Nonetheless, a low-carbohydrate/high-protein diet is likely to lead to lower postprandial glucose concentrations, and thus should be used unless there is a medical need to change diets. Because diabetic remission is an important goal, frequent monitoring (both of body weight and glycemic control) and access to controlled amounts of low-carbohydrate/high-protein food is the best strategy.

REFERENCES

1. Mazzaferro EM, Greco DS, Turner AS, et al. Treatment of feline diabetes mellitus using an alpha-glucosidase inhibitor and a low-carbohydrate diet. J Feline Med Surg 2003;5(3):183–9.
2. Bennet N, Greco D, Peterson M, et al. Comparison of a low carbohydrate-low fibre diet and a moderate carbohydrate-high fibre diet in the management of feline diabetes mellitus. J Feline Med Surg 2006;8:73–84.
3. Frank G, Anderson W, Pazak H, et al. Use of a high-protein diet in the management of feline diabetes mellitus. Vet Ther 2001;2:238–46.
4. Nguyen P, Leray V, Dumon H, et al. High protein intake affects lean body mass but not energy expenditure in nonobese neutered cats. J Nutr 2004;134:2084S–6S.
5. Nguyen P, Dumon H, Martin L, et al. Weight loss does not affect energy expenditure or leucine metabolism in obese cats. J Nutr 2002;132:1649S–51S.
6. Vasconcellos RS, Borges NC, Goncalves KN, et al. Protein intake during weight loss influences the energy required for weight loss and maintenance in cats. J Nutr 2009;139:856–60.
7. Hoenig M, Thomaseth K, Waldron M, et al. Insulin sensitivity, fat distribution, and adipocytokine response to different diets in lean and obese cats before and after weight loss. Am J Physiol Regul Integr Comp Physiol 2007;292:R227–34.
8. Rand JS, Fleeman LM, Farrow HE, et al. Canine and feline diabetes mellitus: nature or nurture? J Nutr 2004;134:2072S–80S.
9. Scarlett JM, Donoghue S. Associations between body condition and disease in cats. J Am Vet Med Assoc 1998;212:1725–31.
10. Prahl A, Guptill L, Glickman NW, et al. Time trends and risk factors for diabetes mellitus in cats presented to veterinary teaching hospitals. J Feline Med Surg 2007;9:351–6.
11. Lund EM, Armstrong PJ, Kirk CA, et al. Prevalence and risk factors for obesity in adult cats from private US veterinary practices. Intern J Appl Res Vet Med 2005;3:88–96.

12. McCann TM, Simpson KE, Shaw DJ, et al. Feline diabetes mellitus in the UK: the prevalence within an insured cat population and a questionnaire-based putative risk factor analysis. J Feline Med Surg 2007;9:289–99.
13. Rand JS, Marshall R. Diabetes mellitus in cats. Vet Clin North Am Small Anim Pract 2005;35:211.
14. Appleton DJ, Rand JS, Sunvold GD. Insulin sensitivity decreases with obesity, and lean cats with low insulin sensitivity are at greatest risk of glucose intolerance with weight gain. J Feline Med Surg 2001;3(4):211–28.
15. State of Pet Health, Banfield Pet Hospital 2012 Report.
16. Cameron KM, Morris PJ, Hackett RM, et al. The effects of increasing water content to reduce the energy density of the diet on body mass changes following caloric restriction in domestic cats. J Anim Physiol Anim Nutr (Berl) 2011;95:399–408.
17. Nguyen PG, Dumon HJ, Siliart BS, et al. Effects of dietary fat and energy on body weight and composition after gonadectomy in cats. Am J Vet Res 2004;65:1708–13.
18. Zoran DL, Buffington CA. Effects of lifestyle changes and dietary choices on the wellbeing of cats: a carnivore that has moved indoors. J Am Vet Med Assoc 2011;239:596–606.
19. Laflamme DP, Hannah SS. Increased dietary protein promotes fat loss and reduces loss of lean body mass during weight loss in cats. J Feline Med Surg 2005;3:62–9.
20. Wei A, Fascetti AJ, Villaverde C, et al. Effects of water content in a canned food on voluntary food intake and body weight in cats. Am J Vet Res 2011;72:918–23.
21. Coradini M, Rand JS, Morton JM, et al. Effects of two commercially available feline diets on glucose and insulin concentrations, insulin sensitivity and energetic efficiency of weight gain. Br J Nutr 2011;106:S64–77.
22. Backus RC, Cave NJ, Keisler DH. Gonadectomy and high dietary fat but not high dietary carbohydrate induce gains in body weight and fat of domestic cats. Br J Nutr 2007;98(3):641–50.
23. Michel K, Scherk M. From problem to success: feline weight loss programs that work. J Feline Med Surg 2012;14:327–36.
24. Slingerland LI, Fazilova VV, Plantinga EA, et al. Indoor confinement and physical inactivity rather than the proportion of dry food are risk factors in the development of feline type 2 diabetes mellitus. Vet J 2009;179(2):247–53.
25. de-Oliveira LD, Carciofi AC, Oliveira MC, et al. Effects of six carbohydrate sources on diet digestibility and postprandial glucose and insulin responses in cats. J Anim Sci 2008;86:2237–46.
26. Martin LJ, Siliart B, Lutz TA, et al. Postprandial response of plasma insulin, amylin and acylated ghrelin to various test meals in lean and obese cats. Br J Nutr 2010;103:1610–9.
27. Thiess S, Becskei C, Tomsa K, et al. Effects of high carbohydrate and high fat diet on plasma metabolite levels and on IV glucose tolerance test in intact and neutered male cats. J Feline Med Surg 2004;6:207–18.
28. Mori A, Lee P, Takemitsu H, et al. Decreased gene expression of insulin signaling genes in insulin sensitive tissues of obese cats. Vet Res Commun 2009;53:315–29.
29. Wei A, Fascetti AJ, Liu KJ, et al. Influence of a high protein diet on energy balance in obese cats allowed ad libitum access to food. J Anim Physiol Anim Nutr (Berl) 2011;95:359–67.
30. Hewson-Hughes AK, Gilham MS, Upton S, et al. The effect of dietary starch level on postprandial glucose and insulin concentration in cats and dogs. Br J Nutr 2011;106:S105–9.

31. Hewson-Hughes AK, Hewson-Hughes VL, Miller AT, et al. Geometric analysis of macronutrient selection in the adult domestic cat, Felis catus. J Exp Biol 2011; 214:1039–51.
32. Farrow H, Rand J, Sunvold G. The effect of high protein, high fat or high carbohydrate diets on postprandial glucose and insulin concentrations in normal cats. J Vet Intern Med 2012;16:360 [abstract].
33. Appleton DJ, Rand JS, Priest J, et al. Dietary carbohydrate source affects glucose concentrations, insulin secretion, and food intake in overweight cats. Nutr Res 2004;24:447–67.
34. Bonagura JD, Twedt DC. Kirk's current veterinary therapy XIV. St. Louis (MO): Elsevier; 2009.
35. Norsworthy GD. The feline patient. 4th edition. Ames (IA): Wiley Blackwell; 2011. p. 997.
36. Hoenig M, Pach N, Thomaseth K, et al. Evaluation of long term glucose homeostasis in lean and obese cats by use of continuous glucose monitoring. Am J Vet Res 2012;73:1100–6.
37. Ceriello A, Colagiuri S. International Diabetes Federation guideline for management of postmeal glucose: a review of recommendations. Diabet Med 2008;25:1151–6.
38. Gin H, Rigalleau V. Postprandial hyperglycemia and diabetes. Diabete Metab 2000;26:265–75.
39. American Diabetes Association. Postprandial blood glucose. Diabetes Care 2001;24(4):775.
40. Elliott KF, Rand JS, Fleeman LM, et al. A diet lower in digestible carbohydrate results in lower postprandial glucose concentrations compared with a traditional canine diabetes diet and an adult maintenance diet in healthy dogs. Res Vet Sci 2011. http://dx.doi.org/10.1016/j.rvsc.2011.07.032.
41. Appleton DJ, Rand JS, Sunvold GD. Plasma leptin concentrations are independently associated with insulin sensitivity in lean and overweight cats. J Feline Med Surg 2002;4:83–93.
42. Roomp K, Rand J. Intensive blood glucose control is safe and effective in diabetic cats using home monitoring and treatment with glargine. J Feline Med Surg 2009;11(4):668–82.
43. Roomp K, Rand J. Detemir results in similar glycaemic control to glargine in diabetic cats. J Feline Med Surg 2009.
44. Marshall RD, Rand JS. Treatment of newly diagnosed feline diabetic cats with glargine insulin improves glycemic control and results in a higher probability of remission than protamine zinc or lente insulins. J Feline Med Surg 2009;11:683–91.
45. Bouchard GF, Sunvold GD. Effect of dietary carbohydrate source on postprandial plasma glucose and insulin concentration in cats. In: Reinhart GA, Carey DP, editors. Recent advances in canine and feline nutrition. Iams nutrition symposium. Wilmington (OH): Orange Frazer Press; 2000. p. 91.
46. Sunvold GD, Bouchard GF. The glycaemic response to dietary starch. In: Reinhart GA, Carey DP, editors. Recent advances in canine and feline nutrition, vol. 2. Wilmington (OH): Orange Frazer Press; 1998. p. 123–31.
47. Gottlieb S, Rand JS, Marshall RD. Diabetic cats in remission have mildly impaired glucose tolerance. J Vet Intern Med 2011 [abstract].
48. Reusch C, Zini E, Hafner M, et al. Predictors of clinical remission in cats with diabetes mellitus. J Vet Intern Med 2010;24:1314–21.

Remission in Cats
Including Predictors and Risk Factors

Susan Gottlieb, BVSc, MANZCVS, BSc(Vet), BAppSc[a],*,
Jacquie S. Rand, BVSc, DVSc, MANZVS, DACVIM[b]

KEYWORDS

- Diabetes • Remission • Feline • Cats

KEY POINTS

- Early treatment of diabetes and obtaining good glycemic control is crucial to achieving remission.
- Frequent monitoring of blood glucose concentrations and appropriate adjustment of insulin dose is vital.
- Glargine and detemir have been associated with the highest rates of remission.
- A low-carbohydrate diet improves remission rates.
- Corticosteroid administration before the diagnosis of diabetes is a positive predictor for remission; however, administration once remission is achieved is a risk factor for relapse.
- Negative predictors for remission include a plantigrade stance and increased cholesterol concentrations.
- Age is positively associated with remission.

WHAT IS DIABETIC REMISSION?

Diabetic remission in cats has previously been defined as the ability to maintain euglycemia for a minimum of 2 weeks after insulin therapy has been stopped.[1] Another study has defined it as the ability to maintain euglycemia without insulin therapy for at least 4 consecutive weeks without the reappearance of clinical signs of diabetes.[2] Remission improves the quality of life for the cat, and is an important goal of treatment.

PATHOPHYSIOLOGY OF REMISSION

The ability to achieve good glycemic control early in newly diagnosed diabetic cats is important because it allows faster resolution of beta cell dysfunction associated

Disclosures: Nil.
Funding sources: S.G., Purina, Abbott; J.R., Abbott, Purina, Iams, Hills, Waltham.
[a] The Cat Clinic, 189 Creek Road, The University of Queensland, Brisbane, Mt Gravatt, QLD 4022, Australia; [b] Centre for Companion Animal Health, School of Veterinary Science, The University of Queensland, QLD, Australia
* Corresponding author. 26 Great George Street, Paddington, QLD 4167, Australia.
E-mail address: susanalisongottlieb@gmail.com

with glucose and lipotoxicity, and increases the probability of remission.[1] Insulin administration facilitates recovery of beta cell dysfunction by minimizing hyperglycemia, thus facilitating the return of endogenous secretion of insulin. However, even when remission is achieved, beta cell function is usually not normal, as shown by impaired glucose tolerance, and cats in diabetic remission have been shown to have a reduced number of pancreatic islet cells.[2] Most diabetic cats that achieve remission continue to have impaired glucose tolerance,[3] and should be considered prediabetic.

MANAGING DIABETES TO INCREASE THE CHANCE OF REMISSION

Treatment with insulin is reported to be the most successful way to achieve good blood glucose control and give the best chance of obtaining remission. However, an early study reported an 18% remission rate in cats only treated with the oral hypoglycemic agent glipizide.[4] However, 56% of cats in this study had worsening of their diabetes and required treatment with insulin, and, of the remaining cats, a further 12% progressed to insulin treatment after failure of the glipizide to control their blood glucose concentration. Given the importance of gaining early glycemic control to maximize the chance of remission, insulin treatment is considered the most suitable treatment of overtly diabetic cats.

The use of glargine has been shown to achieve significantly higher remission rates compared with protamine zinc insulin (PZI) or Lente insulin.[1] One study comparing remission rates between 3 different insulins found that 100% of cats enrolled that were treated with glargine achieved remission within 4 months of treatment, compared with 25% of cats receiving Lente and 38% of cats receiving PZI.[1] All cats were fed a low-carbohydrate, high-protein canned food with approximately 6% of energy from carbohydrate. This study may have been limited by the small numbers of cats in each group (8 cats per group).

Another retrospective study involved 90 cats that received either glargine or PZI in combination with a low-carbohydrate diet. Of the cats surviving to discharge, use of glargine was more likely to result in remission compared with the use of PZI (72% vs 56% remission rate).[2] Remission rates in an earlier study using PZI with a low-carbohydrate diet (12% metabolizable energy) were reported to be 68%.[5] A study based on owners following an insulin dosing protocol designed to achieve intensive blood glucose control using glargine, home blood glucose monitoring, and a low-carbohydrate diet reported remission rates of 64% in cats previously treated with other insulin.[6] However, cats started in the intensive program within 6 months of diagnosis had a remission rate of 84%, compared with a remission rate of 35% for cats started on the program longer than 6 months after diagnosis, despite excellent glycemic control being achieved with the program. This finding highlights the importance of early institution of rigorous glycemic control in increasing the probability of remission. A similar study involving intensive control of blood glucose using detemir (Levemir; Novo Nordisk) and home monitoring found almost identical results (81% remission rate in cats changed to the intensive protocol within 6 months of diagnosis and 42% if changed later).[7] One study found that cats with a lower mean 12-hour blood glucose concentration 17 days after beginning insulin therapy were more likely to achieve remission, likely because these cats had greater beta cell function.[1] There are differences between these studies that may have influenced the outcome of these results. In the study by Zini and colleagues,[2] all cats were newly diagnosed diabetics, but treatment plans varied and diet was not reported, whereas, in the studies by Roomp and Rand,[6,7] all cats enrolled in the trial followed the same strict treatment protocol designed to achieve euglycemia, but most cats had been previously treated with other insulin.

Diet has been reported to be an important management factor contributing to remission in diabetic cats; studies achieving good remission rates have used a combination of insulin and a low-carbohydrate diet.[1,5–7] However, the highest remission rates (>80%) have only been reported using a diet with less than or equal to approximately 6% of metabolizable energy from carbohydrate[1,6,7] along with glargine or detemir. Although a high fiber diet has been reported to improve glycemic control in humans, in cats, low-carbohydrate diets with low to moderate fiber have been associated with higher remission rates compared with a moderate-carbohydrate and high-fiber diet.[5] However, further studies are required to evaluate the benefit of increasing fiber in low-carbohydrate diets.

Frequent monitoring of blood glucose concentrations and appropriate adjustment of insulin dose is likely important in achieving remission. In the 3 studies achieving remission rates greater than 80%, blood glucose was either monitored daily by clients[6,7] or weekly by the veterinarian[1] in the initial stabilization period. In 2 studies, owners measured blood glucose a minimum of 3 times daily and averaged 5 times daily in the initial stabilization period.[6,7] In the other study, cats were initially monitored for 3 days in the hospital and then weekly with serial blood glucose measurements in hospital over 12 hours during the stabilization phase. In all three studies, dosing algorithms designed to achieve rigorous glycemic control were used, and dose was increased if peak blood glucose concentration was greater than 10 mmol/L (180 mg/dL)[1] or more than normal fasting glucose concentrations.[6,7] See the article by Roomp and Rand elsewhere in this issue for details of dosing algorithms.

OTHER FACTORS ASSOCIATED WITH REMISSION

One study reported that increased age was associated with greater chance of remission, which was thought to mimic the finding in human studies that people diagnosed older than 65 years of age have less severe disease and metabolic deterioration.[2] However, another study reported no correlation between age at diagnosis and likelihood of remission.[6]

It has been reported that corticosteroid use in the 6 months before diagnosis of diabetes was significantly associated with higher remission rates, and, in 1 study, all cats with previous corticosteroid use achieved remission.[6] One explanation for this is that cats with diabetes associated with corticosteroid administration have a more abrupt onset of clinical signs, and therefore may be diagnosed more quickly. Early instigation of therapy reduces the duration of hyperglycemia and so reduces damage to the beta cells.[6] Another consideration is that drug-induced diabetes mellitus is considered to be a different type of diabetes from type 2 diabetes, so the underlying pathologic processes may be more easily reversible.[8] An alternative is that, as in some humans, the insulin resistance associated with steroid administration unmasks underlying defects in beta-cell function associated with another disease process such as type 2 diabetes or pancreatitis.[8] This process likely also occurs in cats, given that only a minority of cats develop diabetes following steroid administration. Regardless of the underlying mechanism, diabetic remission occurs when the remaining beta-cell function is sufficient to maintain euglycemia. It is presumed that this happens when insulin sensitivity improves over time following cessation of steroid administration, and beta-cell function improves following control of blood glucose concentrations with insulin, leading to resolution of glucose toxicity. Steroid administration has been also been linked to relapse in diabetic cats in remission,[3] likely because most cats in remission continue to have impaired glucose tolerance and reduced beta-cell function, and should be considered prediabetic.

Some factors have been identified with reduced remission rates in cats. In one study, 79% of cats that did not achieve remission with a protocol of rigorous glycemic control using glargine and low-carbohydrate diet had signs of peripheral neuropathy at the time of diagnosis,[6] likely because peripheral neuropathy occurs as a clinical sign later in the course of diabetes in cats, so greater damage to beta cells would have occurred by this later stage of diagnosis, associated with prolonged hyperglycemia. Higher cholesterol has also been reported as a negative indicator for remission, thought to be caused by the toxic effects of hypercholesterolemia on beta cells and the role it may play in preventing beta-cell recovery.[9] It might also be just a reflection of poorer glycemic control associated with inadequate therapy, and continuing glucose toxic damage to beta cells.

RELAPSE

In one study, 29% of cats that achieved diabetic remission relapsed into overt diabetes and required insulin treatment to be reinstituted; none of these cats achieved remission for a second time.[2] Another study reported that 26% of cats that achieved remission relapsed, and, of these cats (9 in total), 2 were able to achieve remission for a second time using a protocol designed to achieve intensive blood glucose control.[6] In the study that achieved 100% remission in 8 cats treated with glargine, 3 of these cats relapsed.[1] In a current study by the authors investigating diabetic cats in remission, 27% of cats relapsed and no cat achieved remission for a second time.[3] Investigation into risk factors for relapse is ongoing; however, corticosteroid administration and more severe glucose intolerance have been linked to higher relapse rates.[3] Most cats relapsed if blood glucose concentration took 5 hours or longer (normal ≤3 hours) to return to less than or equal to 6.5 mmol/L (117 mg/dL) in a glucose tolerance test (1 g/kg of glucose). Most cats with more severe levels of impaired fasting glucose (>7.5 mmol/L; 135 mg/dL) similarly relapsed. Impaired fasting glucose is defined as glucose concentrations greater than normal, but less than those considered diabetic, and in cats could be defined as between 6.6 and 10 mmol/L (119–180 mg/dL). It likely indicates more severe impairment of beta-cell function, which is no longer adequate to maintain fasting glucose concentrations in the normal range.

SUMMARY

With new treatment modalities, diabetic remission in cats has become common, and should now be considered a primary goal of therapy in newly diagnosed diabetic cats. Early institution of treatment designed to achieve rigorous glycemic control has been associated with the highest remission rates (>80%). This treatment involves an appropriate choice of long-acting insulin (glargine or detemir) and diet selection (<10% of energy from carbohydrates and high protein content), together with close monitoring of blood glucose concentrations and appropriate dose adjustment designed to achieve a rigorous glycemic control. To maximize the probability of achieving remission, it is important to understand the pathophysiology of remission in cats and how different treatments or management strategies help regain and preserve beta-cell function. Certain factors also influence a cat's ability to achieve remission, such as the underlying disease process causing diabetes, duration of diabetes, and previous corticosteroid administration.

REFERENCES

1. Marshall RD, Rand JS, Morton JM. Treatment of newly diagnosed diabetic cats with glargine insulin improved glycaemic control and results in higher probability of remission than protamine zinc and Lente insulins. J Feline Med Surg 2009;11: 683–91.
2. Zini E, Hafner M, Osto M, et al. Predictors of clinical remission in cats with diabetes mellitus. J Vet Intern Med 2010;24:1314–21.
3. Gottlieb SA, Rand JS, Marshall RD. Diabetic cats in remission have mildly impaired glucose tolerance [abstract]. Proceedings of Australian College of Veterinary Scientists Science Week. 2012.
4. Feldman EC, Nelson RW, Feldman MS. Intensive 50-week evaluation of glipizide administration in 50 cats with previously untreated diabetes mellitus. J Am Vet Med Assoc 1997;210:772–7.
5. Bennet N, Greco DS, Peterson ME, et al. Comparison of a low carbohydrate-low fibre diet and a moderate carbohydrate-high fibre diet in the management of feline diabetes mellitus. J Feline Med Surg 2006;8:73–84.
6. Roomp K, Rand J. Intensive blood glucose control is safe and effective in diabetic cats using home monitoring and treatment with glargine. J Feline Med Surg 2009; 11:668–82.
7. Roomp K, Rand J. Evaluation of detemir in diabetic cats managed with a protocol for intensive blood glucose control. J Feline Med Surg 2012;14:566–72.
8. American Diabetes Association. Diagnosis and classification of diabetes mellitus. Diabetes Care 2011;34(S1):S62–9.
9. Zini E, Osto M, Franchini M, et al. Hyperglycaemia but not hyperlipidaemia causes beta call dysfunction and beta cell loss in the domestic cat. Diabetologia 2009;52: 336–46.

Management of Diabetic Cats with Long-acting Insulin

Kirsten Roomp, MSc, Dr rer nat[a],
Jacquie S. Rand, BVSc, DVSc, MANZVS, DACVIM[b],*

KEYWORDS

• Diabetes • Insulin • Cats • Glargine • Detemir

KEY POINTS

- Glargine and detemir are associated with the highest remission rates reported in cats and the lowest occurrences of clinical hypoglycemic events.
- Overall, glycemic control using glargine/detemir is superior to protamine zinc insulin because of the long duration of action of these insulin analogues, which reduces periods of hyperglycemia.
- However, it should be noted that no insulin type has been effective in controlling hyperglycemia in all cats, even with twice-daily administration.
- There is a narrow window of opportunity of treatment for diabetic cats; initiating effective treatment within days of diagnosis leads to remission rates greater than 90% using nonintensive blood glucose control protocols with glargine/detemir.

AIMS OF THERAPY

The use of long-acting insulin and high-protein, low-carbohydrate diets have made the goal of achieving remission in most diabetic cats a realistic one, preventing a lifetime of insulin injections, potential health complications, and high costs for owners. Long-acting insulin, in conjunction with low-carbohydrate diets, facilitates achieving excellent glycemic control. Controlling hyperglycemia assists in the resolution of glucose toxicity, which, over time, is responsible for reducing beta cell mass. Eventually, chronic glucose toxicity makes remission impossible because insufficient insulin-secreting tissue remains in the pancreas. It is important to initiate effective therapy as quickly as possible, not only to prevent possible complications, such as nephropathy or ketoacidosis, but to also achieve optimal glycemic control and increase the probability of remission.

[a] Luxembourg Centre for Systems Biomedicine, University of Luxembourg, Campus Belval, 7, avenue des Hauts fourneaux, Esch-Belval 4362, Luxembourg; [b] Centre for Companion Animal Health, School of Veterinary Science, Seddon Sth Bldg #82, Slip Road, The University of Queensland, Queensland 4072, Australia
* Corresponding author.
E-mail address: j.rand@uq.edu.au

Vet Clin Small Anim 43 (2013) 251–266
http://dx.doi.org/10.1016/j.cvsm.2012.12.005
0195-5616/13/$ – see front matter Crown Copyright © 2013 Published by Elsevier Inc. All rights reserved.
vetsmall.theclinics.com

THERAPY WITH LONG-ACTING INSULINS
Types of Long-acting Insulin

Currently, 3 types of long-acting insulin have been used in diabetic cats (**Table 1**).

Glargine (Lantus) is a long-acting human insulin analogue, which gained approval for humans by the Food and Drug Administration (FDA) in the United States in 2000. In this insulin, several amino acid changes have been made (asparagine at position A21 has been replaced by glycine, and 2 arginines have been added to the B chain at positions 31 and 32), which cause it to remain soluble in acidic solution but form precipitates in neutral subcutaneous tissue.[1] Several studies have demonstrated that glargine is effective at controlling blood sugar levels in diabetic cats and achieving high remission rates.[2–4]

Detemir (Levemir) is another long-acting human insulin analogue, which was approved by the FDA for human use for the US market in 2005.[5] In it, the B30 amino acid threonine has been removed and 14-carbon, myristoyl fatty acid is covalently bound to lysine at position B29. Detemir reversibly binds to albumin via its fatty chain, which increases the duration of action of the insulin.[1] Detemir has been shown to work as effectively as glargine in diabetic cats, both in terms of blood glucose control and remission rates.[6]

The development of protamine zinc insulin (PZI) dates back to the 1930s. It has both protamine (strongly basic protein) and zinc (metal ion) added to prolong its duration of action. PZI was removed from the human market in the 1990s.[7] PZI has been used extensively in feline diabetes. For cats, animal origin preparations of PZI were discontinued in 2008 and have been replaced by human recombinant PZI, which has been shown to be equally effective in cats.[8,9] PZI is also available from some compounding pharmacies in the United States, although the use of insulin from such a source is not recommended because of the possibility of variability in consistency and supply and the increased expense for the owner.

Dosage Adjustment Protocols

Dosing protocol on glargine/detemir and glucose monitoring every 1 to 2 weeks

When adjusting the dose based on serial blood glucose measurements every 3 to 4 hours over 12 hours every week (or less optimally every 2 weeks), the dosing algorithm in **Table 2** has been used successfully. Glargine and detemir are always dosed twice daily. Weekly serial glucose curves are continued for the first 4 months of therapy, which is when remission is most likely to occur.

When glucose meters calibrated for feline blood are unavailable, it is recommended that glucometers calibrated for human blood be used. The type of meter used, feline or

Table 1
Long-acting insulin types and their attributes

Insulin	Brand Name	Manufacturer	Unit per Milliliter	Type	Size	Solution/ Suspension
Glargine	Lantus	Sanofi-Aventis	U-100	rDNA origin, human insulin analogue	3-mL Cartridge, 10-mL Vial	Aqueous solution
Detemir	Levemir	Novo Nordisk	U-100	rDNA origin, human insulin analogue	3-mL Cartridge, 10-mL Vial	Aqueous solution
PZIR	ProZinc	Boehringer Ingelheim	U-40	rDNA origin, human insulin	10-mL Vial	Aqueous suspension

Table 2
Dosing protocol on glargine or detemir and glucose monitoring every 1 to 2 weeks using whole-blood human glucometers

Parameter Used for Dosage Adjustment	Change in Dose
Begin with 0.5 IU/kg if the blood glucose is >360 mg/dL (>20 mmol/L) or 0.25/kg of ideal weight if blood glucose is lower. Do not increase in the first week unless minimum response to insulin occurs, but decrease if necessary. Monitor response to therapy for first 3 d. If no monitoring occurs in the first week, begin with 1 IU per cat BID.	
If preinsulin blood glucose concentration is >216 mg/dL (>12 mmol/L) provided nadir is not in hypoglycemic range Or If nadir blood glucose concentration is >180 mg/dL (>10 mmol/L)	Increase by 0.25–1.0 IU depending on degree of hyperglycemia and total insulin dose
If preinsulin blood glucose concentration is ≥180–≤216 mg/dL (≥10–≤12 mmol/L) Or Nadir blood glucose concentration is 90–160 mg/dL (5–9 mmol/L)	Same dose
If preinsulin blood glucose concentration is 198–252 mg/dL (11–14 mmol/L). Or If nadir glucose concentration is 54–72 mg/dL (3–4 mmol/L).	Use nadir glucose, water drunk, urine glucose, and next preinsulin glucose concentration to determine if insulin dose is decreased or maintained
If preinsulin blood glucose concentration is <180 mg/dL (<10 mmol/L) Or If nadir blood glucose concentration is <54 mg/dL (<3 mmol/L)	Reduce by 0.5–1.0 IU depending on blood glucose concentration and total dose; If total dose is 0.5–1.0 IU SID, stop insulin and check for diabetic remission
If clinical signs of hypoglycemia are observed	Reduce by 50%

Abbreviation: SID, once a day.

If a serum chemistry analyzer or plasma-equivalent meter calibrated for cats is used (eg, AlphaTRAK from Abbott Animal Health), increase the target blood glucose concentration by about 1 mmol/L, 18 mg/dL, or adapt the normal range reported for cats as the target nadir glucose concentration (eg, change 3–4 to 4–5 mmol/L, change 54–72 to 72–90 mg/dL).

human and whole blood or plasma, will determine the exact cut points used to adjust insulin dose. If a serum chemistry analyzer or plasma-equivalent meter calibrated for feline blood is used (eg, AlphaTRAK, Abbott Animal Health, Abbott Laboratories, Abott Park, Illinois), the measurements at the low end of the range need to be adjusted and are 30% to 40% higher than for a whole-blood meter calibrated for human blood. The doses, when using such measuring devices, should be changed as follows: the lower limit of the range should be adjusted accordingly by adding approximately 18 mg/dL (1 mmol/L) to the value listed in the protocol in **Table 2**. For example, a target value of more than 54 mg/dL (>3 mmol/L) becomes more than 72 mg/dL (>4 mmol/L) when using a serum chemistry analyzer or a meter calibrated for feline use. Alternatively, use the normal range for feline blood glucose concentrations as a target when using a meter calibrated for feline blood. Most of the major human brands of glucometers now report plasma-equivalent values and these are intermediate between those measured by whole-blood meters calibrated for human blood and plasma-equivalent meters calibrated for feline blood. Be aware that test strips sold by the major human companies now provide plasma-equivalent readings, even when used in older whole-blood meters, although their accuracy and precision are not as good in the whole-blood meters. Typically, the maximum dose of glargine or detemir that at cat will require will be 1.7 to 2.5 IU per cat twice daily. However, some cats will only require a maximum dose of 0.5 IU twice daily and others a maximum dose of 9.0 IU twice daily.

In general, with the availability of accurate and precise glucometers calibrated for feline blood, their use is recommended in preference to meters calibrated for human blood because of the greater accuracy for blood glucose measurements around the normoglycemic range. Using meters calibrated for feline blood facilitates the use of target blood glucose concentrations in the normal range reported for cats and avoids some of the confusion with human meters whether they are reading whole blood or plasma. It is very important that the meter only requires a small volume of blood to obtain a reading; in the author's experience (Rand), meters requiring only 0.3 μL provide a reading significantly more often than those that require a droplet of 0.6 μL or more. Although many lancing devices designed for humans are available, experience by the author (Rand) has found that the Abbott lancet successfully creates a blood bleb of sufficient size to obtain a reading with the Abbott AlphaTRAK meter more often than several other lancing devices that have been trialed.

Dosing protocol on glargine/detemir and intensive blood glucose monitoring
Intensive blood glucose control requires dedicated owners that are willing to monitor their cat's blood glucose concentration a minimum of 3 times per day (on average 5 times per day). The advantage of this approach is that it allows for optimal blood glucose control, maximizing the chances for remission.[3]

The exact protocol is described in **Table 3**. The protocol was tested in cats using human whole-blood glucometers.[3,6] If a serum chemistry analyzer or plasma-equivalent meter calibrated for felines is used, the measurements at the low end of the range need to be adjusted and are 30% to 40% higher.

Dosing protocol for PZI
Detailed dosing algorithms for PZI for home use by owners have not been described in the literature. All published protocols relied on owner perceptions of clinical control together with in-clinic glucose measurements, in contrast to home testing plus veterinary examinations. One such protocol[9] is as follows:

- PZI is dosed twice daily.

- Nine-hour blood glucose curves are performed weekly in the veterinary clinic for at least 4 weeks.
- Blood glucose concentrations should be maintained between 100 and 300 mg/dL, with the nadir between 80 and 150 mg/dL.
- If nadir is less than 80 mg/dL, decrease the dose by 25% to 100% depending on the clinical signs.
- If nadir is more than 80 mg/dL to less than 150 mg/dL, the dose remains unchanged.
- If nadir is more than 150 mg/dL, increase the dose by 25% to 100%, depending on the clinical signs.
- After 4 weeks, if the cat is still not well controlled, dose adjustments should continue to be made appropriately until the blood sugar levels reach satisfactory levels.

Administration of small doses of glargine and detemir: dilution and insulin dosing pens

Administering small doses of detemir and glargine to cats is problematic and limits their use when doses of less than 1 IU are required.

Insulin dosing pens, such as the HumaPen Luxura HD (Eli Lilly, Indianapolis, IN) and the NovoPen Junior (United States)/Demi (other countries) (Novo Nordisk, Copenhagen, Denmark), are specifically designed for use in babies and children and deliver accurate and precise insulin doses in 0.5 IU increments. In some cats, particularly those going into remission and regaining some beta cell function, dose adjustments for glargine and detemir are required in increments less than 0.5 IU.

One method of administering small total doses of less than 2 IU is to hold the syringe vertically with the needle pointing down and with consistent pressure on the plunger, count the number of drops in 2 IU of insulin. Once the owner learns to reproduce the consistent pressure to deliver the same number of drops per unit, 2 IU can be drawn up and the required number of drops can be discarded before administration. For example, for some syringe-needle combinations there are 5 drops per unit of detemir, allowing increments of 0.2 IU if the client can consistently reproduce the slow pressure to deliver this number of drops per unit.

Another method frequently used by diabetic cat owners contributing to the German Diabetes-Katzen Forum is to use an insulin syringe ruler. Paper rulers are available for download at the following Web site: http://www.diabetes-katzen.net/insulinruler.pdf. Cat owners can print out paper rulers from computer files containing templates, cut them to size with scissors, laminate them, and then, holding the ruler up next to the insulin syringe, measure dose adjustments of 0.1 IU (**Figs. 1** and **2**). For ease of handling when drawing up a dose using such a ruler, glargine or detemir insulin cartridges can be attached to a vertical surface with Velcro (Velcro USA Inc, Manchester, NH) stickers (**Fig. 3**). Insulin syringes have been reported to be quite inaccurate at a total dose of one unit (1 IU).[10] Clinically, this inaccuracy can be dangerous. The position relative to the top of the needle at which the scale is printed on the syringe varies between syringes within a given brand, causing some of the difficulties in achieving a consistent dose. When comparing 20 to 30 syringes from one batch, it is generally easy to see that the relative position of the scale is not identical in all syringes. Anecdotal observations by diabetic pet owners are that differences can be 0.25 IU, in some cases almost 0.5 IU. Using the same ruler for each new syringe might help reduce the variation in the dose associated with variations in graduation markings between different syringes. However, clients should use only one brand of syringe for a given ruler; using the same ruler between different brands of syringes or different sized syringes is dangerous because the barrel diameters may be different.

Table 3
Dosing protocol for glargine or detemir and intensive blood glucose monitoring with a minimum of 3 blood glucose measurements per day (average 5) using whole-blood human glucometers

Parameter Used for Dosage Adjustment	Change in Dose
Phase 1: Initial dose and first 3 d on glargine	
Begin with 0.25 IU/kg of ideal weight BID	
Or	
If the cat received another insulin previously, increase or reduce the starting dose taking this information into account. Glargine has a lower potency than lente insulin or PZI in most cats.	
Cats with a history of developing ketones that remain >16.6 mmol/L (>300 mg/dL) after 24–48 h	Increase by 0.5 IU
If blood glucose is <2.8 mmol/L (<50 mg/dL)	Reduce dose by 0.25–0.5 IU depending on if cat is on low or high dose of insulin
Phase 2: Increasing the dose	
If nadir blood glucose concentration is >16.6 mmol/L (>300 mg/dL)	Increase every 3 d by 0.5 IU
If nadir blood glucose concentration is 11.1–16.6 mmol/L (200–300 mg/dL)	Increase every 3 d by 0.25–0.5 IU depending on if cat is on low or high dose of insulin
If nadir blood glucose concentration is <11.1 mmol/L (<200 mg/dL) but peak is >11.1 mmol/L (>200 mg/dL)	Increase every 5–7 d by 0.25–0.5 IU depending on if cat is on low or high dose of insulin
If blood glucose is <2.8 mmol/L (<50 mg/dL)	Reduce dose by 0.25–0.5 IU depending on if cat is on low or high dose of insulin

If blood glucose at the time of the next insulin injection is 2.8–5.5 mmol/L (50–100 mg/dL)	Initially test which of the alternate methods is best suited to the individual cat: 1. Feed cat and reduce the dose by 0.25–0.5 IU depending on if cat is on low or high dose of insulin 2. Feed the cat, wait 1–2 h; when the glucose concentration increases to >5.5 mmol/L (>100 mg/dL), give the normal dose. If the glucose concentration does not increase within 1–2 h, reduce the dose by 0.25 IU or 0.5 IU (as above). 3. Split the dose: feed cat and give most of dose immediately and then give the remainder 1–2 h later, when the glucose concentration has increased to >5.5 mmol/L (>100 mg/dL). If all of these methods lead to increased blood glucose concentrations, give the full dose if preinsulin blood glucose concentration is 2.8–5.5 mmol/L (50–100 mg/dL) and observe closely for signs of hypoglycemia. In general for most cats, the best results in phase 2 occur when insulin is dosed as consistent as possible, giving the full normal dose at the regular injection time.

Phase 3: Holding the dose: aim to keep blood glucose concentration within 2.8–11.1 mmol/L (50–200 mg/dL) throughout the day

If blood glucose is <2.8 mmol/L (<50 mg/dL)	Reduce dose by 0.25–0.5 IU depending on if cat is on low or high dose of insulin
If nadir or peak blood glucose concentration is >11.1 mmol/L (>200 mg/dL)	Increase dose by 0.25–0.5 IU depending on if cat is on low or high dose of insulin and the degree of hyperglycemia

Phase 4: Reducing the dose: phase out insulin slowly by 0.25–0.5 IU depending on dose

When the cat regularly (every day for at least 1 wk), has its lowest blood glucose concentration in the normal range of a healthy cat and stays less than 5.5 mmol/L (100 mg/dL) overall	Reduce dose by 0.25–0.5 IU depending on if cat is on low or high dose of insulin
If the nadir glucose concentration is 2.2–<2.8 mmol/L (40–<50 mg/dL) at least 3 times on separate days	Reduce dose immediately by 0.25–0.5 IU depending on if cat is on low or high dose of insulin
If the cat decreases <2.2 mmol/L (<40 mg/dL) once	Reduce dose immediately by 0.25–0.5 IU depending on if cat is on low or high dose of insulin
If peak blood glucose concentration is >11.1 mmol/L (>200 mg/dL)	Immediately increase insulin dose to last effective dose

Phase 5: Remission: euglycemia for a minimum of 14 d without insulin

If a serum chemistry analyzer or plasma-equivalent meter calibrated for cats is used (eg, AlphaTRAK from Abbott Animal Health), increase the target blood glucose concentration by about 1 mmol/L, 18 mg/dL, or adapt the normal range reported for cats as the target nadir glucose concentration (eg, change 2.8 to 3.8 mmol/L; change 50 to 68 mg/dL).

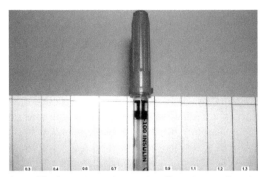

Fig. 1. An insulin syringe filled to 0.8 IU using an insulin syringe ruler. The ruler has been calibrated for BD Micro-Fine+ Demi 0.3-mL U-100 syringes (Becton Dickinson, Franklin Lakes, NJ), containing half unit markings, widely available in Germany, Switzerland, and Austria. The ruler is available for download at the following address: http://www.diabetes-katzen.net/insulinruler.pdf. Note that in Europe, a comma is commonly used instead of a decimal point. The syringes themselves are printed with 0,3 mL, and the packaging for the syringes is also labeled 0,3 mL.

Detemir is a relatively stable insulin and can be mixed with other shorter-acting insulin (eg, lispro or neutral protamine Hagedorn [NPH]). A special diluting medium is also available from Novo Nordisk; but in some countries (United States and Australia), the company will not supply veterinarians. Detemir can also be diluted with sterile water or saline (Shaun O'Mara, 2012 Novo Nordisk, personal communication). However, diluting with saline or water also dilutes the antimicrobial additive (metacresol). Therefore, because of the risk of bacterial contamination, it is recommended that the dilution be done just before the administration of insulin. Having said that, veterinarians in the past have previously diluted other insulin in the bottle and kept it refrigerated and discarded it in about 30 days. Based on experience with other insulin, with time, stability and action seemed to be adversely affected. Therefore, because of the risk of bacterial contamination and unknown changes in time with efficacy, diluting detemir in the bottle is not recommended.

For glargine, neither dilution nor mixing is recommended by the manufacturer and leads to formation of a cloudy precipitate in the syringe. However, human patients

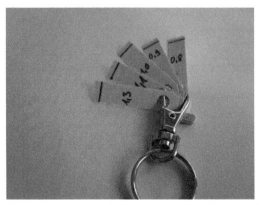

Fig. 2. Measuring ruler strips on a key chain for easy handling. Note that in Europe, a comma is commonly used instead of a decimal point. In this picture, the ruler is labeled with commas (eg, 1,3 IU rather than 1.3 IU).

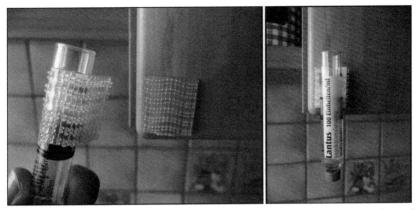

Fig. 3. Velcro sticky-back tape allows insulin cartridges to be temporarily attached to a flat, vertical surface (eg, above counter kitchen cabinet), which leaves both hands free: one for the syringe, one for the measuring ruler.

are mixing glargine with other insulin; a study reported no adverse effect on glycemic control as measured by continuous glucose monitoring.[11] Glargine is a relatively stable insulin; therefore, it would be expected that it could also be diluted with insulin or saline just before injection. Be aware that it will form a cloudy precipitate in the syringe. Mixing in the bottle is not recommended because of problems with accuracy of dosing when the insulin is a precipitate, bacterial contamination and the unknown effect on stability and efficacy.

In general, mixing glargine and detemir with a shorter-acting insulin will change the action profile, mainly of the shorter-acting insulin compared with giving separately. Mixing detemir with a rapid-acting insulin analogue like insulin aspart will reduce and delay the maximum effect of the rapid-acting insulin compared with that observed following separate injections.[12] Mixing glargine with rapid-acting lispro also markedly flattens the early pharmacodynamic peak of lispro.[13]

Storage of glargine and detemir

Glargine is marketed for human use with a 28-day shelf life at room temperature after opening. It is fairly fragile but is chemically stable in solution for 6 months if kept refrigerated.

Detemir is marketed with a 6-week shelf life at room temperature after opening. The US FDA microbiology group has a policy of not recommending longer expiration periods on multiple-use injectable medication vials, even if a preservative is present, because of the risk of bacterial contamination.

Glargine and detemir preparations contain the antimicrobial preservative metacresol, which is thought to be bacteriostatic, not bactericidal. It is most effective at room temperature, hence the recommendation by the manufacturer to keep the vial at room temperature after opening. The FDA thinks the vials have a reasonable probability of becoming contaminated with microbes through multiple daily punctures to withdraw medication past the arbitrary expiration date. However, in veterinary practice, owners of diabetic cats routinely use refrigerated glargine or detemir for up to 6 months or more with no evidence of problems. Owners should be instructed to immediately dispose of any insulin appearing cloudy or discolored because this can represent bacterial contamination or precipitation.

Urine testing

Although suboptimal, the level of glycosuria can be used to guide dosing decisions in cats receiving insulin, such as glargine and detemir. Adjusting the insulin dose based on the level of glycosuria is more successful with glargine or detemir than with lente insulin because lente has an inadequate duration of action, which inevitably results in glycosuria, and this is unassociated with the appropriateness of dose. However, the absence of glycosuria is less meaningful for indicating remission when using glargine or detemir than it is with lente insulin because glargine- or detemir-treated cats with excellent glycemic control typically have no glycosuria, even when they still require insulin. A urine glucose concentration of 3+ or more (scale 0–4+) generally indicates the need for a dose increase (increase dose by 0.5–1.0 IU). A negative urine glucose reading indicates excellent diabetic control or remission (decrease dose by 0.5–1.0 IU).

Urine glucose testing should only be considered if the blood glucose measurement is absolutely not possible.

Fructosamine

Fructosamine reflects blood glucose levels over the period of 2 to 3 weeks and measures the levels of glycated proteins in the serum.[14] Therefore, fructosamine is most useful when the indicators for glycemic control are conflicting, for example, the owner reports signs of good clinical control at home or, alternatively, is unaware of how the cat is progressing clinically at home, and blood glucose concentrations measured in the hospital are high. In these cases, fructosamine is a useful indicator of the mean blood glucose control achieved at home.

Using fructosamine to guide insulin-dosing decisions is not recommended because it is not an accurate guide to recent blood glucose concentrations. Blood glucose monitoring, ideally at home by the owner using a glucometer, is preferred.

Low-Carbohydrate Diet

Cats are obligate carnivores, and it has been demonstrated that glycemic control increases when diabetic cats are fed a low-carbohydrate, high-protein diet (<15% metabolizable energy).[15,16] Wet-food diets more often have a lower carbohydrate content than dry-food diets and are also beneficial in that they have been shown to facilitate weight loss in obese cats.[17–20] The highest remission rates described in diabetic cats have been achieved in studies using glargine or detemir, in which cats were fed a high-protein, low-carbohydrate wet-food diet with 6% or less energy from carbohydrates.[3,4,6] Although the choice of an optimal insulin increases the probability of good glycemic control and remission, the choice of diet also has an important effect.[16] The use of low-carbohydrate food (12% compared with 26% energy from carbohydrate) resulted in statistically higher remission rates (68% compared with 41%) despite similar protein levels.[21] There have been no comparative studies using diets with lower carbohydrate levels, such as those reported to be associated with remission rates of more than 80% in newly diagnosed diabetic cats (≤6% of energy from carbohydrate).

COMPLICATIONS
Hypoglycemia

The only prospective study comparing the frequency of clinical hyperglycemic events in glargine (8 cats) and PZI (8 cats) found that one case occurred in the PZI group and no cases in the glargine group. Blood glucose curves were initially performed weekly in this study and the overall length of the study was 4 months.[4]

A detailed examination of both biochemical and clinical hypoglycemia was made in 2 studies using intensive blood glucose control and glargine (55 cats) or detemir

(18 cats). In these studies, euglycemia was the goal of the dose adjustment algorithm and each cat's blood glucose concentrations were measured an average of 5 times per day (minimum 3 times per day) until stabilization. In the glargine cohort, the median length of time on protocol for insulin-dependent cats was 10 months and 2 months for cats that achieved remission. In the detemir cohort, the median length of time on the protocol for insulin-dependent cats was 10 months and 1.7 months for cats that went into remission. Although biochemical hypoglycemia was frequently observed, only a single episode of mild clinical signs of hypoglycemia was observed in each cohort, which resolved with home treatment by the owner.[3,6]

In a large prospective study of cats receiving PZI (133 diabetic cats [120 newly diagnosed and 13 previously treated]), whereby blood glucose curves were measured on days 7, 14, 30, and 45 (last day of study), the dose was adjusted with the intent to maintain peak blood glucose concentrations between 100 and 300 mg/dL and the blood glucose nadir between 80 and 150 mg/dL. Biochemical hypoglycemia was defined as a blood glucose nadir less than 80 mg/dL and identified in 151 (22%) out of 678 nine-hour serial blood glucose determinations and in 85 (64%) out of 133 diabetic cats. Clinical hypoglycemia was observed in 2 cats, which required veterinary treatment; there were 26 further episodes of owner- or veterinarian-reported clinical signs that were consistent with clinical hypoglycemia. However, these events were not confirmed by blood glucose measurements.[9]

Based on these reports, it suggests that PZI has a higher probability of causing clinical hypoglycemia than glargine or detemir. Also, the frequency of clinical hypoglycemic episodes was not higher using intensive blood glucose control regimens with frequent blood glucose measurements aimed at achieving euglycemia, presumably because low blood glucose concentrations were quickly identified and the insulin dose adjustments made appropriately.

Ketoacidosis

Ketosis and ketoacidosis were not observed in any of the studies described with any of the protocols described previously.[3,4,6,9] However, it should be noted that diabetic ketosis and ketoacidosis are reported in approximately 60% to 80% of diabetic cats at diagnosis based on plasma beta hydroxybutyrate measurements, although ketonuria is present in a smaller percentage of cats. Care should be taken to identify such animals, give a sufficient insulin dose, and stabilize the animal before sending it home.

Both glargine and detemir have a lower potency than insulins, such as NPH and porcine lente insulin. Care should, therefore, also be taken when switching a cat from a more potent (NPH or porcine lente insulin) to a less potent insulin (glargine or detemir) to avoid the development of ketosis. For example, if the cat typically has hyperglycemia and nadir glucose concentrations are 100 mg/dL (5.5 mmol/L) or more, with porcine lente insulin, an equivalent dose of glargine or detemir should be given and increased within 24 to 48 hours if needed.

Handheld point-of-care blood ketone monitors are highly effective tools for identifying ketotic cats.[22-24] They are more sensitive at detecting ketosis because they allow the identification of increased beta hydroxybutyrate concentrations in the blood before increased concentrations can be measured in the urine by dipstick, which measures predominantly acetoacetic acid. The time between increased blood concentrations of beta hydroxybutyrate and a positive urinary dipstick reading is, on average, 5 days; earlier detection of ketosis facilitates earlier treatment.[25] These monitors are also relatively inexpensive and can be used as glucometers with different test strips. Thus, they can be easily used by owners at home to monitor their cat's blood glucose and beta hydroxybutyrate concentrations.

Insulin Resistance

Acromegaly

Acromegaly in diabetic cats is thought to be common. In a study of 184 variably controlled diabetics, 59 showed a marked increase in insulinlike growth factor 1 (IGF-1) (>1000 mg/dL). Of the 18 cats that were available for subsequent imaging studies, 17 had a confirmed diagnosis of acromegaly.[26] Although the actual prevalence among diabetic cats is unknown, acromegaly should be considered in any cat in which the insulin dose with glargine or detemir is more than 1.5 IU/kg. In these cats, it is recommended that IGF-1 be measured and if increased, brain imaging should be considered for a definitive diagnosis. Rarely, some cats with confirmed acromegaly are insulin sensitive and have even achieved remission without specific treatment of acromegaly (Stijn Niessen, 2012).

Cats with acromegaly are typically insulin resistant.[27] In the authors' experience, most cats with acromegaly will require doses of more than 2 IU/kg of glargine or detemir. In fact, cats with such high exogenous insulin requirements invariably also have elevated IGF-1 concentrations when these are measured.

Some animals with acromegaly will require more than 100 IU glargine or detemir per day and may, in some cases, still be hyperglycemic. Cats requiring such high doses of insulin may benefit from combining glargine and detemir with doses of regular insulin to reduce hyperglycemia. Regular insulin is also somewhat less expensive than glargine or detemir, which reduces the financial burden on owners of acromegalic cats. Alternatively, glargine can be administered subcutaneously and intramuscularly simultaneously. When given intramuscularly or intravenously, glargine acts like regular insulin and can also be used this way for the treatment of diabetic ketoacidosis (Detemir does not act like regular insulin via these routes[28]). Cats with acromegaly can achieve remission if the tumor is removed with surgery and less commonly if treated with radiation (refer chapter on Hypersomatotrophism by Niessen SJM, Church DB and Forcada Y elsewhere in this issue).

Hyperthyroidism

Hyperthyroidism is a common endocrine disorder in older cats. Typically, diabetic cats with concurrent hyperthyroidism will not require substantially higher doses of insulin but are resistant to achieving remission or will relapse from diabetic remission. In fact, hyperthyroidism is commonly associated with relapse from diabetic remission (observed in the German Diabetes-Katzen Forum) and a cat's thyroid status should be evaluated should such a relapse occur.

Hyperthyroid diabetic cats (even those receiving medication and, thus, euthyroid) may be more difficult to regulate than nonhyperthyroid diabetic cats.

Insulin-induced rebound hyperglycemia (Somogyi effect)

An evaluation of the prevalence of the Somogyi effect in a cohort of 55 cats undergoing intensive blood glucose control with glargine showed that blood glucose curves that were consistent with insulin-induced rebound hyperglycemia were very rare despite the frequent occurrence of biochemical hyperglycemia.[29]

The fluctuations of blood glucose concentration that were commonly observed in the first weeks, and more rarely months, following the initiation of treatment with glargine, and which might be mistaken for the Somogyi effect, generally resolved with time using consistent dosing.

The dose of glargine or detemir should be reduced if the cat develops asymptomatic or clinical hypoglycemia but not when the blood glucose concentration is high and poorly responsive to insulin.

REMISSION
Remission Rates Comparison

There is only one controlled prospective study in 24 newly diagnosed diabetic cats that compared remission rates between glargine, PZI, and porcine lente insulin. Blood glucose curves were initially performed weekly, and insulin dose adjustments based on an algorithm were also performed weekly. Cats were fed a low-carbohydrate diet (<8%–10% metabolizable energy). The reported remission rate for glargine was 100% (8 out of 8 cats), and this was significantly higher than the remission rate for PZI (38%, 3 out of 8 cats) and porcine lente insulin (25%, 2 out of 8 cats).[30]

The largest study for cats treated with glargine involved 55 previously treated diabetic cats. In this cohort, 91% of the cats had been previously treated with another insulin, predominantly porcine lente insulin, for a median of 15 weeks. Most cats were also fed a very-low-carbohydrate wet-food diet (<6% metabolizable energy) on the first insulin, yet did not go into remission. On switching to glargine, they continued to be fed a very-low-carbohydrate diet. Cats were monitored using home blood glucose measurements at least 3 times daily. The insulin dose was adjusted using an algorithm aimed at achieving euglycemia. Provided the protocol was initiated within 6 months of diagnosis, high remission rates (84%) were achieved. For cats that began on the protocol more than 6 months after diagnosis, a much lower remission rate was achieved (35%). The overall remission rate for all cats, regardless of when the protocol was initiated after diagnosis, was 64%.[3]

For detemir, a cohort of 18 diabetic cats, previously mainly treated with porcine lente insulin, was evaluated using an insulin dosing protocol aimed at achieving euglycemia and fed a very-low-carbohydrate wet-food diet. The remission rates were very similar to those achieved with glargine: the overall remission rate was 67%. Again, there was a difference between cats that initiated the protocol shortly after diagnosis and those that did not; for cats that began the protocol before or after 6 months of diagnosis, remission rates were 81% and 42%, respectively.[6]

No significant differences in terms of remission rate could be identified between glargine and detemir (see **Table 3**).[3,6]

Further recent studies examining the efficacy of PZI in newly diagnosed and previously treated diabetic cats did not explicitly examine remission rates.[8,9]

Relapse

Very few studies have examined the rate of relapse in cats that are in diabetic remission, presumably because of the relatively short time period that many such studies are run. Two studies that have examined the rate of relapse in previously treated diabetic cats treated with glargine or detemir found relapse rates of 26% and 25%, respectively **Table 4**.[3,6]

Frequent causes of relapse are hyperthyroidism and chronic pancreatitis. Very few such cats achieved a second remission because additional glucose toxicity of a further diabetic episode has destroyed too much beta cell mass for a second remission to be possible.

The more quickly effective treatment with insulin begins and the return to euglycemia is achieved, the more likely a second remission will become. It is advisable that cats whose blood glucose concentrations increase and are consistently at more than 120 mg/dL be treated with insulin, beginning with small doses that can be ramped up quickly.

Table 4
Remission rates in diabetic cats comparing different insulins and different time points of initiating treatment

Insulin Type	Newly Diagnosed, Using 1–2 Weekly Blood Glucose Monitoring (%)	Previously Treated with Other Insulin, <6 mo Since Diagnosis, Using Intensive Blood Glucose Control Protocol (%)	Previously Treated with Other Insulin, >6 mo Since Diagnosis, Using Intensive Blood Glucose Control Protocol (%)
Glargine	100	84	35
Detemir	n/a	81	42
PZI	38	n/a	n/a

Abbreviation: n/a = not available.

SUMMARY

- Glargine and detemir are associated with the highest remission rates reported in cats and the lowest occurrences of clinical hypoglycemic events.
- Overall, glycemic control using glargine/detemir is superior to PZI because of the long duration of action these insulin analogues, which reduces periods of hyperglycemia.
- However, it should be noted that no insulin type has been effective in controlling hyperglycemia in all cats, even with twice-daily administration.
- There is a narrow window of opportunity of treatment for diabetic cats; initiating effective treatment within days of diagnosis leads to remission rates more than 90% using nonintensive blood glucose control protocols with glargine/detemir. After this, if intensive blood glucose control is initiated with glargine/detemir within the first 6 months, remission rates are reported to be 81% to 84%. If intensive blood glucose is started more than 6 months after diagnosis, remission rates decrease to 35% to 42%.

REFERENCES

1. Vigneri R, Squatrito S, Sciacca L. Insulin and its analogs: actions via insulin and IGF receptors. Acta Diabetol 2010;47(4):271–8.
2. Boari A, Aste G, Rocconi F, et al. Glargine insulin and high-protein-low-carbohydrate diet in cats with diabetes mellitus. Vet Res Commun 2008; 32(Suppl 1):S243–5.
3. Roomp K, Rand J. Intensive blood glucose control is safe and effective in diabetic cats using home monitoring and treatment with glargine. J Feline Med Surg 2009;11(8):668–82.
4. Marshall RD, Rand JS, Morton JM. Treatment of newly diagnosed diabetic cats with glargine insulin improves glycaemic control and results in higher probability of remission than protamine zinc and lente insulins. J Feline Med Surg 2009; 11(8):683–91.
5. Triplitt CL. New technologies and therapies in the management of diabetes. Am J Manag Care 2007;13(Suppl 2):S47–54.
6. Roomp K, Rand J. Evaluation of detemir in diabetic cats managed with a protocol for intensive blood glucose control. J Feline Med Surg 2012;14(8):566–72.
7. Tripathy B. RSSDI (Research Society for the Study of Diabetes in India): Textbook of diabetes mellitus. 2nd Edition. New Delhi, India: Jaypee Brothers Medical Pub; 2012.

8. Norsworthy G, Lynn R, Cole C. Preliminary study of protamine zinc recombinant insulin for the treatment of diabetes mellitus in cats. Vet Ther 2009;10(1–2):24–8.
9. Nelson RW, Henley K, Cole C. Field safety and efficacy of protamine zinc recombinant human insulin for treatment of diabetes mellitus in cats. J Vet Intern Med 2009;23(4):787–93.
10. Keith K, Nicholson D, Rogers D. Accuracy and precision of low-dose insulin administration using syringes, pen injectors, and a pump. Clin Pediatr (Phila) 2004;43(1):69–74.
11. Kaplan W, Rodriguez LM, Smith OE, et al. Effects of mixing glargine and short-acting insulin analogs on glucose control. Diabetes Care 2004;27(11):2739–40.
12. Cengiz E, Swan KL, Tamborlane WV, et al. The alteration of aspart insulin pharmacodynamics when mixed with detemir insulin. Diabetes Care 2012;35(4):690–2.
13. Cengiz E, Tamborlane WV, Martin-Fredericksen M, et al. Early pharmacokinetic and pharmacodynamic effects of mixing lispro with glargine insulin: results of glucose clamp studies in youth with type 1 diabetes. Diabetes Care 2010; 33(5):1009–12.
14. Lutz TA, Rand JS, Ryan E. Fructosamine concentrations in hyperglycemic cats. Can Vet J 1995;36(3):155–9.
15. Bennett N, Greco DS, Peterson ME, et al. Comparison of a low carbohydrate-low fiber diet and a moderate carbohydrate-high fiber diet in the management of feline diabetes mellitus. J Feline Med Surg 2006;8(2):73–84.
16. Frank G, Anderson W, Pazak H, et al. Use of a high-protein diet in the management of feline diabetes mellitus. Vet Ther 2001;2(3):238–46.
17. Zoran DL. The carnivore connection to nutrition in cats. J Am Vet Med Assoc 2002;221(11):1559–67.
18. Nguyen P, Martin L, Siliart B, et al. Weight loss in obese cats: evaluation of a high protein diet. Nutr Rev 2009;45(10):225–31.
19. Nguyen P, Leray V, Dumon H, et al. High protein intake affects lean body mass but not energy expenditure in nonobese neutered cats. J Nutr 2004;134(Suppl 8):2084S–6S.
20. Vasconcellos RS, Borges NC, Goncalves KN, et al. Protein intake during weight loss influences the energy required for weight loss and maintenance in cats. J Nutr 2009;139(5):855–60.
21. Kirk CA. Feline diabetes mellitus: low carbohydrates versus high fiber? Vet Clin North Am Small Anim Pract 2006;36(6):1297–306, vii.
22. Zeugswetter FK, Rebuzzi L. Point-of-care beta-hydroxybutyrate measurement for the diagnosis of feline diabetic ketoacidaemia. J Small Anim Pract 2012;53(6): 328–31.
23. Weingart C, Lotz F, Kohn B. Measurement of beta-hydroxybutyrate in cats with nonketotic diabetes mellitus, diabetic ketosis, and diabetic ketoacidosis. J Vet Diagn Invest 2012;24(2):295–300.
24. Di Tommaso M, Aste G, Rocconi F, et al. Evaluation of a portable meter to measure ketonemia and comparison with ketonuria for the diagnosis of canine diabetic ketoacidosis. J Vet Intern Med 2009;23(3):466–71.
25. Rand J. Feline diabetes mellitus. In: Mooney CT, Peterson ME, editors. BSAVA manual of canine and feline endocrinology. 4th edition. United Kingdom: British Small Animal Vet. Assoc.; 2012. p. 133–47.
26. Niessen SJ, Petrie G, Gaudiano F, et al. Feline acromegaly: an underdiagnosed endocrinopathy? J Vet Intern Med 2007;21(5):899–905.
27. Feldman EC, Nelson RW. Acromegaly and hyperadrenocorticism in cats: a clinical perspective. J Feline Med Surg 2000;2(3):153–8.

28. Rand J, Gunew M, Menrath V. Intramuscular glargine with or without concurrent subcutaneous administration for treatment of feline diabetic ketoacidosis: a preliminary study. J Vet Emerg Crit Care 2013. [EPub ahead of print].
29. Roomp K, Rand J. The Somogyi effect is rare in diabetic cats managed using glargine and a protocol aimed at tight glycemic control. In: Journal of Veterinary Internal Medicine. Proceedings of: 26th Annual ACVIM Forum. San Antonio (TX): 2008. p. 790–1.
30. Marshall RD, Rand JS, Morton JM. Glargine and protamine zinc insulin have a longer duration of action and result in lower mean daily glucose concentrations than lente insulin in healthy cats. J Vet Pharmacol Ther 2008;31(3):205–12.

Management of Cats on Lente Insulin: Tips and Traps

Sarah M.A. Caney, BVSc, PhD, MRCVS

KEYWORDS

- Diabetes mellitus • Insulin • Lente • Diabetic remission • Glucose curve

KEY POINTS

- The majority of diabetic cats are non-ketotic, and their diabetes is analogous to human type 2 diabetes mellitus, characterized by insulin resistance, obesity, and pancreatic amyloid deposition.
- Many cases of diabetes are straightforward to stabilize using Lente insulins, although it may take several weeks or months to identify an optimal insulin regime.
- Detailed survival statistics for cats treated with Lente insulin are not available.
- Median survival times for diabetic cats treated with Lente, Ultralente, or protamine zinc insulins are approximately 20 months.

INTRODUCTION

The majority of diabetic cats are non-ketotic, and their diabetes is analogous to human type 2 diabetes mellitus, characterized by insulin resistance, obesity, and pancreatic amyloid deposition.[1] This article focuses on routine management of these cases. Ketoacidotic diabetic cats need to be treated urgently, with attention paid to electrolyte imbalances (potassium and phosphate), fluid therapy, and reversing the hyperglycemia and ketoacidosis.

The goals of diabetic stabilization are as follows:

1. If possible, achieve diabetic remission.
2. Resolve clinical signs associated with diabetes mellitus (polyuria, polydipsia, polyphagia, and weight loss are the major ones).
3. Maintain blood glucose levels below the renal threshold (12–14 mmol/L or 215–255 mg/dL) for the majority of the time; this should be associated with prevention/minimization of ketoacidosis and the development of other long-term complications of diabetes, such as peripheral neuropathies (**Fig. 1**).

Disclosures: None.
Conflict of Interest: None.
Vet Professionals Limited, Midlothian Innovation Centre, Pentlandfield, Roslin, Midlothian EH25 9RE, UK
E-mail address: sarah@vetprofessionals.com

Vet Clin Small Anim 43 (2013) 267–282
http://dx.doi.org/10.1016/j.cvsm.2012.11.001
0195-5616/13/$ – see front matter © 2013 Elsevier Inc. All rights reserved.

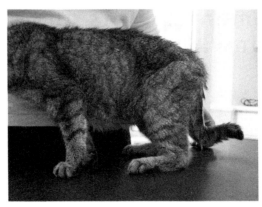

Fig. 1. Peripheral neuropathies can develop as a complication of diabetes. Most often this is associated with a plantigrade and/or palmigrade stance.

4. Avoid hypoglycemia by maintaining blood glucose levels above 5 mmol/L (90 mg/dL).

Aggressive treatment increases the chances of diabetic remission. Efforts should, therefore, concentrate on the following:

- Follow the recommendations made for insulin therapy and dietary management (discussed later). Resolution of glucose toxicity greatly increases the chance of achieving diabetic remission. Glucose toxicity describes the situation whereby prolonged hyperglycemia suppresses insulin secretion by the β-cells of the pancreas. As glucose toxicity resolves, the β-cells may recover some ability to produce and secrete insulin, leading to improved glycemic control and diabetic remission in some patients.
- When possible, withdraw any diabetogenic drugs a cat may be receiving (eg, glucocorticoids or progestagens) or replace them with non-diabetogenic alternatives (eg, antihistamines or cyclosporine for allergic skin disease, inhaled corticosteroids for asthma, or budesonide in place of prednisolone for inflammatory bowel disease).
- Manage obesity, when present. Obesity causes insulin resistance and is an important risk factor for development of feline diabetes (**Fig. 2**).[2–4] A weight

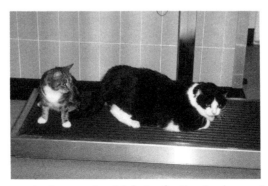

Fig. 2. Obesity is recognized as a major risk factor for the development of feline diabetes.

loss regime resulting in 1% loss of body weight per week is recommended. A low-carbohydrate diet fed at an appropriate caloric intake for weight loss is often an ideal choice for overweight diabetic cats.

- Identify and support pancreatitis, when present.
- Identify and address other underlying conditions. All inflammatory, infectious, and neoplastic conditions have the potential to increase insulin resistance and de-stabilize diabetic control.[5] Successful resolution of these underlying conditions may be enough to result in diabetic remission. For example, periodontal disease is common in middle-aged to older cats and, if present, should be addressed early in the course of treatment of diabetes.
- Identify and manage concurrent illnesses that may be linked to the diabetes. For example, urinary tract infections (UTIs) are a potential complication of diabetes and increase insulin requirements and complicate stabilization. Reported prevalence of bacterial UTIs in cats with diabetes mellitus has varied from 7% to 14.3%.[6–10] Unfortunately, it is common for many of these UTIs to be clinically silent, that is, not associated with typical signs of lower urinary tract disease. Sediment examination may not always show bacteria with increased numbers of leukocytes and erythrocytes.[7,9,10] Therefore, urine culture is recommended as a priority in all newly diagnosed diabetic cats and those whose diabetic control has recently deteriorated.
- Increase physical activity—diabetes is more common in inactive cats. Increased physical activity in other species, including dogs, increases insulin effectiveness and is especially beneficial in aiding weight loss in obese cats.[11] Care providers should be encouraged to play with their cats for 10 minutes each day and to place food in multiple sites around the house to encourage cats to move around during the day.

Typically, approximately 15% to 30% of diabetic cats treated with Lente insulin are reported to achieve remission and are able to maintain normoglycemia without insulin therapy or use of other glucose-lowering drugs.[6] There is evidence that early intensive management with long-acting insulin (glargine or detemir) and dietary management can increase this rate to greater than 80% in some situations.[12–14] Diabetic remission is also possible for patients presenting with diabetic ketoacidosis.[15] Remission typically occurs within 1 to 3 months of initiation of treatment, although relapse occurs transiently or permanently in approximately 25% of these patients. Remission from relapse is generally harder to achieve. Most patients in diabetic remission have reduced pancreatic function as a result of β-cell loss and damage resulting from hyperglycemia (glucose toxicity) as well as any underlying pancreatic pathology that contributed to the diabetes development in the first place. Other clinical problems are often present in these cases and may account for a patient's predisposition to diabetic relapse through increasing insulin requirements. Common concurrent illnesses include gingivitis, obesity, hyperthyroidism, concurrent diabetogenic drugs, and renal disease.

DIETARY MANAGEMENT OF DIABETES MELLITUS

Studies have shown benefits to glycemic control by feeding diabetic cats a low-carbohydrate diet.[12,13,16–19] These studies reported diabetic remission rates between 33% and 100% when using a combination of dietary management and insulin therapy. There are several specially formulated veterinary prescription diets available for this purpose. Wet diets are generally recommended versus dry diets because they often contain lower carbohydrate levels. The lower energy density and greater water content are also useful for managing obesity. Use of low-carbohydrate diets may reduce or eliminate the need for insulin therapy in the long term. In patients where the diet is changed after diagnosis of diabetes, it is important to make any dietary change slowly and to monitor the patients carefully because insulin requirements can change quickly. Low-carbohydrate diets are suitable for use in diabetic cats of all weights—whether they need weight loss or gain. The protein content can be problematic, however, for cats with concurrent renal failure, especially those with International Renal Interest Society (IRIS) stage 4 disease, when azotemia is often associated with inappetance. Low-carbohydrate, prescription veterinary diets for diabetic cats are typically lower in phosphorus than non-prescription, low-carbohydrate diets.

Because cats have a prolonged post-prandial glycemia, timing of meals is not critical for management of most feline diabetic patients and it is generally best to feed cats in the way they are used to being fed (eg, ad lib) rather than changing the regime. In those cats used to being fed meals, it is common to give a proportion of the daily food requirements at the time of (or shortly after) insulin injections with the remainder given at the estimated peak action times of the Lente insulin. Many diabetic cats are polyphagic with Lente insulin, and this usually persists in spite of good clinical stabilization of their diabetes.

INSULIN THERAPY

Insulin therapy is required to stabilize most diabetic cats. Considerable individual variation occurs in duration of action and response to insulin—even when only considering Lente preparations.[20] Intermediate-acting products, such as Lente insulins, should generally be used twice daily. Occasionally cats need Lente insulin 3 times daily to control their diabetes.

There is currently one Lente insulin with a veterinary license for cats (Caninsulin [Vetsulin in the United States], MSD Animal Health [Whitehouse Station, NJ]) and this is a porcine insulin zinc suspension with an insulin concentration of 40 IU/mL. Caninsulin provides good to excellent clinical control of diabetes in a majority of patients. Lente preparations licensed for treatment of diabetic humans and other intermediate-acting preparations, such as neutral protamine Hagedorn (NPH), typically have an insulin concentration of 100 IU/mL. Protamine zinc insulin (ProZinc, Boehringer Ingelheim GmbH, Ingelheim am Rhein, Germany) (40 IU/mL) is an alternative to Caninsulin in those countries where it is available (currently licensed only in North America for veterinary use). NPH and human licensed Lente insulins are alternatives where Caninsulin/Vetsulin is not available, but the human-licensed glargine and detemir provide superior glycemic control in most cats.

Most cats require small doses of insulin. Non-ketotic diabetic cats should be started on insulin at a dose of approximately 0.25 to 0.5 units per kg body weight per injection (maximum starting dose 3 IU per cat). The dose of insulin should not be increased more often than every 3 to 5 days because it takes several days for the effects of a new dose to settle out. Usually the author does not alter the dose of insulin more often than every 1 to 2 weeks.

For those cats receiving low doses of insulin, it is possible to dilute the insulin preparations, but this may alter stability and shelf life, cannot provide a guaranteed concentration of insulin, and constitutes off-label usage. Dilution of insulins may produce unpredictable results and is, therefore, not recommended. Availability of a licensed product with an insulin concentration of 40 IU/mL (eg, Caninsulin) is helpful in most diabetic cats because it allows accurate visualization of low doses. When using 40-IU/mL preparations, it is essential to also use 40-IU/mL syringes. Use of a magnifying glass or reading spectacles can be helpful for care providers with poor eyesight, especially when low doses are prescribed. In some locations, Caninsulin is available in a pen doser, which accurately dispenses insulin in 0.5 IU increments (VetPen, MSD Animal Health). Accurate dosing of insulin is essential in those cats receiving low doses and those with sensitive insulin requirements. Accidental overdose causing hypoglycemia is a particular risk in these cats.

INITIAL MONITORING OF DIABETES MELLITUS: THE STABILIZATION PERIOD

The response to therapy should be monitored using clinical and laboratory parameters. The author prefers to manage routine diabetic patients as outpatients. Care providers are asked to monitor and record details regarding

- Time of insulin injection
- Dose of insulin injected
- Type of diet offered
- Amount of food offered and eaten (and time of feeding if food is not offered ad lib)
- Amount of water drunk over a 24-hour period: this measurement is often the most helpful parameter in indicating diabetic control (**Table 1**). Depending on whether their diet is primarily wet or dry food, uncontrolled diabetics often drink more than 80 to 100 mL/kg/d; those with excellent control may drink less than 20 mL/kg/d. If it is not possible for a care provider to measure water consumption accurately, a subjective assessment of thirst is still helpful. In multi-animal households, total household water consumption can still be useful because any changes are usually a result of the diabetic cat.
- Urine volume (where possible)—for example, weighing the litter tray can give an indication of whether a cat is polyuric
- Demeanor: diabetic cats should remain bright and alert. Well-controlled diabetic cats remain bright and alert with an acceptable thirst and healthy and stable body weight. Any change in demeanor may be an indication of ketosis, hypoglycemia,

Table 1
Example of usefulness of measurement of water consumption in cats

Time Point	24-h Water Consumption	Comment
Diabetes mellitus just diagnosed	370–510 mL (92.5–127.5 mL/kg/d)	Toots is severely and persistently polydipsic.
Diabetes well controlled	120–180 mL (30–45 mL/kg/d)	Toots' water intake has dropped dramatically. Serum fructosamine results confirm that the diabetes is now well controlled. Although fed a totally wet diet, Toots water intake is still noticeable due to IRIS stage 2 chronic kidney disease in addition to her diabetes mellitus.
UTI	260–290 mL (65–72.5 mL/kg/d)	Toots' increase in water intake prompted veterinary assessment at which point a UTI was diagnosed by culture of a cystocentesis urine sample. Once treated, Toots' diabetes mellitus once again came under control.

Data extracted from records relating to Toots: a 13-year-old female neutered domestic short hair cat with diabetes mellitus and chronic kidney disease (Sarah M.A. Caney, BVSc, PhD, MRCVS, unpublished data, 2006).

or other concurrent problems and should prompt consultation with a veterinarian. Signs of hypoglycemia include weakness, ataxia, tremors, and seizures. Care providers should be instructed in signs to look for and actions to take, which include not injecting any more insulin, providing the cat with food, and, if the cat does not eat, applying glucose or sugar solution to the gums. It is sensible to provide carers with glucose powder or solution to keep at home in the event of hypoglycemia.

- Monitoring glucose and ketone levels in urine samples collected by the care provider at home—for example, once or twice a week in the first few months of treatment. A variety of kits are available to facilitate home collection of urine samples (**Fig. 3**). The main value in monitoring urine samples is detection of ketosis (always a cause for concern and requiring prompt re-evaluation of the patient) and absence of glucose (possible evidence of diabetic remission). Both of these findings should prompt immediate contact with a veterinary surgeon for further advice and treatment. A small amount of day-to-day variation in the amount of glucose present in morning urine samples is not cause for concern. A negative urine glucose reading raises suspicion of diabetic remission. In these patients, daily urine glucose monitoring is recommended in addition to other measures, such as reducing or stopping the insulin and performing a blood glucose curve (BGC) (discussed later).

Veterinary check-ups should be done at least once a week in the initial stages of stabilization. These assessments should include

1. History and analysis of data presented by the care provider. In addition to collecting clinical data, this is an opportunity to provide support and reassurance to the care provider.
2. Physical examination, including a weight check and body condition score. Weight gain is a good indication of diabetic control in underweight diabetic cats. In obese diabetic cats, steady weight loss (approximately 1% per week) is recommended.

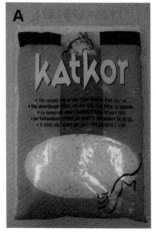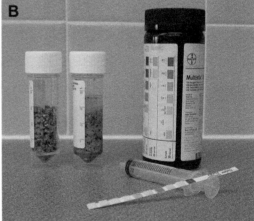

Fig. 3. Urine collection and analysis can be helpful in the diagnosis and assessment of diabetes. Several kits are available for care providers to use as non-absorbent cat litter—(A) Katkor litter is shown. Alternatively, absorbent cat litter, which has been urinated on, can be mixed with a small amount of water before doing a dipstick for glucose. Although not quantitative, this test can indicate whether or not glycosuria is present, as in this case (B).

Blood pressure should be assessed soon after diagnosis and thereafter every 6 months if normotensive. Systemic hypertension is common in middle-aged and elderly cats. A link between diabetes and systemic hypertension has not been confirmed.[21,22]

3. Laboratory assessment of glycemic control. This can be done via mini-BGC or a single sample collected at the estimated peak time of insulin activity (4–6 hours post-injection for Lente insulins). BGCs are discussed in more detail later. If there has been no clinical progress with diabetic control at this first check, however, the author usually increases the dose by 0.5 IU to 1 IU per injection and reassesses the cat after a further week.

Fructosamine assessment is of some value in the diagnosis and monitoring of diabetic cats. Fructosamine is a glycosylated serum protein molecule produced by a non-enzymatic reaction between glucose and the amino groups of plasma proteins. The concentration of fructosamine depends on plasma glucose concentrations for the preceding 1 to 2 weeks and the circulating half lives of plasma proteins (for example, albumin has a half life of approximately 3 weeks). Fructosamine levels are elevated when the blood glucose concentration is high for a prolonged period and an elevation in serum fructosamine indicates that there has been significant hyperglycemia during the previous 1 to 3 weeks. Fructosamine estimation is, therefore, helpful for differentiating stress hyperglycemia from hyperglycemia associated with diabetes when diagnosing new cases and monitoring long-term control in existing patients. Depending on the magnitude of the hyperglycemia, fructosamine levels may exceed the reference range after as few as 3 days.[23] In those cats with less marked hyperglycemia (less than 20 mmol/L or 360 mg/dL) fructosamine measurement may be less helpful, with normal results possible in cats with diabetes.[23] Studies using experimental induction of hyperglycemia in healthy cats have shown that fructosamine results may vary markedly for any given glucose concentration, meaning that fructosamine results cannot be used to accurately extrapolate mean blood glucose levels and, hence, glycemic control.[23] Serum fructosamine estimation is still of some value, however, in evaluating glycemic control in addition to historical, clinical, and other laboratory parameters. Fructosamine levels should be interpreted in line with the reference ranges used by the laboratory in question. In general terms, levels above 400 to 450 μmol/l are generally associated with poor control of the diabetes.[24,25]

Levels of fructosamine can be affected by several factors—there is an artifactual reduction in fructosamine levels in hyperthyroid cats due to accelerated protein turnover, so this test needs to be interpreted with care in these cats.[26,27] Hypoproteinemia also depresses fructosamine levels but, in contrast to dogs, serum fructosamine levels are not affected by hyperlipidemia, hypertriglyceridemia, or azotemia.[28] Although the age of a cat does not seem to affect fructosamine levels, other factors have been shown to have an affect on this parameter.[29] For example, healthy neutered male cats tend to have higher fructosamine levels than healthy neutered female cats and there is a positive correlation between body condition score and body weight with serum fructosamine levels.[29] Cats categorized as lean have lower fructosamine levels than those classed as normal or obese.[29]

If it is clear that the diabetes is not well controlled, then there is little value in assessing fructosamine levels. In general, the author assesses fructosamine every 3 to 6 weeks in the first few months of stabilization with 3-month to 6-month assessments thereafter, depending on the patient. Over time, a patient's insulin requirements may change depending on several factors, including presence of concurrent illness.

BLOOD GLUCOSE CURVES IN DIABETIC CATS RECEIVING LENTE INSULIN

A mini-BGC or full BGC is often helpful 1 to 2 weeks after any change in the insulin regime. The main aims of a blood glucose curve are

- To determine the time of peak action of the insulin. Most cats receiving Lente insulins have a peak action of approximately 3 to 6 hours post-injection. For cats receiving twice-daily Lente, the ideal nadir in glucose is 5 to 6 hours postinjection.
- To determine the duration of the insulin's action, which indicates if the insulin a cat is receiving is lasting long enough or whether a different preparation of insulin or more frequent injections may be appropriate. For most cats receiving Lente insulin, the duration of action is 8 to 10 hours. In an ideal case, the blood glucose remains below the renal threshold (12–14 mmol/L or 215–255 mg/dL) for the majority of the time.
- To determine the trough (nadir) glucose measurement, which is the lowest the blood glucose levels fall after insulin is given. In an ideal situation, the blood glucose falls to approximately 5 mmol/L to 9 mmol/L (90–160 mg/dL) and spends the majority of the 24-hour period below 14 mmol/L (255 mg/dL). If an insufficient response to insulin is seen, a higher dose may be required. It is important that the blood glucose levels are not reduced too low (hypoglycemia defined as 3.5–4.9 mmol/L or 65–90 mg/dL or lower) because this greatly increases the risk of clinical hypoglycemia, which can cause severe clinical signs (seizures or coma) or death. If this is the case, then the dose of insulin needs to be reduced.

A major limitation of the usefulness of the BGC is stress-associated hyperglycemia, which commonly occurs in cats. Use of ear pin-pricks and/or intravenous catheters can be helpful in reducing stress. Care also needs to be taken to avoid iatrogenic anemia through over-sampling with BGC in hospitalized patients. Iatrogenic anemia is avoided by using an ear or footpad for blood sampling and measurement of glucose using a portable glucose meter. Portable glucose meters are available as calibrated for feline blood (eg, AlphaTRAK, Abbott Animal Health, Abbott Park, IL, USA), and meters requiring small amounts of blood (eg, 0.3 μL) are recommended for cats.

Examples of problems that can be identified on BGC are summarized in **Table 2**.

Care providers can be trained to collect small blood samples with cats at home, or cats can be admitted to a veterinary hospital for assessment. Many pocket-sized glucometers are available. Monitors requiring tiny volumes of blood (eg, less than 1 μL) are ideal, and those requiring less than 0.6 μL are more often associated with successful measurements than those requiring large volumes. Monitors or portable glucose meters should be calibrated against hospital glucometers or laboratory equipment to ensure they are producing acceptable results.

Options for performing a BGC:

1. Detailed BGC. Blood samples are collected before administration of insulin and then every 1 to 2 hours for 12 hours (or until the blood glucose reaches pre-insulin levels). Occasionally, Lente insulin may have a duration of 24 hours in some cats.[20] A BGC indicates how effective the dose of insulin is in lowering blood glucose levels, the timing of the blood glucose nadir, and the duration of action of the insulin.
2. Typical protocol for a mini-BGC:
   - Care provider injects morning insulin with cat at home at 7:30 AM.
   - Cat admitted to the hospital at 8:30 AM. Blood collected for glucose analysis.
   - Further blood samples collected every 2 hours during the day until the blood glucose is greater than 14 mmol/L (255 mg/dL).

Table 2
Examples of problems that can be identified on a BGC

Problem	Interpretation	Suggested Action
Pre-insulin glucose <10 mmol/L (180 mg/dL)	There is a possibility of diabetic remission.	Withhold insulin and monitor.
Blood glucose nadir >9 mmol/L (>160 mg/dL)	Insulin dose is too low.	Increase the dose by 1 IU per injection.
Blood glucose nadir 3.5–4.9 mmol/L (65–90 mg/dL)	Risk of hypoglycemia	Reduce insulin dose (eg, by 1 IU per injection and repeat BGC after 1 wk).
Evidence of Somogyi overswing: hypoglycemia (glucose <3.5 mmol/L; <65 mg/dL) followed by hyperglycemia (glucose >17 mmol/L; >300 mg/dL)	The insulin dose is too high. Rapid and/or large falls in blood glucose are associated with a rebound hyperglycemia, which can persist for many hours.	Reduce the insulin dose by 50%.
Blood glucose nadir ≤3 h post-injection	Duration of insulin is too short.	Consider increasing frequency of insulin injections or changing to a different insulin preparation and regime.
Blood glucose above renal threshold (12–14 mmol/L, 215–255 mg/dL) for more than 40% of the time in spite of appropriate nadir blood glucose	Duration of insulin is too short.	Consider increasing frequency of insulin injections or changing to a different insulin preparation and regime.
Blood glucose nadir ≥18 h post-insulin	Duration of action is too long for twice daily injections—there is a danger of insulin overlap if twice daily injections continued.	Consider once daily injections if the duration is 18–24 h; alternatively, consider a change to a different insulin preparation and regime.
Blood glucose below renal threshold (12–14 mmol/L, 215–255 mg/dL) when second daily injection due	Duration of action is too long for twice daily injections—there is a danger of insulin overlap if twice-daily injections continued.	Consider once-daily injections if the duration is 18–24 h; alternatively, consider a change to a different insulin preparation and regime.

3. Strategic-sample BGC. In this situation, a single or a few samples are collected at times estimated or known to be helpful in assessing glycemic control, for example, approximately 4 to 6 hours after administration of Lente insulin, when the insulin is estimated to be at its peak action. In situations when a more detailed BGC has been done in the past, timing of strategic samples can be done according to information gained from these BGC, but there is considerable day-to-day variation in the exact timing of the trough.
4. Continuous glucose monitoring systems (CGMSs) have been described in cats and, where available, offer an alternative option for assessing glycemic control. CGMSs assess the real-time glucose levels in interstitial fluid of patients. These devices involve subcutaneous placement of a sensor attached to a monitor, and results show good agreement with blood glucose measurements.[30]

Once a BGC has been performed, subsequent monitoring can largely be done using strategically timed samples over the day. For example, if the trough glucose is occurring 6 hours after insulin therapy, then future monitoring can involve a sample pre-insulin and 6 hours later. More frequent measurements are valuable, however, in the initial stages of stabilization or if excellent clinical control has not been achieved. Studies have shown that there can be large day-to-day variations in BGC results in cats—even when the insulin dose and food offered were unchanged.[30,31] Day-to-day variations are similarly large, whether the BGC is done in the clinic or with a cat at home in a presumably stress-free environment.[31] Similar variability is documented in human diabetic patients—even when activity levels, meal composition and size, stress, and medications remain constant.[32–34] For these reasons, decisions regarding dose adjustments should not be solely based on BGC results.

BGC results may vary for several reasons, including

- Differences in activity levels
- Differences in stress levels
- Variability in the equipment used to measure blood glucose levels (this includes inappropriate handling or use of the equipment)
- Variation in the injection site used
- Inadvertent variation in the dose administered
- Any problems with the injection technique
- Variation in the amount and type of food offered and eaten
- Presence of underlying disease. Waxing and waning of underlying diseases, such as pancreatitis, can lead to varying insulin requirements from day to day.

DOSE ADJUSTMENTS IN DIABETIC CATS

The dose of insulin can be increased in those cats that do not seem to be responding to insulin but this should not be done too rapidly because accumulation of insulin can occur leading to potentially life-threatening hypoglycemia. The author's recommendation is to be cautious in the magnitude of the dose increase (for example, 0.5 or 1.0 units depending on the patient) and to do this no more frequently than every 3 days. Typically, the author increases the insulin dose once a week in cats managed as outpatients. Once the dose seems to be producing a good response (clinically and on the basis of spot glucose measurements), it is often useful to perform a 12-hour glucose curve measuring the blood glucose every 1 to 2 hours until it has returned to pre-insulin levels.

Insulin requirements are not always constant in any diabetic cat—they vary from day to day, according to many factors, including a cat's environment (eg, a hospital is more stressful than home), activity levels, and resolution of glucose toxicity. Any alteration in dose of insulin should be made gradually on the basis of trends over several days (although the development of hypoglycemia is an exception). The clinician should assimilate all data relating to the patient before advising any change in insulin dose—for example, assessing body weight, water consumption, and other historical and physical data.

DIABETIC REMISSION

Possible indications of diabetic remission include

- Absence of glycosuria—especially if this is a persistent finding
- Low blood glucose (<10 mmol/L or 180 mg/dL) before insulin injection
- Low or normal serum fructosamine readings

If suspected, insulin treatment should be stopped and the patient monitored closely. Urine glucose monitoring from home is a simple way of assessing patients. If glycosuria returns, a cautious dose of insulin may be required and a BGC should be used to titrate the dose.

LONG-TERM CARE OF STABLE DIABETIC CATS

In those cats that do well clinically, frequency of monitoring can be reduced to once every 3 to 6 months. Checks should include a full history; physical examination, including weight and body condition score; complete blood cell count; and serum biochemistry. It is helpful to measure blood pressure and perform serum fructosamine and urinalysis and culture periodically (eg, every 6 months), even in those cats that remain clinically stable. UTIs are not always clinically obvious—a proportion of patients suffering from these show no clinical signs referable to the urinary tract or pyuria/bacteria on microscopic examination.[7,9,10] Annual serum thyroxine measurement is also justified because hyperthyroidism is a common co-morbidity that can adversely affect control.[22,35]

MANAGEMENT OF COMPLEX CASES

Continued clinical signs of diabetes, evidence of hypoglycemia or ketosis, and development of complications associated with long-term diabetes (eg, polyneuropathy [see **Fig. 1**]) are indications of poor control.

Early problems with stabilization are common. They are usually straightforward to identify and remedy.

- Care provider factors accounting for problems with stabilization. A thorough review of the care provider insulin storage and administration regime is important in eliminating simple causes of poor stabilization at home. In some cases it is helpful to ask the care provider to demonstrate exactly how they prepare and give their cat its insulin injections. Care provider causes of problems include
  - Not adhering to a routine—for example, giving injections at a different time each day or giving varying amounts and/or types of food. Encouraging care providers to set reminders on a personal digital assistant or cell phone can help with this.
  - Under-dosage resulting from use of insulin, which has been improperly stored or improperly mixed before withdrawal. For example, although many insulin preparations, including Caninsulin, may remain stable for several weeks at room temperature, optimal long-term stability requires storage in a refrigerator. Insulin bottles should be stored upright; otherwise, insulin may stick to the rubber bung. Manufacturers recommend that insulin preparations be renewed once a month; most clinicians recommend renewing Lente supplies at least every 2 months. Care providers should be shown how to gently mix insulin suspensions by rolling rather than shaking the bottle.
  - Under-dosage resulting from using 100-IU syringes with a 40-IU/mL insulin, such as Caninsulin.
  - Under-dosage resulting from failure to see and remove air bubbles from the syringe before injecting.
  - Incorrect injection technique, including injecting the incorrect dose or injecting through the skin. Many care providers benefit from lengthy tutorials on handling syringes, loading the correct dose of insulin, and injecting this into

a cat. Shaving the fur from possible injection sites may help care providers learning how to inject their cat.

- Insulin-related factors accounting for problems with stabilization. Other than the first of these factors, investigation and resolution generally depend on serial blood glucose measurements:
  - ○ Insulin out of date
  - ○ Inappropriate dose of insulin
  - ○ Inappropriate dose frequency
  - ○ Inappropriate insulin preparation for the patient—for example, duration of action too short to achieve adequate control in a practical way
- Other factors that may account for problems with stabilization:
  - ○ Use of out-of-date test strips for home monitoring of blood or urine glucose
  - ○ Poor insulin absorption from subcutaneous site of administration. Although convenient, the scruff may not be the best site to inject because fibrosis after previous injections may influence absorption and this area has a poor blood supply, making absorption less predictable. Care providers should be encouraged to vary the precise injection site and choose locations other than the scruff, for example, the flank, lateral thorax, over the shoulder, and above the elbow.
  - ○ Reduction in insulin requirements and/or resolution of diabetes associated with reduced glucose toxicity and β-cell exhaustion. Initial monitoring of cats with diabetes requires close attention to the possibility of diabetic remission.
  - ○ Different insulin requirements at home compared with the hospital. This applies to those cases when initial stabilization is done with the cat hospitalized. An un-stressed cat in its home environment may have lower insulin requirements than when stressed and in a hospital or, conversely, if more active at home may have higher insulin requirements than in the hospital.

In cases of cats when a detailed interview of the care provider and physical examination do not provide a straightforward answer, further investigations are required. If the insulin being used has been open for more than 1 month, it is advisable to change to a new bottle before pursuing more expensive investigations. Measurement of water intake and blood glucose measurement are the first investigations to consider. These tests will help to identify whether the insulin is effective in lowering the blood glucose duration of action of the insulin is adequate.

INSULIN RESISTANCE

A variety of physiologic and pathologic conditions are associated with insulin resistance. Concurrent diseases of an inflammatory, infectious, hormonal, or neoplastic nature may all contribute to poor stabilization via secretion of diabetogenic hormones (glucagon, adrenaline, cortisol, and growth hormone). Concurrent illnesses increase the requirements for insulin although this increase is usually subtle and may be variable. Affected cats may, therefore, demonstrate variable or generally poor control of their diabetes. Initial consideration of concurrent disease or complicating factors should aim to rule out the following as causes of poor stabilization:

1. Dioestrus and pregnancy (female cats)
2. Severe obesity
3. Administration of diabetogenic drugs (eg, glucocorticoids and progestagens)
4. Infections—urinary, oral, and skin are most common

5. Ketoacidosis
6. Concurrent chronic diseases (eg, pancreatitis, chronic kidney disease, hyperthyroidism, or liver disease)
7. Presence of anti-insulin antibodies—considered a rare complication in feline diabetics

Careful history taking, thorough physical examination, and laboratory analysis (hematology, serum biochemistry, urinalysis, urine culture, and thyroxine) should be performed. Abdominal imaging (radiography and ultrasound) and measurement of feline pancreatic lipase immunoreactivity may also be of value in the diagnosis of pancreatitis. An improvement in control of diabetes is usually seen once concurrent diseases are stabilized, although this is not always the case, and chronic pancreatitis can be particularly difficult to diagnose and manage.

Insulin resistance is usually defined as present in cats remaining hyperglycemic and glycosuric in spite of their receiving greater than 1.5 units of Lente insulin per kg body weight per dose. It is important to document insulin resistance by performing a glucose curve and to eliminate the causes (discussed previously) before proceeding and performing further diagnostic tests.

Acromegaly and hyperadrenocorticism are important causes of severe insulin resistance.[36–40] Other endocrine tumors (islet cell glucagonoma and pheochromocytoma) are potential causes of marked insulin resistance. Clinical examination and thorough history taking may be helpful in identifying some cases. Clinical pathology is useful in eliminating some of the causes (discussed previously) but it is also specifically worthwhile to consider adrenal ultrasonography and pituitary imaging (MRI/CT) to identify pituitary macroadenomas and unilateral or bilateral adrenomegaly (**Fig. 4**). ACTH stimulation and/or dexamethasone suppression tests can be used to aid identification of hyperadrenocorticism and insulin-like growth factor 1 may be helpful in the diagnosis of acromegaly.

In cases of cats when treatment of the primary disease is not possible or when the cause of the insulin resistance remains undiagnosed, management of glycemic control usually requires at least twice-daily insulin therapy. A combination of short-acting and longer-acting insulin in a 1:2 ratio may also be of value (eg, one-third of the dose regular insulin and two-thirds as Lente). The short-acting insulin may help overcome the insulin resistance and lower the hyperglycemia.

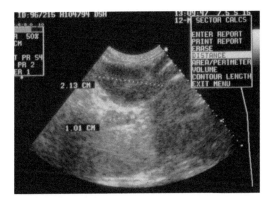

Fig. 4. Advanced imaging can be helpful in diagnosing causes of marked insulin resistance, as in this cat with an adrenal mass associated with hyperadrenocorticism.

SUMMARY

Many cases of diabetes are straightforward to stabilize using Lente insulins, although it may take several weeks or months to identify an optimal insulin regime. One study reported that a majority of cats treated with Caninsulin were stable or in diabetic remission by week 16.[6] None of these cats received dietary management of their diabetes, however, which was expected to have greatly helped outcomes. Intensive treatment increases the chances of diabetic remission. Detailed survival statistics for cats treated with Lente insulin are not available. Median survival times for diabetic cats treated with Lente, Ultralente, or protamine zinc insulins are approximately 20 months.[5]

REFERENCES

1. Rand S, Marshall RD. Diabetes mellitus in cats. Vet Clin North Am Small Anim Pract 2005;35:211–24.
2. Panciera DL, Thomas CB, Eicker SW, et al. Epizootiologic patterns of diabetes mellitus in cats: 333 cases (1980-1986). J Am Vet Med Assoc 1990;197:1504–8.
3. Biourge V, Nelson RW, Feldman EC, et al. Effect of weight gain and subsequent weight loss on glucose tolerance and insulin response in healthy cats. J Vet Intern Med 1997;11:86–91.
4. Appleton DJ, Rand JS, Sunvold GD. Insulin sensitivity decreases with obesity, and lean cats with low insulin sensitivity are at greatest risk of glucose intolerance with weight gain. J Feline Med Surg 2001;3:211–28.
5. Goossens MM, Nelson RW, Feldman EC, et al. Response to insulin treatment and survival in 104 cats with diabetes mellitus (1985-1995). J Vet Intern Med 1998;12:1–6.
6. Michiels L, Reusch C, Boari A, et al. Treatment of 46 cats with porcine lente insulin—a prospective, multicentre study. J Feline Med Surg 2008;10:439–51.
7. Bailiff NL, Nelson RW, Feldman EC, et al. Frequency and risk factors for urinary tract infection in cats with diabetes mellitus. J Vet Intern Med 2006;20:850–5.
8. Bailiff NL, Westropp JL, Nelson RW, et al. Evaluation of urine specific gravity and urine sediment as risk factors for urinary tract infections in cats. Vet Clin Pathol 2008;37:317–22.
9. Mayer-Roenne B, Goldstein RE, Erb HN. Urinary tract infections in cats with hyperthyroidism, diabetes mellitus and chronic kidney disease. J Feline Med Surg 2007;9:124–32.
10. Litster A, Moss S, Platell J, et al. Occult bacterial lower urinary tract infections in cats—urinalysis and culture findings. Vet Microbiol 2009;136:130–4.
11. Zinker BA, Allison RG, Lacy DB, et al. Interaction of exercise, insulin, and hypoglycemia studied using euglycemic and hypoglycaemic insulin clamps. Am J Physiol 1997;272:E530–42.
12. Roomp K, Rand J. Intensive blood glucose control is safe and effective in diabetic cats using home monitoring and treatment with glargine. J Feline Med Surg 2009;11:668–82.
13. Marshall RD, Rand JS, Morton JM. Treatment of newly diagnosed diabetic cats with glargine insulin improves glycaemic control and results in higher probability of remission than protamine zinc and lente insulins. J Feline Med Surg 2009;11:683–91.
14. Roomp K, Rand J. Evaluation of determir in diabetic cats managed with a protocol for intensive blood glucose control. J Feline Med Surg 2012;14:566–72.

15. Sieber-Ruckstuhl NS, Kley S, Tschuor F, et al. Remission of diabetes mellitus in cats with diabetic ketoacidosis. J Vet Intern Med 2008;22:1326–32.
16. Frank G, Anderson W, Pazak H, et al. Use of a high-protein diet in the management of feline diabetes mellitus. Vet Ther 2001;2(3):238–46.
17. Mazzaferro E, Greco D, Turner A, et al. Treatment of feline diabetes mellitus using an alpha-glucosidase inhibitor and a low-carbohydrate diet. J Feline Med Surg 2003;5(3):183–90.
18. Bennett N, Greco D, Peterson M, et al. Comparison of a low carbohydrate-low fiber diet and a moderate carbohydrate-high fiber diet in the management of feline diabetes mellitus. J Feline Med Surg 2006;8(2):73–84.
19. Roomp K, Rand JS. Evaluation of detemir in diabetic cats managed with a protocol for intensive blood glucose control [abstract]. J Vet Intern Med 2009;23(3):697.
20. Marshall RD, Rand JS, Morton JM. Glargine and protamine zinc insulin have a longer duration of action and result in lower mean daily glucose concentrations than lente insulin in healthy cats. J Vet Pharmacol Ther 2008;31:205–12.
21. Sennello KA, Schulman RL, Prosek R, et al. Systolic blood pressure in cats with diabetes mellitus. J Am Vet Med Assoc 2003;223:198–201.
22. Mitchell N. Ocular findings in cats with diabetes mellitus. Dissertation for DVOphthal, Royal College of Veterinary Surgeons 2011.
23. Link KR, Rand JS. Changes in blood glucose concentration are associated with relatively rapid changes in circulating fructosamine concentrations in cats. J Feline Med Surg 2008;10:583–92.
24. Thoresen SI, Bredal WP. Clinical usefulness of fructosamine measurements in diagnosing and monitoring feline diabetes mellitus. J Small Anim Pract 1996; 37:64–8.
25. Reusch CE, Liehs MR, Hoyer M, et al. Fructosamine. A new parameter for diagnosis and metabolic control in diabetic dogs and cats. J Vet Intern Med 1993;7: 177–82.
26. Graham PA, Mooney CT, Murray M. Serum fructosamine concentrations in hyperthyroid cats. Res Vet Sci 1999;67:171–5.
27. Reusch CE, Tomsa K. Serum fructosamine concentration in cats with overt hyperthyroidism. J Am Vet Med Assoc 1999;215:1297–300.
28. Reusch CE, Haberer B. Evaluation of fructosamine in dogs and cats with hypo- or hyperproteinaemia, azotaemia, hyperlipidaemia and hyperbilirubinaemia. Vet Rec 2001;148:370–6.
29. Gilor C, Graves TK, Lascelles DD, et al. The effects of body weight, body condition score, sex and age on serum fructosamine concentrations in clinically healthy cats. Vet Clin Pathol 2010;39:322–8.
30. Ristic JM, Herrtage ME, Walti-Lauger SM, et al. Evaluation of a continuous glucose monitoring system in cats with diabetes mellitus. J Feline Med Surg 2005;7:153–62.
31. Alt N, Kley S, Haessig M, et al. Day-to-day variability of blood glucose concentration curves generated at home in cats with diabetes mellitus. J Am Vet Med Assoc 2007;230:1011–7.
32. Bantle JP, Weber MS, Rao SM, et al. Rotation of the anatomic regions used for insulin injections and day-to-day variability of plasma glucose in type I diabetic subjects. JAMA 1990;263:1802–6.
33. Moberg E, Kollind M, Lins PE, et al. Day-to-day variation of insulin sensitivity in patients with type I diabetes: role of gender and menstrual cycle. Diabet Med 1995;12:224–8.

34. Boden G, Chen X, Urbain JL. Evidence for a circadian rhythm of insulin sensitivity in patients with NIDDM caused by cyclic changes in hepatic glucose production. Diabetes 1996;45:1044–50.

35. Blois SL, Dickie EL, Kruth SA, et al. Multiple endocrine diseases in cats: 15 cases (1997-2008). J Feline Med Surg 2010;12:637–42.

36. Peterson ME, Steele P. Pituitary-dependent hyperadrenocorticism in a cat. J Am Vet Med Assoc 1986;189:680–3.

37. Goossens MM, Feldman EC, Nelson RW, et al. Cobalt 60 irradiation of pituitary gland tumors in three cats with acromegaly. J Am Vet Med Assoc 1998;213:374–6.

38. Elliott DA, Feldman EC, Koblik PD, et al. Prevalence of pituitary tumors among diabetic cats with insulin resistance. J Am Vet Med Assoc 2000;216:1765–8.

39. Norman EJ, Mooney CT. Diagnosis and management of diabetes mellitus in five cats with somatotrophic abnormalities. J Feline Med Surg 2000;2:183–90.

40. Abraham L, Helmond SE, Mitten RW, et al. Treatment of an acromegalic cat with the dopamine agonist L-deprenyl. Aust Vet J 2002;80:479–83.

Practical Use of Home Blood Glucose Monitoring in Feline Diabetics

Sara L. Ford, DVM[a],*, Heather Lynch, LVT[b]

KEYWORDS

- Feline diabetes • Diabetes management • Home blood glucose monitoring
- Diabetes mellitus • Feline diabetic remission

KEY POINTS

- Handheld glucometer technology has made accurate home blood glucose monitoring (home monitoring) possible for owners of diabetic cats.
- Improvements in treatment and monitoring options change therapy goals from simply controlling observable clinical signs, and preventing consequences of overt hyperglycemia or hypoglycemia, to controlling the cat's blood glucoses in a near-normal range, and attempting to achieve resolution of the diabetic state.
- Home monitoring allows for tight glycemic control and reversal of pancreatic glucose toxicity and significantly increases the likelihood of diabetic remission.
- In the absence of home monitoring, the owner and veterinarian are unlikely to be aware of the day-to-day variation in blood glucose values, because cats are tolerant to both hypoglycemia and hyperglycemia, often with a paucity of recognizable clinical signs.
- Acute and chronic complications of diabetes can be avoided with home monitoring, leading to enhanced quality of life for the cat and owner.

INTRODUCTION

Recently, the management of feline diabetes has become more interesting and rewarding; recommendations for monitoring and treatment of diabetes in cats have changed significantly. In the last 10 years, improvements in handheld glucometer technology have made at-home monitoring of blood glucose (BG) possible for most owners of diabetic cats. In May 2010, the American Animal Hospital Association (AAHA) published the *AAHA Diabetes Management Guidelines for Dogs and Cats*, making the following statement: "Home monitoring of BG is ideal and strongly encouraged to obtain the most accurate interpretation of glucose relative to clinical signs." The guidelines went on to say, "Most owners are able to learn to do this with a little

[a] American College of Veterinary Internal Medicine (Internal Medicine), VCA Emergency Animal Hospital & Referral Center, San Diego, CA; [b] Tatum Point Animal Hospital, Phoenix, AZ
* Corresponding author.
E-mail address: drsaraford@aol.com

Vet Clin Small Anim 43 (2013) 283–301
http://dx.doi.org/10.1016/j.cvsm.2012.12.003
0195-5616/13/$ – see front matter © 2013 Elsevier Inc. All rights reserved.

encouragement and interpretation of glucose results is much easier for the clinician."[1] We have had the opportunity to train hundreds of owners to successfully perform this task and have seen the positive results. Appropriate application of home BG monitoring in veterinary patients is a powerful tool to improve case outcome. This situation is particularly true in the feline diabetic, in which insulin requirements are variable or transient, food intake is often inconsistent, and vomiting results in lost calories. Home monitoring provides real-time values, allowing the clinician to be confident with intensive insulin therapy, achieving tighter glycemic control with reduced risk of hypoglycemia and increased chance of diabetic remission.

A NEW STANDARD OF CARE

Veterinary professionals strive to provide companion animals with the best quality of life possible. Until recently, veterinary professionals have depended on the cat owner's observation of the cat at home and in-hospital BG testing to determine both the cat's level of glycemic control and quality of life. Inconsistent owner observation skills and limitations of in-hospital testing reduce the ability of the clinician to reliably achieve optimum case results. Even the most astute owner finds it difficult to predict what their pet's BG is. Mild weakness, dizziness, or lethargy is not something a cat can easily communicate to its owner. By the time most clinical signs of hyperglycemia or hypoglycemia develop, the BG is usually dangerously high or life-threateningly low. Using home monitoring removes the guess work for both the owner and the clinician.

STANDARD OF CARE IN CATS: AIMING HIGHER

The management of diabetes mellitus in the cat has always been clinically challenging. Opinions as to the best way to treat and monitor diabetic cats are numerous and varied, but one thing is certain: administration of insulin without the knowledge of the real-time BG concentration has dangerous and potentially life-threatening consequences.

Home BG monitoring is the standard of care for human diabetics, and the administration of insulin is contraindicated without self- monitoring.[2,3] In humans, the treatment goal is to control BG within a narrow range (fasting BG = 70–130 mg/dL or 3.9–7.2 mmol/L). This level of control is achieved with multiple BG measurements and usually several doses of insulin daily. Additional goals in human patients include avoiding the progression of the devastating vascular consequences of prolonged hyperglycemia, namely, diabetic retinopathy, nephropathy, vasculitis, peripheral neuropathy, stroke, and heart attack. Human patients who are able to achieve tight glycemic control have a significantly lower incidence of these complicating conditions.[4] The severity of the long-term negative effects of diabetes is a strong impetus for most human diabetics to follow rigorous monitoring regimes in an attempt to minimize complications.

Historically, the goal for the management of diabetes in the cat has been a practical one: to control the patient's clinical signs (most notably, polyuria, polydipsia, and polyphagia), as well as to avoid a ketoacidotic state and insulin-induced hypoglycemia.[5] Sinister systemic effects of the hyperglycemic state are well documented. However, because veterinary patients typically are not treated as diabetics for decades, as humans are, many of the negative effects of chronic hyperglycemia do not have time to develop.[5] Because of this situation, veterinarians have long accepted a mild to moderate hyperglycemic state in their diabetic patients, because the risks associated with it are considered to be less than the risk of a possible insulin overdose. Home monitoring, along with recent innovations in the combined use of longer-acting insulin (glargine [Lantus, Sanofi-Aventis, Paris, France], detemir [Levemir, Novo Nordisk, Princeton, NJ, USA], and ProZinc [Boehringer Ingelheim Vetmedica, St Joseph, MO, USA]) and low-carbohydrate, high-protein diets,[6] has created the potential to expand our definition of well-controlled diabetic to one that more closely resembles the standard of care in humans. Home monitoring is the crux of this therapy, because it allows the clinician the freedom to prescribe insulin doses necessary to narrow the acceptable BG range in the patient and simultaneously to reduce the risk of unrecognized insulin overdosage. These improvements in treatment and monitoring options allow the veterinarian to increase their expectations of therapy goals from controlling observable clinical signs and preventing catastrophic consequences of extreme hyperglycemia to controlling the cat's BGs in a lower, near-normal range (80–200 mg/dL or 4.4–11.1 mmol/L) and attempting to achieve resolution of the diabetic state.[7]

Management goals
- Resolution of clinical signs
- Achievement of glycemic control (BG <180 mg/dL; 10 mmol/L)
- Lowest BG 80 mg/dL or greater (4.4 mmol/L)
- Prevent clinical hypoglycemia
- Reverse pancreatic glucose toxicity and regain endogenous insulin secretion
- Prevent chronic complications
  - Diabetic neuropathy
  - Relapsing chronic pancreatitis
  - Progression of renal azotemia
  - Development of bacterial, viral, and fungal infections
- Remission of diabetic state

THREE COMPELLING REASONS TO USE HOME BG MONITORING

1. Home monitoring improves quality of life.

Long-term complications associated with hyperglycemia can significantly affect a cat's quality of life. Diabetic neuropathy, a common effect of chronic hyperglycemia in cats, results in weakness of the hind limbs, which progresses to difficulty walking, jumping, and climbing stairs. In severe cases of polyneuropathy, forelimb weakness is also present. This weakness is often reversible once glycemic control is established and maintained. Poor glycemic control results in an osmotic diuresis, polyuria, and the potential for dehydration, which can exacerbate pancreatitis and renal azotemia. The feeling of constant thirst, hunger, and needing to urinate interfere with quality of life. Patients who have their glucose monitored at home can be safely placed on higher dosages of insulin, thereby achieving better glycemic control. Diabetic remission in the cat is more likely with tight glycemic control (BG ≤200 mg/dL or ≤1.1 mmol/L), which can more consistently be achieved safely with daily home monitoring.[7] Diabetic remission is promptly recognized, with home monitoring reducing the potential for a cat entering remission to suffer an insulin overdose. Achieving a near-normal quality of life at home with tight glycemic control also improves the cat owner's impression of the cat's prognosis, which decreases risk of euthanasia.

2. Home BG monitoring decreases risks of insulin overdose.

Exogenous insulin is the mainstay of treatment of feline diabetes. In humans, exogenous insulin by injection is contraindicated without home BG monitoring.[2] Home BG monitoring has been adopted as the standard of care for children and adults alike for many reasons, the most important of which is patient safety. The most common adverse reaction to insulin is hypoglycemia. Insulin administration in the face of hypoglycemia carries with it significant morbidity and mortality. Home monitoring similarly improves safety for veterinary patients. It both protects the client from administering the insulin when the cat is hypoglycemic, or in danger of becoming so, and provides the veterinarian with more insight into the effect that insulin has on the cat.

3. BG is variable without cause.

One of the most important reasons for home monitoring in cats with diabetes is the dynamic nature of the disease: with all other variables kept constant, BG concentrations in diabetic cats vary significantly on a day-by-day and hour-by-hour basis. Significant variations between day-to-day BG concentrations have long posed difficulty for clinicians dealing with diabetics. In one study, insulin dose in individual diabetic dogs varied by 68% to 103% when serial BG curves were performed over 2 consecutive days in hospital.[8] When the investigators compared the curves in diabetic dogs from 1 day to the next, recommendations for insulin adjustment were opposite one another 27% of the time (ie, on day 1 the clinician would have recommended increasing insulin dose, but on day 2 the recommendation would have been to lower the dose). This finding led the investigators to conclude that there was day-to-day variability of BG concentrations of a magnitude that would significantly affect the clinician's recommendations for insulin dose administration on a day-to-day basis.[8] Daily monitoring addresses this problem and helps to resolve what has been the greatest challenge for clinicians in achieving and maintaining glycemic control in diabetic dogs and cats: to discover the dose of insulin that prevents prolonged hyperglycemia (BG >300 mg/dL or $\geq$16.7 mmol/L) without causing potentially acutely dangerous episodes of hypoglycemia (BG $\leq$60 mg/dL or $\leq$3.3 mmol/L). A study of day-to-day variation of BG concentrations was performed in cats with similar findings, and, in contrast to the dog study, it was performed at home and therefore presumed to be associated with less stress. The curves were generated using a consistent meal size and insulin dose. Cats with good glycemic control had more reproducible curves than cats with poorer glycemic control. Limitations of this study include that insulin injection sites were varied and an intermediate-acting insulin (Caninsulin/Vetsulin, MSD Animal Health) was used.[9] In addition, several studies have shown that cats have increased variation in BG concentrations when stress is induced.[10]

It follows that their BG concentration would also be affected by other variables similarly to humans and dogs.

Variables known to influence BG concentrations in most species include stress, excitement, exercise, diet quality (glycemic index of and amount of carbohydrates) and quantity, and the amount of insulin absorbed from the subcutaneous tissue, which is dependent on patient's temperature, as well as environmental temperature. Varying the injection site leads to different absorption. For this reason, it is not advisable to rotate the location of the patient's injection site. If local inflammation associated with repeat injections occurs, the injection site should be changed to a new site, rather than rotated between sites (**Fig. 1**).

Variability in glucose also occurs in the absence of an explainable cause. Inconsistent glucose concentrations are a source of frustration for veterinarians and owners. After daily glucose monitoring is instituted, the magnitude of the fluctuations becomes apparent even when known variables are consistent. Every day is not the same. In the absence of home monitoring, the owner or veterinarian is unlikely to be aware of the inconsistent values, because cats are tolerant to both hypoglycemia and hyperglycemia, with a paucity of recognizable clinical signs.

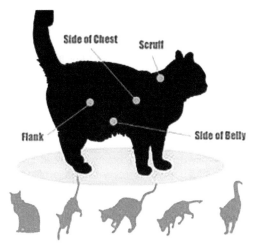

Fig. 1. Potential insulin injection sites in the cat.

USING HOME MONITORING IN PRACTICE
Make Capillary Blood Sampling Routine

The most important aspect of creating a home BG monitoring program in a veterinary practice is developing the ability to easily and consistently collect capillary blood samples. This skill should be developed by the entire staff.

The best way to develop this skill is to adopt capillary blood collection as the preferred method of obtaining BG readings in the hospital. This procedure can be performed in the examination room or cage with nonfractious animals, thereby minimizing handling. A recent study[11] suggested that every cat older than 8 years that is examined should have blood collected from the lateral ear margin at the beginning of the evaluation as a routine screening. These investigators suggests that routine screening of BG can reliably identify a prediabetic state in the cat, allowing the clinician to institute dietary changes, or recommend further diagnostic testing. As staff gain experience, they improve their skill and confidence and are better able to both competently demonstrate the method to clients as well as help clients troubleshoot the process if issues arise.

VETERINARY VERSUS HUMAN GLUCOMETERS

There has been debate within the veterinary profession about the use of a human glucometer rather than a veterinary model. We believe that the most important point of monitoring is that clients check BGs at home, regardless of which glucometer is used, because a trend can be established. However, the use of veterinary-purposed glucometers is recommended for several reasons:

1. As was shown in a study in 2009, there are differences in accuracy from meter to meter, and generally the veterinary meter, in this study the AlphaTRAK [Abbott Animal Health, Abbott Park, IL, USA] veterinary-specific handheld BG monitor[12] (http://abbottanimalhealth.com), was more accurate than the human meters.
2. Human glucometers commonly underestimate the BG, depending on the model, by as much as 25% to 30%. The absolute difference in glucose concentrations is greater, the higher the glucose concentration is compared with the normal

reference value. The discrepancy around the normal reference range for BG concentration is large enough to result in inappropriate differences in the insulin dosing plan.[12]

3. The veterinary meter with which we are most familiar (AlphaTRAK BG monitoring system by Abbott) requires small samples (0.3 μL) and is designed with capillary blood draw in animals in mind, making it easier for the owner to consistently collect blood. The other veterinary meter (the iPet) requires a larger sample size at 1.6 μL.

The maker of the veterinary meter (Abbott Animal Health) provides both educational and technical support for their veterinary customers, whereas the makers of human models generally do not support meters used in veterinary patients.

a. An example of this situation is the recent release of a specialized veterinary data management system facilitating downloading BG values available online (AlphaTRAKer [Abbott Animal Health, Abbott Park, IL, USA]), making evaluation of patient data less time-consuming for veterinarians.[13]

CHOOSING THE COLLECTION SITE

One of the first decisions the veterinary team needs to make is to choose which blood collection site works best for the patient.

- In cats, 2 main collections sites are recommended. The best site is the one that the cat tolerates and that consistently yields an adequate blood sample.
- The owner needs to be able to collect the sample at home, and therefore they must be able to safely and simply collect the sample with minimal restraint.

Lateral Ear Margin

The lateral ear margin is the most common collection site used in the cat, and is also generally the best tolerated. The outside of the ear margin rather than the inside is preferred, although a few owners prefer the inside. We have worked with cats that have had capillary samples drawn 2 to 4 times daily from their ears for 2 to 6 years, with minimal scarring or bruising (**Figs. 2–4**).

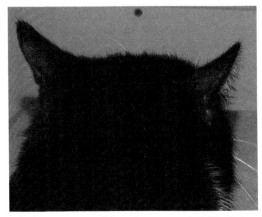

Fig. 2. Harley Konotchick, a 12-year-old, male-neutered, DSH. Twice-daily to four-times-daily testing of the lateral ear margin for 6 years.

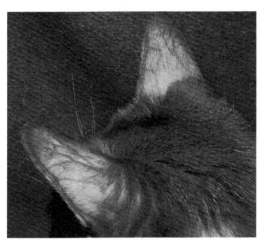

Fig. 3. Example of cat's ears after twice-daily BG testing for 2 years. Note: ears have been shaved at the owner's request for ease of sampling.

Helpful hints

- Capillary blood is being collected, not venous. Do not try to hit the vein on the dorsal surface of the lateral ear margin with the skin prick; it is enough to get close to it. Hitting the vein may result in excessive bleeding or bruising.
- In cats, work on the outside of the ear pinna and hold a cotton ball or gauze square under the pinna to prevent the ear from moving away from the lancet, and to prevent excessive digital pressure occluding vessels, or the lancet piercing the operator's finger.
- Shaving the lateral ear margins and applying a thin layer of petroleum jelly to the ear pinnae before blood collection often assists in the formation of a blood drop after lancing the ear, and improves blood collection success.
- Vasoconstriction occurs with cooler ambient temperatures, making blood collection more difficult. Warming the ear with a warm cloth, moist, warm cotton ball or rice sock for 30 seconds to 1 minute results in vasodilation, hastening blood collection.

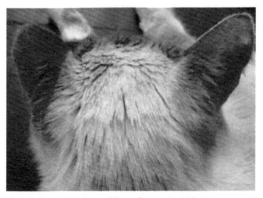

Fig. 4. Sweeney Wildermuth, a 12-year-old, male-neutered, Siamese mix. Example of home testing from right ear only, for 2 1/2 years. Testing from left ear was not possible due to scarring from historic hematoma.

Pisiform (Wrist) Paw Pad

Paw pads yield excellent blood samples; however, collecting from the metacarpal (plantar), metatarsal (palmar), or digital pads, all weight-bearing pads, tends to be uncomfortable and often is not well tolerated by the patient. Use of the weight-bearing pads (metacarpal [plantar], metatarsal [palmar], and digital) is not recommended because of discomfort and the risk of infection with use of a litter box. Using the nonweight-bearing pad, wrist pad, or pisiform pad on the forelimbs alleviates this issue and is generally well tolerated in cats that do not mind having their feet handled (**Figs. 5** and **6**).

Helpful hints

- Try collecting blood from the pisiform or wrist pad with the cat's paw flipped back caudally (as if you were cleaning a horse's hoof). This technique provides excellent access to the pisiform pad in both a standing and a laterally recumbent position, and is less stressful for the cat than trying to access the pad in other positions. Cats that are comfortable or accustomed to lying in the owner's lap on their back can have blood drawn from the pisiform in this position as well.
- Lightly pinch the pad for a few seconds before performing the procedure and continue to pinch the pad until an adequate blood drop forms.
- If the environmental temperature is low, the foot can be warmed, similarly to the ear.

LANCING DEVICES

A lancing device is a spring-loaded device that holds the lancet; when triggered, the lancet pricks the skin with a controlled depth. Whether a lancing device is used in

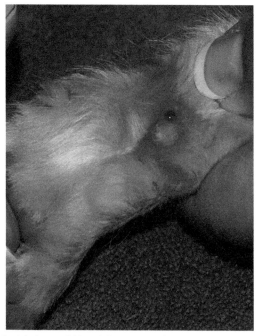

Fig. 5. Pisiform pad with formed blood drop ready for sampling.

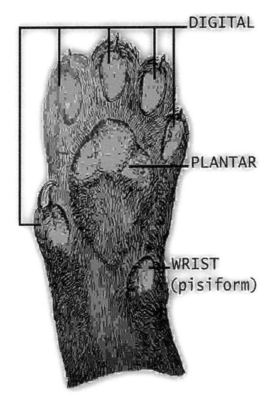

Fig. 6. Pisiform pad anatomy.

capillary blood collection is a personal preference; however, they are particularly help-ful for clients who feel uncomfortable with the alternative of pricking the skin manually or using a free-hand stick for blood sample collection. The lancets used in the lancing device typically fit in all lancing devices. The size or gauge of the lancet is variable. The lancet included in the starter kit for the recommended veterinary glucometer is 28 gauge, and has various depth settings. Lancets in different gauges from 25 to 32 gauge are available for purchase at most pharmacies. If a patient bleeds easily or excessively or if the cat is on anticoagulants and has cardiac disease, a smaller lancet is preferred. On the other hand, in some cats that do not bleed so easily when pierced, larger gauge lancets can be used.

The key to using a lancing device is to make certain that the tissue cannot move away from the lancet or needle. For instance, with ear margins, rolled-up gauze or a cotton ball should be held under the ear pinna to provide firm pressure and allow the lancing device to work and to protect the operator's finger.

Working with the Pet Owner

Successful home monitoring programs require active cat owner participation. Often, the level of owner compliance achieved is directly related to how well they are prepared for success by the veterinary staff at initiation of treatment.

Recognizing that every patient and client is unique and adjusting the blood collec-tion technique to each client and cat's needs is integral to success at home.

Many pet owners attempt home BG monitoring if

- It is positively recommended by the veterinarian
- They understand the benefits
- They receive adequate training and support from the veterinary team

Recommendations for Successful Communication with Cat Owners

1. Diabetes is not a death sentence.[14]

   The owners should understand that, although diabetes is a serious chronic disease, it is manageable. With the owner's help, the veterinarian can in most cases achieve good glycemic control, resolution of clinical signs, and a near-normal life span and quality of life. Newly diagnosed cats that are intensively managed have high remission rates (>80%), and home monitoring facilitates achieving tight glycemic control and recovery of β cells from glucose toxicity.

2. Make a positive recommendation.

   The veterinarian should make a positive recommendation for home monitoring at time of diagnosis of diabetes (similar to recommending urine culture if an infection is suspected or pain medication in conjunction with surgery). This strategy validates the treatment in the eyes of the cat owner as a recommended part of treatment rather than just an option. The veterinarian or staff should explain that home monitoring

   a. Enables the veterinarian to improve their understanding of the day-to-day effect that insulin has on BG

   b. Enables the cat owner to know whether they should give insulin or not

   c. Alerts the cat owner to potential emergencies or loss of glycemic control before the cat develops clinical signs

   d. Is the best way to achieve diabetic remission in the cat

3. Be certain you can collect blood from the cat before client demonstration.

   This point is possibly the single most important part of the treatment plan. If the veterinary staff are unable to draw blood easily during demonstration, the owner loses confidence and often declines the plan. In all cases, the veterinary staff should

   a. Discover the best site to collect blood from the cat away from the owner, before recommending the protocol.

   b. Once the best collection site is located, and it is determined whether the patient is tolerant of the procedure, demonstrate the procedure to the cat owner.

   c. If the cat owner is motivated to initiate home monitoring, have them collect a capillary blood sample successfully from the cat before discharge.

   d. Even if owners have decided not to pursue home monitoring, do not hesitate to collect BG samples in front of them when they come in for visits. Often, if owners see sample collection performed regularly, they become more amenable to trying it themselves.

4. Give the cat owner clear, written instructions.

   Failures in owner compliance, such as owner self-adjustment of insulin, are often directly linked to the absence of a clear directive from the veterinary team. Written discharge instructions should include

   a. The treatment plan

   b. Specific parameters for clinical signs and BG readings that should prompt the pet owner to contact the office (eg, call the office if 2 readings are >350 mg/dL [19.4 mmol/L] or any readings <80 mg/dL [4.4 mmol/L])

   c. The follow-up schedule and goals of treatment

5. Be sure the client understands that a learning curve is associated with glucose monitoring.

Home monitoring should never be portrayed as simple or easy to perform. Instead, cat owners should be prepared for a 7-day to 10-day period when they may experience some difficulty in performing glucose monitoring. If the cat owners realize it may take a few days to acclimate, they feel less frustrated during this adjustment period, increasing the likelihood of compliance to the veterinarian's recommendations.

6. Give the pet owner permission to call or return to the hospital for help.
   Ideally have a trained technician as the primary point of contact and encourage the cat owner to ask for help if they have any issues with the monitoring plan. Follow up with regular calls to check in on the cat and the owner to find out whether they have any questions or concerns.

7. Consider lending a glucometer.
   Consider keeping an extra glucometer in the hospital that can be loaned to an owner of a diabetic who is skeptical as to whether they can perform the protocol. This strategy allows them to attempt the protocol without making the commitment. Owners generally appreciate having the opportunity and generally find that they can perform the procedure. This system can also be useful when the cat owner would like to try a human glucometer, and they can perform side-by-side comparisons. Again, the owner generally returns and purchases the veterinary model, because they tend to be superior in terms of accuracy and ease of blood collection.

At-Home Monitoring Strategies

There are multiple ways to implement home BG monitoring in practice. The strategy chosen depends on the cat, the veterinarian's preference, and the cat owner's schedule/ability to perform the procedure and the therapeutic goals. The most commonly used protocols are given in the following sections:

Spot Check BG Reading

Spot check or casual BG readings as a home monitoring protocol were perhaps the first incarnation of home monitoring in veterinary medicine. The protocol calls for the owner to collect intermittent, single BG readings at various times of day. These readings may be on a predetermined schedule by the veterinarian or at random times, depending on the veterinarian's direction. Often, owners are directed to perform casual BG readings when they believe their cat is acting abnormally, or they suspect hypoglycemia. Although this system is effective in determining hypoglycemia, it offers little insight into the overall effect of insulin on the patient. Adjustment of insulin based on casual BG readings alone is not recommended.

Home BG Curves

BG curves generated at home are accurate and comprehensive

BG curves remain the clinician's fundamental tool when making decisions about insulin efficacy. Possibly the most exciting aspect of home monitoring is having the ability to educate the cat owner to perform this test at home. Performing the curve at home eliminates the stress of transport and being in the hospital environment, and allows generation of a 12-hour to 14-hour BG curve. At home, the curve is not truncated by the hospital or doctor's schedule, and the cat's daily routine relative to feeding and physical activity may be followed. Duplicating the home environment in a caged cat is not possible. Caloric consumption is also difficult to reproduce, because most cats do not eat well, or at all, in the hospital. The key difference here is who collects the data. Empowering the owner to measure glucose at home ensures accurate and complete data, which are not attainable in the hospital setting. As a result, the veterinary clinician is able to more accurately recommend adjustments in the insulin dose.

In-hospital BG curves are inaccurate and not cost-effective

Considering the staff time required to generate a glucose curve in the hospital, it is more profitable to have the owner generate the curve at home. Owners can be asked to perform a glucose curve that is discussed, along with their daily BG log, at each of the recheck visits. According to the AAHA guidelines mentioned earlier, owner compliance with long-term glucose monitoring is excellent and does not affect the frequency of re-evaluation by the veterinarian. Evaluation of long-term home monitoring of BG concentrations in cats with diabetes mellitus supports this finding.[15] In addition, having the client perform in-home BG curves with the veterinarian interpreting them is cost-effective for the hospital when staff time is taken into account. Veterinary practices often do not charge appropriately for all the labor and other costs associated with in-hospital measured curves.

Daily/Multiple Times per Day Home Monitoring

In this system, the owner measures BG, usually 2 times daily and sometimes up to 4 times daily for cases that are difficult to regulate. When feline diabetic remission is the goal, monitoring the BG ideally 4 times a day with a minimum of 3 times a day for the first 8 to 12 weeks provides the best chance of remission. In newly diagnosed diabetic cats, with intensive insulin therapy and home BG monitoring 3 to 4 times a day, there is a high probability of remission within 6 to 8 weeks. This system provides the most information to the clinician and the cat owner, and enables intensive insulin therapy. Ideal postdiagnosis protocol is as follows:

An Intensive Home BG Monitoring Protocol
- Initial stabilization period glucose checked 3 to 4 times/d
  - BG first thing in morning before morning meal and insulin
  - BG in the middle of the day 4 to 8 hours after morning insulin between approximately 11 AM and 4 PM
  - BG 12 hours later in the evening before evening meal and insulin
  - BG at bedtime

Suggested Morning and Evening Diabetic Routine
1. Obtain BG and log the value
2. Administer any preprandial medication as directed
3. Feed
   a. Offer a consistent measured (ideally weighed on a scale) amount of specified diet that the patient eats and the owner has agreed to feed
4. Administer insulin dose based on a customized chart
   a. Administer full dose of insulin if the cat has consumed at least 50% of the diet
   b. If cat consumes less than 50%, insulin dose is reduced by 50%
   c. If the BG is too low (less than 120–149 mg/dL; 6.6–8.3 mmol/L) insulin is not administered and the veterinarian is contacted for advice.

Cat owner education and compliance with the treatment plan are necessary to achieve durable glycemic control. Even with home monitoring, keen observation for recurrence of clinical signs or changes in the cat's status is a vital component of successful management. The clinician should be sure to provide the client with a written treatment plan, educational and reference materials, and in-clinic support as necessary to be certain that they understand and can perform the treatment plan as prescribed.

Clients should be advised to record the following (including the time of the events): BG value, food/water intake, insulin dose, and any change in their cat's clinical status at home (ie, vomiting, changes in appetite, elimination habits, or other concerns).

The therapeutic goals are cat-driven, owner-driven, and veterinarian-driven, but, if diabetic remission is the goal, then the BG should not be higher than 200 mg/dL (11 mmol/L) or lower than 3.5 to 4.4 mmol/L or 63–80 mg/dL (using the veterinary glucometer). Home monitoring puts these seemingly lofty goals within reach, thereby improving quality of life for both the cat and owner. Home monitoring of BG values can be simply and safely mastered by most owners, which results in a longer and healthier life for their cat, and a more satisfied owner and veterinarian.

Insulin Dosage Chart: Veterinary-Directed Insulin Prescription

With the implementation of daily home monitoring, there exists the possibility of instituting a treatment plan similar to that used by human diabetics who measure and adjust their insulin dose according to the BG reading daily. In humans, this protocol has resulted in improved glycemic control.[16] This adjustment of the insulin dose based on a real-time BG measurement allows marked improvement in glycemic control in veterinary patients, without increasing the risk of clinical hypoglycemia.[7,17] The variability in BG values with and without explainable cause makes this approach successful. Use of a dosing algorithm has been successfully performed in veterinary medicine in at least 1 large-scale study that was performed in Europe.[17] However, there is concern that differences in owner understanding, observation, and compliance coupled with the fact that veterinary patients cannot consistently express subtle changes in their physical state to their owner cause some concern that client adjustment of dose may not be in the best interest of the patient. One solution to this issue is to implement an insulin dosage chart, whereby the cat owner is given a chart by the clinician that predefines the insulin dose to be administered at a given range of BGs. This strategy maximizes the benefits of improved glycemic control with reduced risk of hypoglycemia (because the insulin dose decreases proportionately to the BG reading) and prevents the owner from making independent decisions about how to adjust the dose. Essentially, the insulin dosage chart is an expanded prescription label controlled by the veterinarian. Subsequent insulin dose adjustments are based on regular physical examinations by the veterinarian, resolution of clinical signs, evaluation of patient daily BG logs, BG curve, and recommended diagnostic testing.

Creating the insulin dose chart
1. Establish home monitoring and exogenous insulin therapy at recommended starting dose for the chosen insulin and patient status (**Table 1**).
   a. Insulin choice and starting dose are clinician-driven, patient-driven, and owner-driven.
2. Collect 7 to 14 days' worth of data using the home monitoring protocol described earlier.
   a. Instruct the client to keep a daily log, as described earlier.
3. Have the client perform an at-home BG curve before recheck.
   a. Once-daily or twice-daily monitoring of BG concentration does not replace the need for BG curves in the overall evaluation of insulin efficacy, peak effect, and duration of action.
4. Evaluate the client's BG log and curve with respect to the prescribed insulin dose.
   a. Many handheld glucometers, including veterinary models, have data transfer capabilities, enabling easier evaluation of raw data.
5. Create an insulin dosage chart based on the results of the BG log evaluation (**Table 2**).

Table 1
Diabetic cat example. Sample starting insulin dose chart. Fixed insulin dosage chart

	BG (mg/dL [mmol/L])	Eats 50%–100% (28.35 g [1 oz] or 0.25 cup low carbohydrate dry)	Eats <50%
Too high	>500 (>27.8)	2 units	1 unit
	450–500 (25–27.8)	2 units	1 unit
	375–449 (20.9–24.9)	2 units	1 unit
Acceptable	300–374 (16.7–20.8)	2 units	1 unit
	250–299 (13.9–16.6)	2 units	1 unit
Good	200–249 (11.1–13.8)	2 units	1 unit
Nondiabetic range	150–199 (8.3–11)	1 unit	0.5 units
	100–149 (5.6–8.2)[a]	0	0
Too low	60–99 (3.3–5.5)[a]	0	0
	<60 (<3.3)	1. Recheck immediately to verify 2. If alert, feed and recheck in 30 min 3. If weak, give Karo syrup, recheck in 30 min, call hospital	1. Recheck immediately to verify 2. If alert, feed and recheck in 30 min 3. If weak, give Karo syrup, recheck in 30 min, call hospital

Insulin: glargine, detemir, or ProZinc U-40 (4.5 kg).
Starting dose 0.25 U/kg-0.5 U/kg subcutaneously twice daily (immediately after eating).
[a] If BG is <150 mg/dL (8.3 mmol/L), recheck BG 1 h after feeding and dose according to the chart.

Table 2
Diabetic cat example. Variable insulin dosage chart

	BG (mg/dL [mmol/L])	Eats 50%–100% (28.35 g [1 oz] or 0.25 cup low carbohydrate dry)	Eats <50%
Too high	>500 (>27.8)	4 units	2 units
	450–500 (25–27.8)	3.5 units	1.5 units
	375–449 (20.9–24.9)	3 units	1.5 units
Acceptable	300–374 (16.7–20.8)	2.5 units	1 unit
	250–299 (13.9–16.6)	2 units	1 unit
Good	200–249 (11.1–13.8)	1.5 units	1 unit
Nondiabetic range	150–199 (8.3–11)	1 unit	0
	100–149 (5.6–8.2)[a]	0	0
Too low	60–99 (3.3–5.5)[a]	0	0
	<60 (<3.3)	1. Recheck immediately to verify 2. If alert, feed and recheck in 30 min 3. If weak, give Karo syrup, recheck in 30 min, call hospital	1. Recheck immediately to verify 2. If alert, feed and recheck in 30 min 3. If weak, give Karo syrup, recheck in 30 min, call hospital

Insulin: glargine, detemir, or ProZinc U-40 (4.5 kg).
Starting dose 0.25 U/kg-0.5 U/kg subcutaneously twice daily (immediately after eating).
[a] If BG is <149 mg/dL (8.2 mmol/L), recheck BG 1 h after feeding and dose according to the chart.

6. **Table 3** describes the algorithm used to create and adjust insulin dosage charts, with tight glycemic regulation and remission as a treatment goal.

Note: insulin dose changes should be made based on preinsulin glucose concentration for glargine and detemir, and nadir (lowest) glucose concentrations for all insulin types. Initially, clients should measure BG concentrations 3 to 5 times per day. For glargine and detemir, ideally, this measurement should be taken before each insulin injection, 2 measurements between these times, and before bed, although, realistically, the 2 additional measurements tend to be when the owner gets home from work, and before bed.

We prefer and routinely use a veterinary-directed algorithm that makes changes in the insulin dosage chart based on the BG readings. We have not used and are not comfortable with a protocol in which the owner changes the dose.

The Veterinary-Directed Home BG Monitoring Protocol is as follows.

Admittedly the editor, Dr Rand, is an advocate of the following protocol. Alternatively, if the owner is experienced and reliable, and is at home to monitor the cat, the veterinarian may choose to use an insulin dose adjustment protocol in which the owner is given an algorithm and makes incremental changes in the insulin dose based on the BG reading. This system was used successfully in both European remission studies:

i. Feed the cat, and if it eats well, reduce the dose by 0.25 to 0.5 IU per injection depending on if the cat on is on a low (<3 IU) or high (≥3 IU) dose of insulin.
ii. Feed the cat, wait 1 to 2 hours, and when the glucose concentration increases to more than 7.5 to 8.3 mmol/L (135–149 mg/dL), give the normal dose. If the glucose concentration does not increase within 1 to 2 hours, reduce the dose by 0.25 IU or 0.5 IU per injection (as above).
iii. Split the dose: feed the cat, and give most of the dose immediately, and then give the remainder 1 to 2 hours later, when the glucose concentration has increased to more than 7.5 to 8.3 mmol/L (135–149 mg/dL).
iv. If all these methods lead to increased BG concentrations, give the full dose if preinsulin BG concentration is 3.6 to 8.3 mmol/L (65–149 mg/dL) and observe closely for signs of hypoglycemia.
v. In general, for most cats, the best results in the stabilization phase occur when insulin dose is as consistent as possible, giving the full normal dose at the regular injection time.

Regardless of which system of monitoring is instituted, the owner should be given specific acceptable BG parameters and report any BG readings outside those parameters to the veterinarian on the same day. In addition, the owner should understand that monitoring is performed to enhance the veterinarian's capability to manage the cat's condition, not to replace regular rechecks with the veterinarian.

Long-Term Evaluation and Follow-Up

Monitoring plans should be individualized to the cat's condition. The clinician should focus on the cat's physical condition and clinical response to therapy, and data from the history such as weight, history, physical examination, and client observations regarding thirst, urine output, energy level, and behavior should be evaluated at every veterinary check.[1] Home monitoring logs containing daily insulin dose, all BG measurements, and the owner's clinical observations (eg, water consumption, wetness of litter box, signs consistent with hypoglycemia) should be evaluated. It is particularly important to assess insulin dose and clinical signs about the

Table 3
Veterinarian-directed protocol to induce diabetic remission in the cat

Parameter Used for Dosage Adjustment	Initial Dose on Insulin Dosage Chart–Veterinarian Directed
Step 1: Initial dose and first 3 d on glargine, ProZinc, or detemir	Try not to increase dose for 1 wk
If the cat received another insulin previously, increase or reduce the starting dose taking this information into account. Glargine has a lower potency than lente insulin and protamine zinc insulin in most cats	0.25 IU/kg of ideal weight BID
Ketonuria or history of ketones and BG >300 mg/dL (16.7 mmol/L) (after 24–48 h)	Increase by 0.5 IU/cat BID
If BG is <80 mg/dL (4.4 mmol/L)	Reduce dose by 0.5–1.0 IU/cat BID
Step 2: Dosage increases	Change insulin dosage chart–veterinarian directed
If nadir (lowest) BG concentration >300 mg/dL (16.7 mmol/L)	Increase every 3 d by 0.5–1.0 IU/cat BID
If nadir (lowest) BG concentration 200–300 mg/dL (11–16.7 mmol/L)	Increase every 3 d by 0.5 IU/cat BID
If nadir (lowest) BG concentration <200 mg/dL (11 mmol/L) but peak is >200 mg/dL (11 mmol/L)	Increase every 5–7 d by 0.5–1.0 IU/cat BID
If BG is <80 mg/dL (4.4 mmol/L)	Reduce dose by 0.5–1.0 IU/cat BID depending on if cat on low or high dose of insulin
Initially insulin not given if glucose <150 (8.3 mmol/L)	<150 mg/dL (8.3 mmol/L) glucose rechecked 1 h after feeding if >150 mg/dL (8.3 mmol/L) insulin given, if <150 mg/dL (8.3 mmol/L) glucose recheck in 1 h, if >150 mg/dL (8.3 mmol/L) insulin given, if <150 mg/dL (8.3 mmol/L) after 2 h dosage reduced by 0.5–1.0 IU/cat BID
BG before feeding and insulin <150 (8.3 mmol/L) than increases 3–4 times greater than 150 mg/dL (8.3 mmol/L) 1–2 h after feeding	Adjust insulin dosage chart parameters to administer insulin down to a BG of 100–110 mg/dL (5.6–6.1 mmol/L)
Step 3: Dosage maintenance goal glucose 80–200 mg/dL (4.4–11 mmol/L)	Change insulin dosage chart–veterinarian directed
If BG is <80 mg/dL (4.4 mmol/L)	Reduce dose by 0.5–1.0 IU/cat BID
If nadir or peak BG concentration >200 mg/dL (11 mmol/L)	Increase dose by 0.5–1.0 IU/cat BID depending on dose of insulin and the degree of hyperglycemia
Step 4: Dosage reduction	Change insulin dosage chart–veterinarian directed
Insulin dosage chart insulin not given if glucose <110 mg/dL (6.1 mmol/L)	Insulin dosage chart phases out insulin administration with normoglycemia
When the cat regularly (every day for at least 1 wk), has its lowest BG concentration in the normal range of a healthy cat, and stays <130–150 mg/dL (7.2–8.3 mmol/L)	Change the insulin dosage chart back to only administer insulin if BG ≥150 mg/dL (8.3 mmol/L)

(continued on next page)

Table 3 *(continued)*	
Parameter Used for Dosage Adjustment	**Initial Dose on Insulin Dosage Chart–Veterinarian Directed**
If the nadir glucose concentration is <80 mg/dL (4.4 mmol/L) at least 3 times on separate days	Reduce dose by 0.5–1.0 IU/cat BID
If the cat decreases <70 mg/dL (3.9 mmol/L) once	Reduce dose immediately by 0.5–1.0 IU/cat BID or 50%
If peak BG concentration >200 mg/dL (11 mmol/L)	Immediately increase insulin dose to last effective dose
Step 5: Remission euglycemia for a minimum of 14 d without insulin	Change insulin dosage chart–veterinarian directed
Insulin administration stopped	Glucose checked 1 h after feeding once a week, if glucose >150 (8.3 mmol/L), restart insulin at last effective dose

Dose changes should be made based on preinsulin glucose concentration, or nadir (lowest) glucose concentrations. Initially, clients should be measuring BG concentrations 3 to 4 times per day.

corresponding BG measurements for that day. Appropriate laboratory measurements should be performed and an attempt should be made to establish the tightest possible glycemic control without negatively affecting quality of life.

What about fructosamine? It is just an average

Fructosamine levels are a measure of the average BG for the previous 3 to 4 weeks, but do not reflect daily fluctuations. Most reference laboratories consider fructosamine levels of less than 500 μmol/L as good glycemic regulation. Fructosamine levels between 500 and 614 μmol/L are considered by reference laboratories as fair regulation, and levels greater than 614 μmol/L are considered as poor regulation. Most of our feline patients that did not achieve diabetic remission that are on chronic twice-daily home monitoring routinely have fructosamine values of less than 400 μmol/L. Once home monitoring is instituted, the degree of variation in BG concentration in a patient with a fructosamine of less than 500 μmol/L is often surprising, and the daily BG concentrations in a cat with fructosamine less than 500 μmol/L are typically not consistent with a definition of good glycemic regulation, despite good clinical control.

Real-time BG values allow for real-time decision making and insulin dosage plans that are based on the cat's BG. Furthermore, availability of real-time BG values prevents the administration of insulin in the face of hypoglycemia, facilitates identification of short duration of insulin action or lack of glucose-decreasing effect, and allows recognition of insulin-induced hypoglycemia or the Somogyi phenomenon, Fructosamine measurements are not contributory in patients whose BGs are being monitored at home at least twice daily, because the clinician has detailed records with multiple data points, and a mean BG is simple to calculate. However, we often continue to measure fructosamine to show what the value is in a patient with good glycemic regulation.

General ongoing evaluation recommendations based on the 2010 AAHA diabetic guidelines, and adjusted for stable patients managed with a home monitoring protocol aimed at achieving remission, are as follows:

- Every 3 months
  - Record body weight, complete history of polyuria, polydipsia, polyphagia, partial anorexia (defined by many as a picky or finicky appetite), and complete physical examination.

- ○ Perform any diagnostic testing clinically indicated by the cat's condition.
- ○ Evaluate biochemical glycemic control; evaluate their daily log and include the BG curve. Availability of real-time BG measurements allows clients to readily identify prolonged or chronic hyperglycemia, and any episodes of hypoglycemia, and to quickly contact the clinician for recommendations.
- At least every 6 months
  - ○ Undertake full laboratory workup, including complete blood count, biochemistry profile, total T4 or free T4, urinalysis, urine culture, and any other recommended diagnostics as appropriate
- Preventative health care as recommended by the veterinarian
  - ○ Dental care
  - ○ Nutritional consult/dietary recommendations
  - ○ Vaccinations
  - ○ Intestinal parasite testing/treatment
  - ○ Heartworm preventative/testing

SUMMARY

Many clients attempt home monitoring if it is recommended by the veterinarian as the standard of care, they understand the benefits, and they receive adequate training and support from the veterinary team. Home monitoring, like any diagnostic test, is a tool to gain helpful information, and does not replace regular rechecks with the veterinarian. However, when used appropriately, it provides invaluable information that helps the client and the veterinarian better understand the cat's disease process and make more informed decisions regarding treatment. This strategy facilitates achieving the best treatment outcome for each cat, which ideally is diabetic remission, and is attainable in most newly diagnosed patients.

REFERENCES

1. Rucinsky R, Cook A, Haley S, et al. AAHA diabetes management guidelines for dogs and cats. J Am Anim Hosp Assoc 2010;46:215–24.
2. Unknown. Levemir drug insert. In: Novo Nordisk USA. Available at: http://www.novo-pi.com/levemir.pdf. Accessed November 5, 2012.
3. Unknown. Living with diabetes: checking your blood glucose. In: American Diabetes Association. Available at: http://www.diabetes.org/living-with-diabetes/treatment-and-care/blood-glucose-control/checking-your-blood-glucose.html. Accessed November 5, 2012.
4. Wang PH, Lau J, Chalmers TC, et al. Meta-analysis of effects of intensive blood glucose control on late complications of type I diabetes. Lancet 1993;341(8856):1306–9.
5. Nelson R, Couto C, Bunch S, et al. Disorders of the endocrine pancreas. In: Small animal internal medicine. 2nd edition. St Louis (MO): Mosby; 1998. p. 735–74.
6. Hall TD, Mahony O, Rozanski EA, et al. Effects of diet on glucose control in cats with diabetes mellitus treated with twice daily insulin glargine. J Feline Med Surg 2009;11(2):125–30.
7. Roomp K, Rand J. Intensive blood glucose control is safe and effective in diabetic cats using home monitoring and treatment with glargine. J Feline Med Surg 2009;11(8):668–82.
8. Fleeman L, Rand J. Evaluation of day-to-day variability of serial blood glucose concentration values in diabetic dogs. J Am Vet Med Assoc 2003;222:317–21.

9. Alt N, Kley S, Haessig M, et al. Day-to-day variability of blood glucose concentration curves generated at home in cats with diabetes mellitus. J Am Vet Med Assoc 2007;203:1011–7.

10. Rand JS, Kinnaird E, Baglloni A, et al. Acute stress hyperglycemia in cats is associated with struggling and increased concentrations of lactate and norepinephrine. J Vet Intern Med 2002;16(2):123–32.

11. Reeve-Johnson MK, Rand JS, Anderson S, et al. Determination of reference values for casual blood glucose concentration in clinically-healthy, aged cats measured with a portable glucose meter from an ear or paw sample. J Vet Intern Med 2012;26(3):755.

12. Cohen TA, Nelson RW, Kass PH, et al. Evaluation of six portable blood glucose meters for measuring blood glucose concentration in dogs. J Am Vet Med Assoc 2009;235(3):276–80.

13. Unknown. About AlphaTRAKer. In: AlphaTRAK Glucose Meter. Available at: http://www.alphatrakmeter.com/alphatraker-what-is.html. Accessed November 5, 2012.

14. Lynch H. Home monitoring of blood glucose: practical tips for incorporating it into your practice. Today's Veterinary Practice 2011;1(3):31–5.

15. Reusch CE, Kley S, Casella M. Home monitoring of the diabetic cat. J Feline Med Surg 2006;8(2):119–27.

16. Selam JL, Koenen C, Weng W, et al. Improving glycemic control with insulin detemir using the 303 algorithm in insulin naïve patients with type 2 diabetes: a subgroup analysis of the US PREDICTIVE 303 study. Curr Med Res Opin 2008;24(1):11–20.

17. Roomp K, Rand J. Evaluation of detemir in diabetic cats managed with a protocol for intensive blood glucose control. J Feline Med Surg 2012;14:566–72.

Pancreatitis and Diabetes in Cats

Sarah M.A. Caney, BVSc, PhD, MRCVS

KEYWORDS

- Acute pancreatitis • Chronic pancreatitis • Diabetes mellitus

KEY POINTS

- Pancreatitis, in particular chronic pancreatitis, is a common co-morbidity in diabetic patients.
- Pancreatitis can complicate management of diabetes through reducing insulin secretion by the pancreas and increasing peripheral insulin resistance; however, in many patients, there is much controversy as to how much this condition affects diabetic stability and patient quality of life, especially in cases of chronic pancreatitis.
- Presence of active pancreatic inflammation is most likely to complicate diabetic control.
- Cats with evidence of acute pancreatitis around the onset of diabetes can achieve diabetic remission, and some may have no demonstrable residual impairment in glucose tolerance.

INTRODUCTION

The prevalence of pancreatitis in the cat population as a whole is unknown because pancreatitis is difficult to diagnose ante mortem. Recent post mortem surveys have shown that between 14% and 67% of cats may have identifiable pancreatic lesions.[1,2] In one study, 45% of clinically healthy cats had evidence of pancreatitis at necropsy.[2] Typically, the pancreatitis identified in these cats has comprised mild, chronic changes. The clinical significance is controversial because the prevalence is so high in apparently healthy cats.

Pancreatitis is an acknowledged concurrent disease in diabetic cats. Post mortem examination of diabetic cats found lesions consistent with pancreatitis in approximately half of diabetic patients, with chronic pancreatitis present in the majority and acute pancreatitis in 5%.[3] The prevalence of chronic pancreatitis lesions in diabetic cats, however, is similar to that reported with a recent post mortem survey of clinically healthy cats, which raises questions over the significance of this finding.[2,3] Management of pancreatitis is indicated with the aim of improving glycemic control and improving patient quality of life.

Disclosures: None.
Conflict of Interest: None.
Vet Professionals Limited, Midlothian Innovation Centre, Pentlandfield, Roslin, Midlothian EH25 9RE, UK
E-mail address: sarah@vetprofessionals.com

Vet Clin Small Anim 43 (2013) 303–317
http://dx.doi.org/10.1016/j.cvsm.2012.12.001
0195-5616/13/$ – see front matter © 2013 Elsevier Inc. All rights reserved.

There is no universally approved system for classification of feline pancreatitis. Pancreatitis is broadly subclassified histologically into acute or chronic categories according to how permanent the changes are:

- Acute necrotizing or suppurative pancreatitis: reversible changes are present in the pancreas and include edema, ischemia, inflammation, and necrosis. Acute pancreatitis is less common than the chronic form, with post mortem surveys reporting up to 15.7% prevalence.[2]
- Chronic (relapsing) pancreatitis: permanent histologic changes are present in the pancreas. This is typically a continuous, progressively worsening condition.[2] Chronic pancreatitis is characterized by mononuclear cell infiltration, fibrosis, and acinar atrophy within the pancreas. Although chronic pancreatitis is usually thought more benign in terms of clinical signs and prognosis, extension of inflammation into endocrine tissue of the pancreas can lead to destruction of islets and impaired β-cell function. Some studies have, therefore, indicated that this condition predisposes to the development of diabetes mellitus (diabetes) and exocrine pancreatic insufficiency.[4–7] In some cases, acute inflammation is superimposed on chronic pancreatitis—so-called acute on chronic pancreatitis or chronic active pancreatitis.

The cause of pancreatitis is often not evident at the time of diagnosis; hence, in many patients, the diagnosis is idiopathic pancreatitis. No significant age, body condition score or gender predisposition for development of pancreatitis has so far been described. A wide range of ages has been reported with pancreatitis and many clinicians believe that middle-aged and older-aged cats (cats over the age of 7 years) are more vulnerable.[8–11] Domestic short-haired and long-haired cats are most frequently reported with pancreatitis.[8–11] Many of the risk factors for development of pancreatitis in dogs, such as feeding a high-fat diet and presence of pre-existing endocrinopathies, are not currently recognized in cats.

Cats with inflammatory bowel disease, especially those with clinical signs, including vomiting, seem more vulnerable to the development of pancreatitis. This may be because vomiting increases the pressure within the duodenum and predisposes to reflux of intestinal contents into the pancreatic duct. In cats, the sphincter of Oddi at the duodenal papilla is a common channel for both the pancreatic and biliary ducts, meaning that any reflux of intestinal contents increases the risk of both pancreatic and hepatic inflammation. The significantly higher levels of bacteria in the lumen of the normal feline duodenum compared with those in dogs increase the probability of movement of bacteria from the bowel to the pancreas and/or liver with pancreaticobiliary reflux.[12]

Presence of concomitant bowel, pancreas, and hepatic inflammation, termed *triaditis*, may be present in some patients. For example, in one post mortem study, 83% of cats with cholangiohepatitis had concurrent inflammatory bowel disease and 50% had concurrent pancreatitis. In 39% of patients with cholangiohepatitis, inflammatory bowel disease and pancreatitis was diagnosed concurrently (triaditis). The pancreatitis in these cases was described as mild. The prevalence of inflammatory bowel disease and pancreatitis was lower (28% and 14%, respectively) in those cats where lymphocytic portal hepatitis was identified at post mortem.[1] The investigators of this study suggested that patients with cholangiohepatitis should be evaluated for bowel and pancreatic disease.

Causes of pancreatitis include

- Blunt abdominal trauma, such as resulting from a road traffic accident or fall from a height[13]
- Pathology affecting the distal common bile duct, such as infectious and inflammatory conditions, calculus formation

- Infectious causes, such as toxoplasmosis, liver flukes, feline infectious peritonitis, feline herpesvirus, and virulent feline calicivirus.[14-19] Experimentally, it has been shown that *Escherichia coli* can spread to the pancreas hematogenously, transmurally from the colon, or via reflux through the pancreatic duct.[20,21] Pancreatitis associated with *Enterococcus hirae* has also been described.[22]
- Pancreaticobiliary reflux. Reflux of infected bile is especially dangerous, resulting in damage to the tight junctions between duct epithelial cells, loss of epithelial cells, and increased vulnerability to development of pancreatitis.[23,24] Reflux associated with an increase in the ductal pressure is more likely to induce acinar necrosis and more severe pathology.[24]
- Hypoxia, ischemia, and/or hypotension
- Pancreaticolithiasis[25]
- Lipodystrophy
- Organophosphate toxicity[26]
- Idiosyncratic drug reactions
- Experimentally, both hypercalcemia and aspirin can induce pancreatitis.[27-30] Both hypercalcemia and oral aspirin result in an increase in the permeability of pancreatic duct cells to larger molecules, including those the size of pancreatic enzymes, and this is a mechanism behind induction of pancreatitis.[27,31]

Concurrent disease is common in patients with pancreatitis; in one study, this applied to 92% of patients overall—all of the cats with chronic pancreatitis and 83% of the patients with acute pancreatitis.[10] Hepatobiliary disease, renal disease, gastrointestinal disease, neoplasia, and diabetes were most common; 15% of the cats with chronic pancreatitis were diabetic in this study. Other studies have shown similar results.[8] Cats with diabetic ketosis or diabetic ketoacidosis may be more vulnerable to concurrent illnesses. In one study of 42 cats with diabetic ketosis or diabetic ketoacidosis, 93% had concurrent illnesses, including pancreatitis.[32]

HOW COMMON IS PANCREATITIS IN CATS WITH DIABETES MELLITUS?

Diabetes is a recognized co-morbidity with pancreatitis. Pancreatitis can lead to development of transient and permanent diabetes through destruction and loss of β cells and through exacerbating or inducing peripheral insulin resistance.

Pancreatic abnormalities are commonly found in cats with diabetes. In one study where post mortem examination was possible in 37 diabetic cats, exocrine pancreatic abnormalities were present in 73%, islet abnormalities in 89%, and both exocrine and endocrine abnormalities in 57%.[3] Exocrine abnormalities were not limited to pancreatitis, although this was present in 51% cats. Chronic pancreatitis was present in 46% of cats and acute pancreatitis in 5%. Other pancreatic abnormalities included exocrine pancreatic adenocarcinoma (19% cats), pancreatic adenoma, and multifocal pancreatic cysts.[3] There was no apparent association between glycemic control or survival time and presence of pancreatic neoplasia in this study. Glycemic control tended to be better in cats without chronic pancreatitis although this did not reach statistical significance.[3] There was no association between survival times and presence of chronic pancreatitis.

A recent study looked at feline serum pancreatic lipase immunoreactivity (fPLI) levels in 29 cats with diabetes compared with a control population of 23 non-diabetic cats with similar signalment.[33] fPLI results were significantly higher in the diabetic cat population, with 83% of the diabetic cats having elevated fPLI results. In 55% of the diabetic cats, the fPLI elevation was described as moderate or marked (fPLI >20 μg/L). Elevated fPLI results were also common in the non-diabetic group, with 66% of these cats having elevated results — a similar result to the prevalence of pancreatitis changes found in a recent post mortem survey of cats.[2] None of the non-diabetic cats had marked elevations in their fPLI and 35% of cats had elevations described as moderate (fPLI 12–20 μg/L). The investigators reported a weaker association between fPLI and serum fructosamine results, although in this small study there was no apparent association between fPLI levels and the degree of diabetic control.[33]

WHAT CLINICAL SIGNS ARE EXPECTED IN CATS WITH PANCREATITIS AND DIABETES MELLITUS?

Clinical signs attributable to pancreatitis vary according to the severity of disease. In some patients, especially those with chronic pancreatitis, no signs directly attributable to pancreatitis may be present. Clinical signs may wax and wane.

Clinical signs associated with pancreatitis are typically non-specific signs and most commonly include[8,10,26]

- Lethargy: present in approximately 50% to 100% of patients
- Reduced appetite: present in approximately 60% to 100% of patients
- Dehydration (acute pancreatitis patients): present in approximately 33% to 90% of patients
- Vomiting: present in approximately 33% to 50% of patients
- Weight loss: present in approximately 20% to 40% of patients

Physical examination does not consistently reveal specific abnormalities, and in many cats with chronic pancreatitis, no abnormalities referable to the pancreatitis can be found. Even in those cats where abnormalities are present, these are typically non-specific. For example, dehydration, tachypnea, dyspnea, hypothermia, and tachycardia may be found in patients with acute pancreatitis. Presence of a cranioventral abdominal mass, found in approximately 20% to 25% of acute pancreatitis cases, is not always associated with pain. There may be evidence of common concurrent diseases, such as thickened bowel loops in those cats with inflammatory bowel disease and altered hepatic palpation (eg, hepatomegaly or more firm feeling liver) in those patients with cholangiohepatitis. Chronic relapsing pancreatitis may be associated with general signs of long-term illness, such as poor hair coat and general failure to thrive.

HOW IS PANCREATITIS DIAGNOSED?

Pancreatitis is notoriously difficult to diagnose without a pancreatic biopsy. Even then, not all biopsies are diagnostic because the disease may be focal or patchy in distribution. Diagnosis of pancreatitis currently relies on assessing the complete picture of patient history, physical examination, and laboratory and imaging data. A presumptive diagnosis can be made in some cases but in others, further investigations and, in particular, pancreatic biopsy may be required. Acute necrotizing pancreatitis and chronic pancreatitis in cats cannot be distinguished from each other solely on the basis of clinicopathologic testing.

Screening hematology and serum biochemistry may reveal a variety of non-specific abnormalities[8,10,26]:

- White cell abnormalities:
  - Leukocytosis: present in approximately 30% to 60% of patients. A left shift and toxic changes may be seen in some patients.
  - Leukopenia: present in approximately 15% of patients

- Red cell abnormalities
  - Non-regenerative anemia: present in approximately 25% of patients
  - Hemoconcentration: present in approximately 15% of patients
- Biochemical abnormalities
  - Hyperbilirubinemia: present in 15% to 65% of patients
  - Elevated liver enzymes: present in 25% to 70% of patients
  - Hyperglycemia: present in up to 65% of patients with acute pancreatitis due to glucose intolerance or diabetes mellitus
  - Hypoglycemia: present in up to 75% of patients with acute pancreatitis
  - Hypercholesterolemia: present in up to 65% of patients, especially if concurrent diabetes
  - Azotemia: present in up to 33% of patients, which may be pre-renal, if acute, or renal, if chronic and associated with concurrent diabetes

Presence of combinations of these non-specific changes, such as hyperbilirubinemia, elevation of liver enzymes, and hyperglycemia, increases the suspicion of pancreatitis. Low ionized calcium levels, less than 1 mmol/L, due to saponification of peripancreatic fat, are associated with a poorer outcome in acute pancreatitis cases.[34]

Analysis of serum amylase and lipase levels is usually of no diagnostic value. Amylase and lipase are not pancreas-specific (also produced by gastric and intestinal mucosa) and are affected by renal disease, where reduced clearance can be associated with up to 2-fold to 3-fold increases in levels. Hepatic and neoplastic disease can also affect amylase and lipase levels. Lipase levels may also be increased after administration of dexamethasone.

In those cases where a peritoneal effusion is present, analysis of fluid and serum lipase activity is helpful in addition to cytology. Cats with pancreatitis have grossly increased amounts of lipase in their peritoneal fluid compared with serum levels. One study of experimentally induced pancreatitis suggested that analysis of fluid amylase levels was also helpful and that levels correlate with the severity of the pancreatitis.[35]

fPLI testing is of value in the diagnosis of pancreatitis and has a reasonable sensitivity and specificity, especially in diagnosing acute pancreatitis cases, which tend to have marked elevations of fPLI.[36,37] Elevations in fPLI can be seen in patients with non-inflammatory pancreatic disease (eg, neoplasia and trauma) and mild to moderate elevations are common in cats with chronic pancreatitis and gastrointestinal and hepatic disease. Marked elevations are more likely to suggest significant pancreatic disease. Therefore, elevations in fPLI should be used as part of the diagnostic repertoire and not as the sole test for pancreatitis. Overall, the sensitivity of the fPLI test in one study was approximately 67% for identification of pancreatic pathology with a specificity of approximately 91%.[36] In a later study by the same investigator, the sensitivity for diagnosing pancreatitis was 79% and the specificity 82% using a diagnostic cutoff of greater than or equal to 5.4 μg/L,[38] with greater than 12 μg/L now suggested as the cut-point indicative of pancreatitis.[38] Feline serum trypsin-like immunoreactivity testing is of value in the diagnosis of exocrine pancreatic insufficiency but of much less value in the diagnosis of pancreatitis, where it has a sensitivity of approximately 30%.[8,36]

Imaging can be of value in the diagnosis of pancreatitis and is also of value in ruling out other concurrent problems. The following radiographic changes, which may be associated with this condition, are often non-specific and seen in the minority of patients.[8,9]

- Loss of detail in the cranial abdomen associated with peritoneal effusion (**Fig. 1**)
- Presence of a cranial abdominal mass

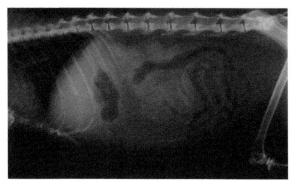

Fig. 1. Abdominal radiography may reveal loss of contrast in the cranial abdomen associated with peritoneal effusion. In this patient, lipase levels were 10 times higher in the ascitic fluid than in the serum.

- Dilated bowel loops
- Gas in the duodenum
- Pleural effusion

Ultrasound can be sensitive in diagnosing pancreatitis if done by a skilled operator and interpreted in line with the clinical signs and additional data. Even under these conditions, however, the sensitivity of ultrasound in identifying pancreatitis ranges from 11% to 67%.[8,9,11,36] Therefore, a normal abdominal ultrasound cannot rule out pancreatitis. In some cats with confirmed acute pancreatitis, the pancreas may be normal or not visible on ultrasound, even with highly qualified sonographers.[9] Repeat examination may be helpful, especially in cases with more subtle abnormalities. In normal cats, the pancreas is small and difficult to identify. Abnormalities compatible with a diagnosis of pancreatitis include

- Enlarged, hypoechoic pancreas sometimes with cavitary lesions. Causes of pancreatic enlargement, such as neoplasia and edema, also need to be considered. Hypoalbuminemia and portal hypertension are potential causes of pancreatic edema.
- Hyperechoic peripancreatic fat and mesentery
- Presence of a peritoneal effusion
- Local lymphadenopathy
- Dilation of the common bile duct
- Dilation of the pancreatic duct has been reported as a change associated with pancreatitis[39]; however, care needs to be taken not to overinterpret this, especially in older cats because the pancreatic duct diameter increases slightly with age.[40]
- In cats with chronic pancreatitis, there may be decreased pancreatic size, variable echogenicity, nodular echotexture, acoustic shadowing due to mineralization, and scarring and irregular widening of the pancreatic ducts[41]
- Other abnormalities (eg, increased thickness of gut wall in patients with inflammatory bowel disease)

Endosonography using a video ultrasound gastroscope has also been described in some cases of pancreatitis and may offer superior imaging in those patients where it is difficult to obtain an image using standard transabdominal ultrasound, for example, due to obesity or gas in intestines.[42]

Scintigraphic imaging of the pancreas after administration of technetium Tc 99m citrate has been described in 5 normal cats and in 10 cats with spontaneous acute pancreatitis confirmed at post mortem after the study. The pancreas is not visible in normal cats but in those with acute pancreatitis, the uptake of radioactivity is increased.[43]

CT imaging of the pancreas has been described in normal cats.[44] Unfortunately, it does not seem to be a sensitive technique for diagnosis of pancreatitis, frequently failing to enable visualization of the pancreas.[8]

In spite of the limitations of pancreatic biopsy (discussed previously), obtaining a sample of pancreas for assessment may be the only way to confirm a diagnosis of pancreatitis. Biopsies can be safely collected via laparotomy or laparoscopy as long as patients are not too ill to cope with anesthesia and surgery. Where appropriate, it is often helpful to collect bowel, lymph node, and liver biopsies for histopathologic analysis (**Fig. 2**).

WHAT IS THE IMPACT OF PANCREATITIS ON ASSESSMENT OF DIABETIC PATIENTS?

Presence of pancreatitis has the potential to complicate assessment as well as management of diabetic cats. Diabetes can be associated with signs of chronic or acute pancreatitis. Depending on the reversibility of the changes affecting the islets, diabetic cats may or may not achieve diabetic remission with appropriate insulin therapy to control glucose toxicity. In some cats with pancreatitis, glucose intolerance is more mild, resulting in glucose concentrations below those considered diabetic but above normal, and these need to be differentiated from transient hyperglycemia of acute stress. Other laboratory findings common to both diabetes and pancreatitis include elevation of liver enzymes and cholesterol, and this too can make diagnosis and differentiation of these two conditions challenging in some patients.

WHAT IS THE IMPACT OF PANCREATITIS ON DIABETIC CONTROL?

The impact of pancreatitis on management depends on the severity of the pancreatic disease and associated complications. In patients with active pancreatic disease, management of diabetes is more complicated and presence of pancreatitis is a negative prognostic indicator. Presence of acute pancreatitis is most likely to be clinically

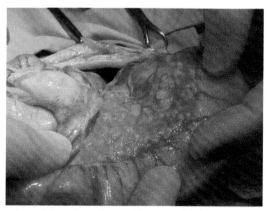

Fig. 2. The pancreas, bowel, lymph nodes, and liver can be assessed and biopsied via exploratory laparotomy. In this case, the pancreas is enlarged and nodular with histologic evidence of chronic active pancreatitis.

significant. Chronic pancreatitis is often associated with gastrointestinal and/or hepatic disease and these latter complications may be more important clinically than the pancreatitis. Specific management of any intercurrent disease is indicated in the diabetic cat to maximize the chances of a successful and sustained positive treatment outcome.

Standard diabetes mellitus treatments, such as insulin and dietary therapy, are still important in patients with concurrent pancreatitis. Resolution of glucose toxicity provides the best chance of achieving diabetic remission. Close monitoring is important to detect problems with stabilization. Most common problems encountered are

- Increased insulin requirements due to insulin resistance and worsening glucose intolerance induced by pancreatitis. This may be manifested as destabilization of a previously well stabilized patient or requirement for high insulin doses (eg, approaching or exceeding 2 IU insulin per kg bodyweight per dose).
- Diabetic remission associated with resolution of underlying pancreatitis. Owner home-monitoring (discussed elsewhere in this issue) is indicated to detect diabetic remission promptly. Owners should be informed that diabetic relapse is possible should the pancreatitis recur.
- Varying insulin requirements due to changes in insulin secretion and insulin resistance associated with waxing and waning pancreatitis. Affected patients may show variations in thirst, urination, blood, and urine glucose levels. Owner home-monitoring is valuable in assessing these patients. These patients can be challenging to manage. For some patients, it is safer to prescribe a cautious dose of insulin (eg, 0.25–0.5 IU insulin per kg bodyweight per dose), such that hypoglycemia is not induced should insulin requirements suddenly decrease.

HOW IS PANCREATITIS MANAGED?

Where indicated, treatment of pancreatitis should aim to provide supportive care (discussed later). Attention should also be given to other co-morbidities, such as hepatic lipidosis. In cats with chronic pancreatitis, the most successful strategy is usually to focus on concurrent gastrointestinal and/or hepatic disease, which is generally of greater clinical significance to the patient. Generic treatment of chronic pancreatitis is often not justified.

Fluid and Electrolyte Abnormalities

Crystalloid therapy (eg, lactated Ringer solution, 0.9% saline) may be required to replace losses and maintain normal hydration. In addition colloids, such as hydroxyl starch or high-molecular-weight dextran (at a dose of 5 mL/kg over 15 minutes, repeated up to 4 times daily), may be helpful in supporting pancreatic perfusion.[45] High-molecular-weight dextrans have been shown beneficial in rodent models of pancreatitis through reducing trypsinogen activation, preventing acinar cell necrosis, and reducing mortality through support of the pancreatic microcirculation.[46] If present, hypocalcemia should be managed with a calcium gluconate infusion at a starting rate of 50 mg/kg to 150 mg/kg over 12 hours to 24 hours, monitoring closely.[47]

Plasma transfusions may be indicated in some patients with acute disease. Plasma is valuable in providing oncotic support, clotting factors, and proteinase inhibitors, such as α-macroglobulin, which helps scavenge activated pancreatic enzymes.[45] Pancreatitis is associated with marked consumption of circulating macroglobulins, including plasma protease inhibitors. Free proteases can trigger acute disseminated intravascular coagulation, shock, and death through activation of kinin, coagulation, fibrinolytic, and complement cascade systems. Administration of 10 mL/kg/d to 40 mL/kg/d fresh plasma is recommended in aliquots of 5 mL/kg.[45] Whole blood is an option in those situations where access to plasma is not possible. Albumin is of value in increasing the oncotic pressure, which helps maintain blood volume and limits edema formation in the pancreas.

Nutritional Requirements

Anorexic patients benefit from nursing support, for example, hand feeding palatable, highly digestible foods. A low-fat diet is not essential in cases of feline pancreatitis; it is more important that the diet is highly digestible and well tolerated by the cat. In patients with concurrent inflammatory bowel disease, a hydrolyzed or single protein source diet may be more appropriate.[45] A canned diet is preferable because it is lowest in carbohydrates and, therefore, most suited to a diabetic cat.[48–53]

More-aggressive nutritional support required in some cases may include appetite stimulation (for example, mirtazapine, 1.9 mg per cat every other day) and placement of feeding tubes. In theory, placing a jejunostomy tube would be the ideal option for cats with pancreatitis; however, these tubes are not easy to place or maintain. In addition, many patients with severe pancreatitis may be classed as high risk for anesthesia. Naso-esophageal feeding tubes can be placed in fully conscious cats and are suitable for short-term support of cats deemed to sick to sedate or anesthetize (**Fig. 3**). A recent study confirmed that nasogastric feeding is often well tolerated by cats with pancreatitis.[54] Those cats requiring long-term support are better managed with esphagostomy or gastrostomy tubes because these also allow feeding of blended cat food rather than specific liquid diets. Enteral nutrition should be pursued unless intractable vomiting is present, in which case, partial or total parenteral nutritional support may be required.[45] Successful use of an endoscopically place percutaneous gastrojejunostomy tube has been described in a cat with pancreatitis and has the advantage of maintaining gut integrity with a lower risk of sepsis than can be seen with parenteral nutrition.[55]

Antioxidant therapy using agents, such as S-adenosylmethionine (eg, 200 mg per cat, once daily orally), has been proposed as a useful adjunctive treatment in patients with pancreatitis, although there is no published evidence to support this.

Management of Abdominal Pain

Pancreatitis may be associated with significant abdominal discomfort and some patients benefit from analgesic support. Clinical signs of pain are not always easy to

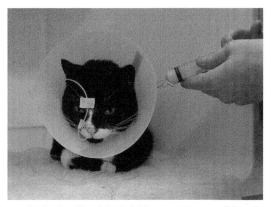

Fig. 3. Naso-esophageal tube feeding is helpful in providing nutritional support for patients too sick for anesthesia.

identify so it may be safer to assume that analgesic treatment is warranted, especially in acute cases. Buprenorphine can be administered sub-lingually by an owner at home or intramuscularly at a dose of 10 μg/kg to 20 μg/kg 2 to 4 times a day. Alternatives include fentanyl patches.

Management of Vomiting

Anti-emetics are indicated in patients suffering from nausea and vomiting. Options include oral mirtazapine (1.9 mg per cat every other day), maropitant (0.5–1.0 mg/kg once daily for 7 days, then every other day, as required), and ondansetron (0.1–0.2 mg/kg intravenously 2 to 4 times daily). H_2 blockers, such as ranitidine (1–2 mg/kg twice daily) or famotidine (0.5–1.0 mg/kg once daily), can also be helpful.

Temporary withdrawal of food, followed by gradual re-introduction, may be necessary in vomiting patients.

Antibiotic Therapy

Although routine antibiotic therapy is not generally recommended for pancreatitis cases, it should be considered in those patients that show signs of sepsis (eg, pyrexia or shock) or breakdown of the gastrointestinal barrier (increased white cells, left shift, or toxic neutrophils). Routine broad-spectrum antibiotics are probably justified in those acute pancreatitis patients with concurrent diabetes mellitus. Diabetic patients may be more vulnerable to acquiring infections and their reduced immune function may make them more vulnerable to more serious consequences. A sensible empiric choice of antibiosis may be amoxicillin and a fluoroquinolone, such as pradofloxacin.

In patients known or suspected to have gastrointestinal disease, metronidazole treatment may be an alternative appropriate choice.[56]

Prevention and Treatment of Disseminated Intravascular Coagulation

Several strategies have been used in acute pancreatitis cases with the aim of reducing the likelihood of disseminated intravascular coagulation from developing and treating this complication when present. Low-molecular-weight heparin (100 IU/kg subcutaneously once daily) is recommended to prevent coagulopathies secondary to systemic inflammatory response syndrome, although no data exist to show any benefit.[45] As discussed previously, plasma transfusions may also be of value in prevention/treatment of disseminated intravascular coagulation. Peritoneal dialysis has been reported to have some success by removing toxic material from the peritoneal cavity and may be recommended. Vitamin K therapy may be helpful in patients suffering from coagulopathies.

Other Treatments

Oral pancreatic enzyme supplements and/or oral feeding of fresh frozen pancreas have been recommended with the aim that these reduce pancreatic enzyme production and release and, hence, provide some symptomatic support from the pain associated with pancreatitis. In human cases, there have been anecdotal reports of a reduction in pain associated with this treatment.

Dopamine treatment (5 μg/kg/min intravenously) has been suggested as a splanchnic vasodilator, which may improve blood flow to the pancreas and reduce pancreatic microvascular permeability through its β-agonist effects. In experimental models of acute hemorrhagic and edematous pancreatitis, dopamine was found to reduce the severity of pancreatic inflammation, even when administered more than 12 hours after onset of acute hemorrhagic pancreatitis. The dopamine, however, did not have any significant effect on pancreatic blood flow and the beneficial effects were probably related to reduction of pancreatic duct and/or microvascular permeability.[57–60] The anti-inflammatory effects of dopamine were mediated by both dopamine and β-adrenergic receptor binding.

Cobalamin supplementation has been suggested in cats with pancreatitis (eg, 0.25 mg per cat subcutaneously every week) because the pancreas is the only source of intrinsic factor in cats. Hypocobalaminemia is frequently reported in cats with inflammatory bowel disease and pancreatitis.[61–63] A recent study of cats with inflammatory bowel disease reported that increased fPLI levels were significantly negatively correlated with serum cobalamin levels.[64] Cobalamin levels were significantly lower in those inflammatory bowel disease patients with elevated fPLI results above 12 μg/L compared with those inflammatory bowel disease patients with normal or only mildly elevated fPLI results.[64]

Glucocorticoids (eg, prednisolone 1–2 mg/kg once or twice daily) are not contraindicated in cases of feline pancreatitis and can be of value in acute management of fulminant cases and in long-term management of those patients with mild chronic pancreatitis and concurrent inflammatory bowel and/or liver disease.[65,66] The dose should be tapered to the lowest effective dose. Addition of glucocorticoids is more complicated in those patients with pre-existing diabetes because it is associated with insulin resistance and, hence, more problematic control. Glucocorticoids also have the potential to induce diabetes in normoglycemic patients and patients with pancreatitis may be especially brittle in this respect. Alternative immunomodulatory agents, such as ciclosporin (5 mg/kg once or twice daily), chlorambucil (2 mg/cat every 2–3 days), or glucocorticoids with a high first-pass metabolism, such as budesonide, should be considered, as appropriate to each patient.[56]

Ursodeoxycholic acid (10–15 mg/kg/d) is often included in treatment of patients with pancreatitis, especially in those where cholestasis is a factor. Ursodeoxycholic acid is a non-toxic, hydrophilic bile acid that stimulates choleresis. It should not be used in patients with bile duct obstruction.

Surgical treatment of pancreatitis is indicated in some cases to relieve obstruction of the bile duct, obtain biopsies, and potentially débride or excise abscesses and necrotic tissue. Because pancreatic disease can be patchy in distribution, multiple biopsies, including of other organs, as appropriate, can be helpful. Pancreaticojejunostomy has been reported to improve pancreatic blood flow, reduce fibrosis, and improve pancreatic histology in cats with experimentally induced chronic obstructive pancreatitis.[67,68] Surgical decompression of the pancreatic duct has also been reported in experimental models of chronic pancreatitis to relieve pain, reduce tissue pressure, improve interstitial pH (which is reduced in ischemia caused by chronic pancreatitis), and improve pancreatic blood flow.[69,70]

SUMMARY

Optimizing outcome in diabetic patients requires attention to all concurrent problems to provide the best quality of life and treatment outcome. Pancreatitis, in particular chronic pancreatitis, is a common co-morbidity in diabetic patients. Pancreatitis can complicate management of diabetes through reducing insulin secretion by the pancreas and increasing peripheral insulin resistance. In many patients, however, there is much controversy as to how much this condition affects diabetic stability and patient quality of life, especially in the case of chronic pancreatitis. Presence of active pancreatic inflammation is most likely to complicate diabetic control. Cats with evidence of acute pancreatitis around the onset of diabetes can achieve diabetic remission, and some may have no demonstrable residual impairment in glucose tolerance. Unfortunately, in other patients, there may be residual impairments of glucose tolerance leaving patients either in a pre-diabetic state or as an insulin-dependent diabetic long-term.

REFERENCES

1. Weiss DJ, Gagne JM, Armstrong PJ. Relationship between inflammatory hepatic disease and inflammatory bowel disease, pancreatitis and nephritis in cats. J Am Vet Med Assoc 1996;209:1114–6.
2. De Cock HE, Forman MA, Farver TB, et al. Prevalence and histopathologic characteristics of pancreatitis in cats. Vet Pathol 2007;44:39–49.
3. Goossens MM, Nelson RW, Feldman EC, et al. Response to insulin treatment and survival in 104 cats with diabetes mellitus (1985-1995). J Vet Intern Med 1998;12: 1–6.
4. Macy DW. Feline pancreatitis. In: Kirk RW, editor. Current veterinary therapy X. Small animal practice. Philadelphia: WB Saunders Co; 1989. p. 893–6.
5. Simpson KW, Shiroma J, Biller D, et al. Ante mortem diagnosis of pancreatitis in 4 cats. J Small Anim Pract 1994;35:93–9.
6. Steiner JM, Williams DA. Serum feline trypsin-like immunoreactivity in cats with exocrine pancreatic insufficiency. J Vet Intern Med 2000;14:627–9.
7. Thompson KA, Parnell NK, Hohenhaus AE, et al. Feline exocrine pancreatic insufficiency: 16 cases (1992-2007). J Feline Med Surg 2009;11:935–40.
8. Gerhardt A, Steiner JM, Williams DA. Comparison of the sensitivity of different diagnostic tests for pancreatitis in cats. J vet Intern Med 2001;15:329–33.
9. Saunders HM, Van Winkle TJ, Drobatz K, et al. Ultrasonographic findings in cats with clinical, gross pathologic, and histologic evidence of acute pancreatic necrosis: 20 cases (1994-2001). J Am Vet Med Assoc 2002;221:1724–30.
10. Ferreri JA, Hardam E, Kimmel SE, et al. Clinical differentiation of acute necrotizing from chronic nonsuppurative pancreatitis in cats: 63 cases (1996-2001). J Am Vet Med Assoc 2003;223:469–74.
11. Swift NC, Marks SL, MacLachlan NJ, et al. Evaluation of serum feline trypsin-like immunoreactivity for the diagnosis of pancreatitis in cats. J Am Vet Med Assoc 2000;217:37–42.
12. Johnston KL, Swift NC, Forsert-van-Hijfte M, et al. Comparison of the bacterial flora of the duodenum in healthy cats and cats with signs of gastrointestinal tract disease. J Am Vet Med Assoc 2001;218:48–51.
13. Westermarck E, Saario E. Traumatic pancreatic injury in a cat: a case history. Acta Vet Scand 1989;30:359–62.
14. Rothenbacher H, Lindquist WD. Liver cirrhosis and pancreatitis in a cat infected with Amphimerus Pseudofelineus. J Am Vet Med Assoc 1963;143:1099–102.
15. Montali RJ, Strandberg JD. Extreperiotoneal lesions in feline infectious peritonitis. Vet Pathol 1972;9:109–21.
16. Van Pelt CS, Crandell RA. Pancreatitis associated with a feline herpesvirus infection. Compan Anim Pract 1987;1:7–10.
17. Duncan RB, Lindsay R, Chickering, et al. Acute primary toxoplasmic pancreatitis in a cat. Feline Pract 2000;28:6–8.
18. Pedersen NC, Elliott JB, Glasgow A, et al. An isolated epizootic of hemorrhagic-like fever in cats caused by a novel and highly virulent strain of feline calicivirus. Vet Microbiol 2000;73:281–300.
19. Hurley KE, Pesavento PA, Pedersen NC, et al. An outbreak of virulent systemic feline calicivirus disease. J Am Vet Med Assoc 2004;224:241–9.

20. Widdison AL, Alvarez C, Chang YB, et al. Sources of pancreatic pathogens in acute pancreatitis in cats. Pancreas 1994;9:536–41.
21. Widdison AL, Karanija ND, Reber HA. Routes of spread of pathogens into the pancreas in a feline model of acute pancreatitis. Gut 1994;35:1306–10.
22. Lapointe JM, Higgins R, Barrette N, et al. Enterococcus hirae enteropathy with ascending cholangitis and pancreatitis in a kitten. Vet Pathol 2000;37:282–4.
23. Arendt T. Penetration of lanthanum through the main pancreatic duct epithelium in cats following exposure to infected human bile. Dig Dis Sci 1991;31:75–81.
24. Arendt T. Bile-induced acute pancreatitis in cats. Role of bile, bacteria and pancreatic duct pressure. Dig Dis Sci 1993;38:39–44.
25. Bailiff NL, Norris CR, Sequin B, et al. Pancreaticolithiasis and pancreatic pseudo-bladder associated with pancreatitis in a cat. J Am Anim Hosp Assoc 2004;40: 69–74.
26. Hill RC, Van Winkle TJ. Acute necrotizing pancreatitis and acute suppurative pancreatitis in the cat. A retrospective study of 40 cases (1976-1989). J Vet Intern Med 1993;7:25–33.
27. Wedgwood KR, Adler G, Kern H, et al. Effects of oral agents on pancreatic duct permeability. A model of acute alcoholic pancreatitis. Dig Dis Sci 1986;31: 1081–8.
28. Frick T, Spycher M, Kaiser A, et al. Electron microscopy of the exocrine pancreas in experimental acute hypercalcemia. Helv Chir Acta 1991;57:713–6 [in German].
29. Frick TW, Spycher MA, Heitz PU, et al. Hypercalcemia and pancreatic ultrastructure in cats. Eur J Surg 1992;158:289–94.
30. Mentes A, Batur Y, Bayol U. Salycylate-induced pancreatic injury in the cat: a preliminary study. Rom J Gastroenterol 2002;11:309–12.
31. Cates MC, Singh SM, Peick AL, et al. Acute hypercalcemia, pancreatic duct permeability, and pancreatitis in cats. Surgery 1988;104:137–41.
32. Bruskiewicz KA, Nelson RW, Feldman EC, et al. Diabetic ketosis and ketoacidosis in cats: 42 cases (1980-1995). J Am Vet Med Assoc 1997;211:188–92.
33. Forcada Y, German AJ, Noble PJ, et al. Determination of serum fPLI concentrations in cats with diabetes mellitus. J Feline Med Surg 2008;10:480–7.
34. Kimmel SE, Washabau RJ, Drobatz K. Incidence and prognostic value of low plasma ionised calcium concentration in cats with acute pancreatitis: 46 cases (1996-1998). J Am Vet Med Assoc 2001;219:1105–9.
35. Zhao P, Yang Z, Tang W. The role of amylase in abdominal fluid in evaluating severity of acute pancreatitis and its prognosis. Zhpngguo Yi Xue Ke Xue Yuan Xue Bao 1996;18:195–8 [in Chinese].
36. Forman MA, Marks SL, De Cock HE, et al. Evaluation of serum feline pancreatic lipase immunoreactivity and helical computed tomography versus conventional testing for the diagnosis of feline pancreatitis. J Vet Intern Med 2004;18:807–15.
37. Steiner JM, Wilson BG, Williams DA. Development and analytical validation of a radioimmunoassay for the measurement of feline pancreatic lipase immunoreactivity in serum. Can J Vet Res 2004;68:309–14.
38. Forman MA, Shiroma J, Armstrong PJ, et al. Evaluation of feline pancreas-specific lipase (SPEC fPLTM) for the diagnosis of feline pancreatitis. ACVIM [abstract: #165]. John Wiley and Sons, Inc 2009.
39. Wall M, Biller DS, Schoning P, et al. Pancreatitis in a cat demonstrating pancreatic duct dilatation ultrasonographically. J Am Anim Hosp Assoc 2001;37:49–53.
40. Moon Larson M, Panciera DL, Ward DL, et al. Age-related changes in the ultrasound appearance of the normal feline pancreas. Vet Radiol Ultrasound 2005; 46:238–42.

41. Hecht S, Henry G. Sonographic evaluation of the normal and abnormal pancreas. Clin Tech Small Anim Pract 2007;22:115–21.
42. Schweighauser AS, Gaschen F, Steiner J, et al. Evaluation of endosonography as a new diagnostic tool for feline pancreatitis. J Feline Med Surg 2009;11:492–8.
43. Ercan MT, Aras T, Aldahr AM, et al. Scintigraphic visualization of acute pancreatitis in cats with 99Tcm-citrate. Nucl Med Commun 1993;14:798–804.
44. Head LL, Daniel GB, Tobias K. Evaluation of the feline pancreas using computed tomography and radiolabeled leucocytes. Vet Radiol Ultrasound 2003;44:420–8.
45. Zoran DL. Pancreatitis in cats: diagnosis and management of a challenging disease. J Am Anim Hosp Assoc 2006;42:1–9.
46. Schmidt J, Fernandez-del Castillo C, Rattner DW, et al. Hyperoncotic ultrahigh molecular weight dextran solutions reduce trypsinogen activation, prevent acinar necrosis and lower mortality in rodent pancreatitis. Am J Surg 1993;165:40–5.
47. Baral RM. Diseases of the exocrine pancreas. In: Little SE, editor. The cat: clinical medicine and management. St Louis (MO): Elsevier Saunders; 2012. p. 513–22.
48. Frank G, Anderson W, Pazak H, et al. Use of a high-protein diet in the management of feline diabetes mellitus. Vet Ther 2001;2(3):238–46.
49. Mazzaferro E, Greco D, Turner A, et al. Treatment of feline diabetes mellitus using an alpha-glucosidase inhibitor and a low-carbohydrate diet. J Feline Med Surg 2003;5(3):183–90.
50. Bennett N, Greco D, Peterson M, et al. Comparison of a low carbohydrate-low fiber diet and a moderate carbohydrate-high fiber diet in the management of feline diabetes mellitus. J Feline Med Surg 2006;8(2):73–84.
51. Marshall RD, Rand JS, Morton JM. Glargine and protamine zinc insulin have a longer duration of action and result in lower mean daily glucose concentrations than lente insulin in healthy cats. J Vet Pharmacol Ther 2008;31:205–12.
52. Roomp K, Rand JS. Evaluation of detemir in diabetic cats managed with a protocol for intensive blood glucose control [abstract]. J Vet Intern Med 2009;23(3):697.
53. Roomp K, Rand J. Intensive blood glucose control is safe and effective in diabetic cats using home monitoring and treatment with glargine. J Feline Med Surg 2009;11:668–82.
54. Klaus JA, Rudloff E, Kirby R. Nasogastric tube feeding in cats with suspected acute pancreatitis: 55 cases (2001-2006). J Vet Emerg Crit Care 2009;19:337–46.
55. Jennings M, Center SA, Barr SC, et al. Successful treatment of feline pancreatitis using an endoscopically placed gastrojejunostomy tube. J Am Anim Hosp Assoc 2001;37:145–52.
56. Trepanier L. Idiopathic inflammatory bowel disease in cats. Rational treatment selection. J Feline Med Surg 2009;11:32–8.
57. Karanjia ND, Lutrin FJ, Chang YB, et al. Low dose dopamine protects against hemorrhagic pancreatitis in cats. J Surg Res 1990;48:440–3.
58. Karanjia ND, Widdison AL, Lutrin FJ, et al. The anti-inflammatory effect of dopamine in alcoholic hemorrhagic pancreatitis in cats. Studies on the receptors and mechanisms of action. Gastroenterology 1991;101:1635–41.
59. Karanjia ND, Widdison AL, Lutrin FJ, et al. The effect of dopamine in a model of biliary acute hemorrhagic pancreatitis. Pancreas 1991;6:392–7.
60. Karanjia ND, Widdison AL, Lutrin FJ, et al. Dopamine in models of alcoholic acute pancreatitis. Gut 1994;35:547–51.
61. Simpson KW, Fyfe J, Cornetta A, et al. Subnormal concentrations of serum cobalamin (vitamin B12) in cats with gastrointestinal disease. J Vet Intern Med 2001;15:26–32.

62. Salvadori C, Cantile C, De Ambrogli G, et al. Degenerative myelopathy associated with cobalamin deficiency in a cat. J Vet Med A Physiol Pathol Clin Med 2003;50:292–6.
63. Ruaux CG, Steiner JM, Williams DA. Early biochemical and clinical responses to cobalamin supplementation in cats with signs of gastrointestinal disease and severe hypocobalaminaemia. J Vet Intern Med 2005;19:155–60.
64. Bailey S, Benigni L, Eastwood J, et al. Comparisons between cats with normal and increased fPLI concentrations in cats diagnosed with inflammatory bowel disease. J Small Anim Pract 2010;51:484–9.
65. Whittemore JC, Campbell VL. Canine and feline pancreatitis. Compend Contin Educ Pract Vet 2005;27:766–76.
66. Xenoulis PG, Steiner JM. Current concepts in feline pancreatitis. Top Companion Anim Med 2008;23:185–92.
67. Zhao P, Tu J, Penninck F, et al. Early derivation operation can restore the pancreas histology and function in chronic obstructive pancreatitis in the cat. Hepatogastroenterology 1998;45:1849–54.
68. Patel AG, Reber PU, Toyama MT, et al. Effect of pancreaticojejunostomy on fibrosis, pancreatic blood flow and interstitial pH in chronic pancreatitis: a feline model. Ann Surg 1999;230:672–9.
69. Reber PU, Patel AG, Lewis MP, et al. Stenting does not decompress the pancreatic duct as effectively as surgery in experimental chronic pancreatitis. Surgery 1998;124:561–7.
70. Reber PU, Patel AG, Toyama MT, et al. Feline model of chronic obstructive pancreatitis: effects of acute pancreatic duct decompression on blood flow and interstitial pH. Scand J Gastroenterol 1999;34:439–44.

Hypersomatotropism, Acromegaly, and Hyperadrenocorticism and Feline Diabetes Mellitus

Stijn J.M. Niessen, DVM, PhD, PGCVetEd, FHEA, MRCVS[a,b,*],
David B. Church, BVSc, PhD, MACVSc, MRCVS[a],
Yaiza Forcada, DVM, MRCVS[a]

KEYWORDS

- Hypersomatotropism • Hyperadrenocorticism • Diabetes mellitus
- Other specific types of diabetes • Pituitary • Adrenal • Pancreas • Insulin resistance

KEY POINTS

- Diabetes mellitus in cats most commonly results from a primary disease process classified as type 2 diabetes, but in a proportion of cats, it is the consequence of another specific disease and classified as "other specific type of diabetes."
- Hypersomatotropism, which can result in acromegaly, usually results in diabetes classed as "other specific type of diabetes—subclass, endocrinopathies." It has been reported to be a primary cause of feline diabetes in up to one-third of insulin-treated diabetic cats presented for assessment of glycemic control in UK primary practices.
- Hyperadrenocorticism-induced diabetes is another example of "other specific type of diabetes" and although seemingly less common, when hyperadrenocorticism occurs, it will cause diabetes in 80% of cases.
- Recognition of these and other specific forms of diabetes, and specifically differentiation from type 2 diabetes, is crucial to enable election of the best possible treatment options and provision of the most accurate prognosis.
- Diagnosis of both feline hypersomatotropism and feline hyperadrenocorticism requires careful consideration of the clinical picture and usually a combination of diagnostic tests.
- Diabetic remission can be achieved when the diabetes is recognized to be a form of an "other specific type of diabetes" associated with insulin resistance, provided it is in an early phase and there is adequate treatment of the underlying etiology.

Funding Sources: The Royal Veterinary College.
Conflict of Interest: Nil.
[a] Department of Veterinary Clinical Sciences, The Royal Veterinary College, University of London, Hawkshead Lane, North Mymms AL9 7TA, Herts, UK; [b] Diabetes Research Group, Institute for Cellular Medicine, Medical School Newcastle, Framlington Place, Newcastle-upon-Tyne, Tyne and Wear NE2 4HH, UK
* Corresponding author. Department of Veterinary Clinical Sciences, Royal Veterinary College, University of London, Hawkshead Lane, North Mymms, Herts AL9 7TA, UK.
E-mail address: sniessen@rvc.ac.uk

INTRODUCTION

When confronted with a diabetic cat in clinical practice, it is tempting to assume we are dealing with a cat with a form of diabetes mellitus akin to human type 2 diabetes mellitus. Indeed, most feline cases will have a form of diabetes that occurs during middle or older age, which can be associated with obesity, inactivity, initial endogenous hyperinsulinemia (ultimately usually followed by endogenous hypoinsulinemia), and insulin resistance, as well as islet cell dysfunction and perhaps amyloid deposition[1,2] (see article by Dr Rand, elsewhere in this issue). Additionally, genetic research has provided further evidence toward a shared pathogenesis of feline diabetes and human type 2 diabetes.[3] Therefore, the immediate classification of these cats as having type 2 diabetes is often justified.

Management of diabetic cats can at times prove challenging,[4] however, and in many of these challenging cases, the etiopathogenesis of the diabetes is not type 2, but rather underlying disease processes better categorized as "other specific types of diabetes." Indeed, various other disorders outside the endocrine pancreas could play a crucial role in the etiology of the disease in a significant proportion of cases. Understanding and recognizing that a patient might not have type 2 diabetes will affect optimal management options and prognosis of the patient in question. This article, therefore, deals with other specific types of diabetes—subclass endocrinopathies in cats, and, more specifically, diabetes induced by excess growth hormone (ie, hypersomatotropism resulting in acromegaly) and cortisol (hyperadrenocorticism).

HYPERSOMATOTROPISM AND ACROMEGALY

Hypersomatotropism (HS) implies a state of production of excess growth hormone, whereas acromegaly is the name of the syndrome that results from that state of excess growth hormone production. Hypersomatotropism might therefore result in acromegaly, although all signs constituting the syndrome of acromegaly might not always be present with hypersomatotropism, especially early on in this slowly progressive disease process. A growth hormone–induced postreceptor defect in insulin action at the level of target tissues is thought to explain why most cats with acromegaly have concurrent diabetes mellitus.[5] The past 6 years have seen a renewed interest in the potential for excess growth hormone to induce and complicate diabetes in the cat. In fact, feline hypersomatotropism is now being recognized as an important cause of feline diabetes, largely as a result of 3 studies. All studies suggested that feline acromegaly occurs in a significant proportion of diabetic cats, especially those with insulin resistance. Estimates of prevalence in the diabetic cat population from 2 studies range from 1 in 3 to 1 in 4[5–7]; however, the method of sample recruitment could have influenced the results of these studies (for details please refer to section on hypersomatotropism prevalence that follows). Nevertheless, even when adhering to a more conservative estimate, this has quite clearly justified the initiation of several studies on various aspects of this endocrinopathy, including more careful evaluation of etiology, clinical presentation, and management aspects.

PREVALENCE OF HYPERSOMATOTROPISM

A screening study in which veterinarians in primary practice were offered free fructosamine measurements in diabetic cats, regardless of level of glycemic control, revealed that 59 (32%) of 184 diabetic cats had insulinlike growth factor-1 (IGF-1; see hypersomatotropism diagnostics section later in this article) concentrations strongly suggestive of acromegaly (>1000 ng/mL).[5] Of these 59 cats, a subpopulation was more closely evaluated with intracranial contrast-enhanced computed tomography (CT) and/or magnetic resonance imaging (MRI), as well as growth hormone (GH) concentration evaluation so as to conclusively establish the diagnosis of hypersomatotropism. The diagnosis was subsequently confirmed in 94% of these more carefully assessed cases, proving the original estimation of prevalence among these cats, made on the basis of raised IGF-1 concentrations only, to be likely close to the prevalence in a similarly selected population. Another study in the United States retrospectively assessed medical records of 74 diabetic cats with an IGF-1 concentration recorded, to determine the specificity and sensitivity of IGF-1 for diagnosis of acromegaly.[8] Of those classed as poorly controlled, 26% had IGF-1 levels consistent with a diagnosis of acromegaly; however, the selection criteria likely overestimated the prevalence among this diabetic cat population, as samples could have been preferentially evaluated for IGF-1 measurement, based on an existing suspicion of acromegaly. In a study of diabetic cats with insulin resistance and poor glycemic control (insulin dose >6 U/cat and mean blood glucose >300 mg/dL), all 16 cats had a pituitary mass on imaging and 12 (75%) were classed as acromegalic based on IGF-1 concentrations or suggestive signs together with normal adrenal function tests.[6] However, the argument of bias applies to a significantly lesser extent to the authors' prevalence studies,[5,7] in which prospectively IGF-1 was determined on serum submitted for fructosamine evaluation. A degree of bias may still persist also with this study type, because fructosamine evaluation might be opted for in light of suboptimal glycemic control, a phenomenon more frequently encountered with feline hypersomatotropism than with uncomplicated type 2 diabetes (the latter group might not even attend a veterinary practice on a regular basis or cease to do so in case of diabetic remission having been achieved). Nevertheless, it could equally be argued that the previously mentioned studies in fact also underestimate the true prevalence of acromegaly, as a rather arbitrary cutoff for IGF-1 was chosen (1000 ng/mL), misclassifying cases with a borderline IGF-1 or an IGF-1 that would have increased following initiation of exogenous insulin therapy (please refer to section on hypersomatotropism diagnostics). Additionally, a proportion of diabetic cats that prove difficult to control might be euthanized on the request of owners and therefore would not benefit from further assessments and inclusion in these screening studies.

In light of these surprising results, a more extensive evaluation of diabetic cats in the United Kingdom was undertaken by the authors' research group, using the same methodology as in the first study, which revealed similarly high prevalence numbers after 4 years of screening of diabetic cats. A total of 1222 diabetic cats had IGF-1 determined and 334 (26.4%) showed an IGF-1 concentration suggestive of hypersomatotropism.[7] All 3 studies highlight the difficulty of establishing unbiased prevalence figures. Nevertheless, the prevalence of hypersomatotropism seems sufficiently high to warrant its consideration when dealing with diabetic cats and particularly when problems with glycemic control arise. In light of the significant impact on prognosis and management, one could even argue that routine screening of diabetic cats for the presence of hypersomatotropism is beneficial, just as we screen for urinary tract infections in diabetics, presence or absence of an adrenal tumor in cases with clinical signs of hyperadrenocorticism, or underlying disease in cases with immune-mediated hemolytic anemia. Given the strong association with poorly controlled diabetes, prompt screening is definitely indicated if cats are not well controlled within 2 to 4 months of institution of therapy, or require a dose of 1.5 IU/kg or more. Early detection could have a beneficial impact on response to treatment, especially if beta cell mass is preserved and remission, therefore, a possibility. If screening is applied, however, the characteristics and dynamics of serum total IGF-1 as a screening tool should be taken into account (please refer to section on hypersomatotropism diagnostics).

ETIOLOGY OF HYPERSOMATOTROPISM

Traditionally, hypersomatotropism or acromegaly in the cat has been seen as a process caused by excess endogenous growth hormone secretion caused by a pituitary adenoma. A more systematic evaluation of pituitary histopathology in a larger number of patients is currently ongoing and suggests that, alongside a vast majority with indeed an acidophilic adenoma, some cases instead display acidophilic hyper-plasia.[5,9] If there are indeed at least 2 underlying etiologic mechanisms, questions arise over a possible interrelationship between them (eg, initial hyperplasia leading to adenomatous change or presence of a suprahypophyseal process or stimulus).[4,5,9,10] In this respect, a comparison to current hypotheses on the etiology of feline hyperthy-roidism can be made.

When hypersomatotropism is present, GH hypersecretion results in excess produc-tion of IGF-1. The combination of excess circulating GH and IGF-1 will eventually result in the clinical syndrome of acromegaly, which is directly related to the physio-logic function of these hormones (**Fig. 1**).

SIGNALMENT AND PRESENTATION OF HYPERSOMATOTROPISM

The basic characteristics of recently reported cats are shown in **Table 1**. Presence of insulin resistant diabetes mellitus has been shown to be a risk factor for presence of hypersomatotropism. Nevertheless, when using a screening approach among dia-betic cats, a significant number of detected patients will appear insulin sensitive at

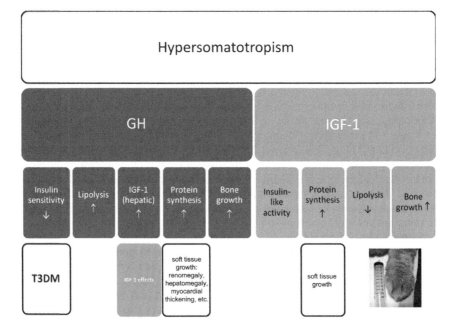

Fig. 1. Overview of pathophysiology of hypersomatotropism. GH, growth hormone; IGF-1, insulin like growth factor 1; T3DM, other specific type of diabetes/type 3 diabetes.

Table 1
Basic characteristics of cats with hypersomatotropism and cats with hyperadrenocorticism

	Hypersomatotropism	Hyperadrenocorticism
Median age, y (range)	11 (4–19)	10 (5–16)
Gender	Male bias	No convincing bias
Breed	Domestic short hair bias	Domestic short hair bias
Weight	Often weight gain (median 5.8 kg, range 3.5–9.2)	Often weight loss
Insulin requirements	Insulin resistance frequent, and ultimately often extreme (median 7 IU twice a day, range 1–35)	Insulin resistance frequent, yet not always and not usually extreme

time of the initial diagnosis. Interestingly, data acquired using that same screening approach suggest that the "typical" acromegalic phenotype is not consistently present, possibly related to the gradual onset of hypersomatotropism-induced changes and/or previous failure to screen assumed "atypical" cases. Interestingly, only 24% of clinicians suspected the presence of hypersomatotropism in diabetic cats found to have an IGF-1 greater than 1000 ng/mL (strongly suggesting the presence of hypersomatotropism), indicating the likely presence of a subtle phenotype in 76% of these cases.[7] Once again it seems tempting to draw comparisons to the feline hyperthyroidism situation, in which we currently more rarely see the classical hyperthyroid cat, possibly owing to increased preparedness to screen for this disease in the elderly cat and/or possible increasing prevalence.[10]

Commonly encountered signs in the acromegalic cats seen are shown in **Table 2** and **Figs. 2–4**.[4,5,9] Weight gain despite poor glycemic control should alert clinicians for the possible presence of hypersomatotropism, because weight loss would normally be expected. The existence of individual nondiabetic acromegalic cases has been mentioned in textbooks,[11] although the true prevalence of such cases is currently unknown.

Cardiomyopathies and nephropathies have been reported to ensue as part of the pathophysiology of acromegaly, presumably being induced by excess GH and IGF-1 concentrations. Because relatively few cases of feline acromegaly have been

Table 2
Commonly encountered clinical signs in feline hypersomatotropism

Clinical Sign	Timing
Polyuria/polydipsia	Early + late stages
Polyphagia (possibly extreme)	Early + late stages
Weight gain	Early + late stages
Enlarged kidneys	Early + late stages
Enlarged liver	Early + late stages
Prognathia inferior (see **Fig. 2**)	Usually only in later stages
Broad facial features (see **Fig. 3**)	Usually only in later stages
Systolic cardiac murmur	Early + late stages
Respiratory stridor (usually in later stages)	Usually only in later stages
Plantegrade stance (reversible with improved glycemic control)	Early + late stages

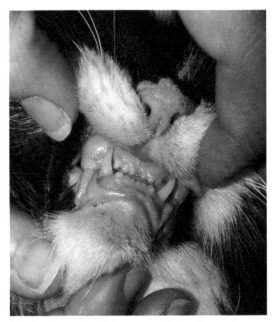

Fig. 2. Prognathia inferior in a cat with hypersomatotropism and acromegaly.

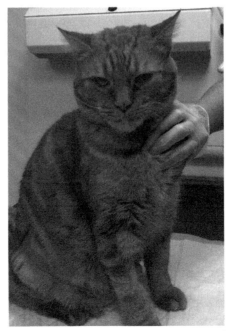

Fig. 3. An acromegalic cat showing an overall big stature, broad facial features, clubbed paws, and prognathia inferior.

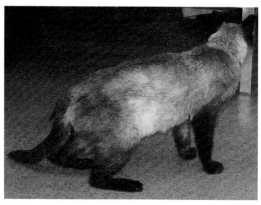

Fig. 4. A plantegrade stance as a consequence of suboptimal glycemic control in a cat with hypersomatotropism-induced diabetes mellitus.

described thus far and most previous cases seem to have an advanced stage of hypersomatotropism-induced acromegaly, however, this assumption warrants further investigation, especially, in view of the high prevalence of concurrent disease, including cardiomyopathies and nephropathies among nonacromegalic diabetic and nondiabetic geriatric cats in general. A recent comparison of routine clinical pathology parameters between acromegalic diabetic cats and nonacromegalic diabetic cats did not reveal a greater incidence of azotemia among acromegalic cats.[12] Pancreatic abnormalities, specifically hyperplasia, do seem particularly prevalent in acromegalic cats based on post mortem examinations of patients seen in the authors' acromegalic cat clinic (**Fig. 5**).[4,10] The overall message should probably be that clinicians ought to remain open minded about the signalment and presentation of the acromegalic cat in this age of rediscovery of this endocrinopathy.

DIAGNOSIS OF HYPERSOMATOTROPISM
Routine Clinical Pathology

Routine clinical pathology will not be decisive in the diagnostic process, although can appraise the clinician of presence of any comorbidities or deleterious consequences of the hypersomatotropism. Diabetes mellitus–induced changes, including hyperglycemia, glycosuria, high cholesterol, and elevation of hepatic enzymes, can be found in hypersomatotropism, although do not help differentiate diabetes secondary to

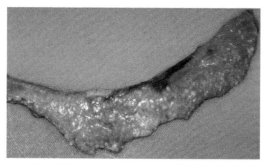

Fig. 5. Nodular hyperplasia of the pancreas in a cat with hypersomatotropism.

hypersomatotropism from type 2 diabetes. A recent comparison study of biochemistry findings in either group, did find significantly higher total protein concentrations in acromegalic diabetic cats, which fits with the bias toward protein synthesis in hypersomatotropism. Influence of dehydration, however, quite common in diabetic animals, causes significant overlap in protein levels between the 2 groups, prohibiting its use as a discriminatory test.[12] Azotemia was previously found in 2 reports[13,14] and was suggested to be related to a GH-induced and/or IGF-1–induced nephropathy, diabetes, and/or hypertension. Interestingly, neither azotemia nor hypertension is commonly seen in the authors' clinic.[5,12] In terms of hematology findings, a nonsignificant trend toward higher hematocrit values was also apparent.[12]

Endocrine Testing: Which Test is Best for Screening?

An overview of the thus far assessed screening tests is shown in **Table 3**. Feline growth hormone (fGH; serum and plasma) and IGF-1 (serum) have been shown to be useful screening tests. A suggested growth hormone cutoff value of 10 ng/mL was shown to result in an acceptable specificity of 95% and sensitivity of 84% when using the fGH assay recently developed by the authors.[9] Feline GH also appeared relatively stable, allowing overnight transport of unseparated samples[9]; however, fGH determination is currently not commercially available. Additionally, both fGH and IGF-1 were shown to yield false-positive results in a minority of cases.[5] Cases of hypersomatotropism with a normal basal fGH concentration have yet to be documented, yet IGF-1 has been documented to be falsely negative in a minority of cases.[4,10,14] The duration of exogenous insulin administration could play an essential role in the latter, because hepatic IGF-1-production is induced via stimulation of insulin-dependent hepatic GH-receptors. An insulin-deficient state can act as an inhibitor of such IGF-1 production, resulting in low IGF-1 concentrations in diabetic patients before institution of exogenous insulin treatment or even during the first few weeks of such treatment. When screening for presence of acromegaly, these specific IGF-1 dynamics should be taken into account and repeat IGF-1 determination should be considered 6 to 8 weeks into the treatment. Alternatively, if one wishes to determine IGF-1 only once, the latter time point is recommended over the immediate time of diagnosis of diabetes mellitus. When a diabetic cat has a mild elevation of IGF-1, yet not in the acromegalic range, the clinician is faced with a dilemma. This mild elevation can be seen in uncomplicated diabetes as well as in genuine hypersomatotropism. A repeat measurement 1 or 2 months later could be considered in such cases; however, if the cat already has evidence of insulin resistance (requiring >1.5–2.0 units per kg per injection on a twice-a-day regimen), values in this grey-zone result, probably justify proceeding immediately with further hypersomatotropism diagnostics, including intracranial imaging.

Given the potential for both false positives and false negatives with either GH or IGF-1 assessment and the need for confirmatory intracranial imaging, research is currently ongoing to evaluate alternative biomarkers for feline hypersomatotropism. Because hypersomatotropism is associated with tissue growth, serum type III procollagen propeptide (PIIIP), a peripheral indicator of collagen turnover, has recently been shown to be elevated in cats with hypersomatotropism. A PIIIP concentration greater than 8 ng/mL was shown to be 100% specific for a diagnosis of hypersomatotropism, with a sensitivity of 75%.[15] Serum ghrelin, an endogenous ligand of the GH secretagogue receptor and therefore susceptible to negative feedback in a state of hypersomatotropism, has thus far not been found useful in differentiating diabetes from hypersomatotropism-induced diabetes, despite such suggestions in human hypersomatotropism.[16] The glucose suppression test (measuring GH before and after

Table 3
Overview and characteristics of endocrine screening tests for feline hypersomatotropism

Screening Test	Protocol	Interpretation	Sensitivity	Specificity
IGF-1	1. Baseline serum sample 2. Alternatively: sample after 8 wk of insulin therapy OR 2 samples: 1 before insulin therapy and 1 after 8 wk of insulin therapy	>1000 ng/mL: HS suspected, pituitary imaging indicated <1000 ng/mL, BUT insulin therapy only recently started/yet to start: repeat test in 8 wk time	☆☆☆☆	☆☆
fGH	1. Baseline serum sample fasted, morning and before receiving insulin that day	<10 ng/mL: HS unlikely >10 ng/mL: HS possible, IGF-1 and/or pituitary imaging indicated	☆☆☆☆	☆☆
IGF-1/fGH combination	1. As per above	As per above, with added specificity	☆☆☆☆	☆☆☆
PIIIP	1. Random serum sample	Only limited data available; >8 ng/mL HS likely, additional fGH, IGF-1 and/or pituitary imaging indicated	☆☆☆	☆☆☆
Glucose suppression test	1. Baseline serum fGH sample, fasted, morning and before receiving insulin that day 2. Inject intravenously 1 g/kg glucose (diluted 1:1 with sterile water) 3. Serum fGH at 30 min, 60 min, and 90 min	Only limited data available; use currently not supported	—	—
Feline ghrelin	1. Baseline fasted, morning and before receiving insulin that day	Only limited data available; use currently not supported	—	—

Abbreviations: The star rating indicates the degree of sensitivity or specificity with: ☆, indicating very poor sensitivity or specificity; ☆☆☆☆, indicating very good sensitivity or specificity; —, not sufficient data available; fGH, feline growth hormone; HS, hypersomatotropism; IGF-1, insulinlike growth factor 1; PIIIP, type III procollagen propeptide.

administration of glucose) is a gold standard test in the diagnosis of human hyperso-matotropism, although little evidence in favor of its use in feline hypersomatotropism has as yet been published.[14,17-19]

THE ROLE OF IMAGING IN HYPERSOMATOTROPISM

Intracranial imaging (with contrast enhancement) has been proven useful in confirming the presence of hypersomatotropism, with MRI probably more sensitive than CT.[5,9,11,13,14,20] Cases with a negative CT and/or MRI have been documented, however, with the diagnosis eventually being confirmed on post mortem examination.[5] Nevertheless, if a structural pituitary abnormality is documented, this indeed provides further circumstantial evidence for the presence of hypersomatotropism, especially if there are concurrent increases in frontal bone thickness and/or evidence of soft tissue accumulation in the nasal cavity, sinuses, and pharynx.[21] However, the demonstration of a pituitary tumor as such does not provide differentiation from a nonfunctional pitu-itary tumor or pituitary dependent hyperadrenocorticism (PDH), especially because pituitary tumors are a relatively common type of brain tumor in the cat.[22] Additionally, cases with subtle (microscopic) acidophilic hyperplasia or microadenoma, instead of obvious (macroscopic) adenoma, might more likely show negative intracranial imaging. Dynamic intracranial imaging studies using timed injection of contrast might be of aid here.

The potential for false-negative results for intracranial imaging raises the question of the appropriate course of action when a negative image result is obtained despite the presence of a documented hormonal imbalance (elevated fGH, IGF-1, presence of diabetes). When imaging is negative, it seems more logical to have the ultimate pre-mortem diagnosis of hypersomatotropism (and subsequent treatment decisions) rely on hormonal assessment. In conclusion, pituitary imaging is too expensive and too invasive (sedation or anesthesia needed) to be considered suitable as a *screening* test, and is ideally used as an attempt *to confirm* the disease or for preradiation or pre-surgical planning. Refinement of our hormonal assessment methods and increasing availability of assays probably constitutes the best way to improve the diagnosis of hypersomatotropism.

TREATMENT OPTIONS FOR HYPERSOMATOTROPISM

Treatment options for hypersomatotropism consist of medical treatment, surgical options, radiotherapy, or palliative treatment. When definitive treatment is instituted, clinicians and owners need to be vigilant for rapid changes in insulin demands should the treatment prove effective. Iatrogenic hypoglycemia is frequently encountered and home blood glucose measurement or, at least, home urine glucose screening should be considered.

Medical Treatment

In contrast to the situation in human hypersomatotropism, medical treatment options aimed at inhibiting the pituitary have not proven very successful in the cat thus far, including the use of somatostatin analogues lanreotide (Ipsen, Paris, France) and sandostatin (Novartis, Basel, Switzerland) (long-acting synthetic somatostatin analogues).[4,10,23,24] The use of dopamine agonists has not resulted in convincing im-provement, yet carries the risk of a range of side effects.[4,24] One study showed that intravenous octreotide alters serum GH levels in a subset of acromegalic cats, sug-gesting that, at least in such subset, medical pituitary inhibition could prove beneficial.[25]

Most recently, hope for effective medical management of feline hypersomatotropism has arisen in a phase 2 clinical trial conducted by the authors using a novel somatostatin analogue (Pasireotide, Novartis), which has yielded undisputable evidence of reduction of insulin requirements in all 8 participating patients with feline hypersomatotropism, as well as diabetic remission in one of them (Stijn Niessen, DVM, PhD, DipECVIM, personal communication, 2012). The effectiveness of this drug suggests that the feline acidophilic adenoma does display somatostatin receptors, contrary to previous beliefs. Receptor mutations or predominance of certain receptor subtypes not targeted by previous somatostatin trials might form the explanation of why those previous trials proved unsuccessful.

Surgery

Hypophysectomy is considered the treatment of choice in human hypersomatotropism. After decades of this procedure being available only in the Netherlands, transphenoidal hypophysectomy has in recent years become available also in the United Kingdom (London), United States (California), and Japan. Analog to the situation in human medicine, success rates are strongly correlated with the experience of the surgeon, as well as the availability of high-quality intensive postoperative care.

The surgical approach is with the patient in a sternal position, through the cat's open mouth and a soft palatial incision to subsequently expose the sphenoid bone through the mucoperiosteum. A small drill ensures exposure of the dura mater surrounding the pituitary fossa (**Fig. 6**).[26] Perioperatively and postoperatively, desmopressin, thyroxine, and glucocorticoid supplementation should be initiated to ensure a smooth recovery of the patient. In the authors' clinic, a constant rate intravenous insulin infusion ensures reasonable glycemia preoperatively, perioperatively, and postoperatively until the patient is eating again, after which traditional insulin protocols are applied. Glucose concentrations must be very closely monitored, however, because severe clinical hypoglycemia can ensue in patients as soon as the first week after surgery. In addition, perioperatively and immediately postoperatively, an intravenous

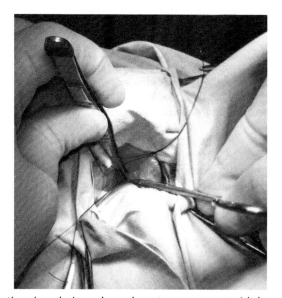

Fig. 6. Intraoperative view during a hypophysectomy on a cat with hypersomatotropism. The soft palatial incision is being closed after removal of the cat's pituitary.

hydrocortisone constant rate infusion ensures glucocorticoid provision until the patient starts eating again, after which prednisolone (0.1 mg/kg/d) or hydrocortisone (0.5 mg/kg/d is started). The induced diabetes insipidus seems only temporary in nature in most patients, whereas secondary hypocortisolism and secondary hypothyroidism require lifelong supplementation.[26]

A recent report described the successful application of hypophysectomy in an acromegalic cat, resulting in an immediate drop of GH levels after surgery, as well as resolution of the diabetes mellitus within 3 weeks.[26] Subsequently, 5 more cases were published all showing diabetic remission rates within 4 weeks after surgery.[27] In the authors' clinic, diabetic remission has been noted as soon as 1 week after surgery. This further substantiates that early diagnosis and subsequent immediate and effective intervention increases the chance for complete diabetic remission hugely, given that sufficient beta-cell function will still be present in many of these cases. Finally, cryohypophysectomy has been reported to be successful in 2 cases.[28]

Radiation Therapy

Radiation therapy is currently still the most widely applied definitive treatment modality for feline hypersomatotropism. Indeed, it is able to reduce the size of the adenoma as well as reduce the excess hormone secretion to a certain degree in a high proportion of cases.[29,30] Evaluation of more refined protocols and "gamma-knife" technology are currently ongoing and might improve results further. Nevertheless, several important less desirable characteristics are associated with this modality: high costs, need for multiple anesthetics, and, most importantly, the response is variable and unpredictable. Some patients will start showing a treatment effect during the radiation course, others will not have a response until a year after treatment. The duration of effect is also variable. In 13 of 14 diabetic cats with hypersomatotropism receiving radiotherapy in 10 fractions, 3 times a week to a total dose of 3700 cGy (representative of many commonly used protocols), diabetic control improved, although diabetic remission occurred in only 6 cats, 3 of whom relapsed 3, 17, and 24 months after treatment.[30] Finally, radiation does not usually normalize GH and IGF-1 concentrations,[9,30] in contrast to hypophysectomy.[26,27]

Palliative Treatment

A more conservative approach ignores the underlying disease mechanism and focuses on gaining more control of the diabetes mellitus and treating possible comorbidities. Eventually most cats tend to need high dosages of insulin and/or combinations of short-acting and long-acting insulin types to ensure an adequate quality of life for both pet and owner. Nevertheless, this approach can result in an adequate level of diabetic control in a minority of cases, although careful and continued assessment of quality of life is indicated, possibly aided by quantitative tools.[31] Home monitoring of blood glucose concentrations can prove very useful to optimize dose. This is particularly relevant, as GH is secreted in a pulsatile fashion, also in case of an acidophilic adenoma, leading to variable insulin resistance and therefore variable insulin requirements. Home monitoring can prevent insulin overdose and clinical hypoglycemia at particular times of lower growth hormone concentrations. A low-carbohydrate canned diet would be advocated, as is the case in regular diabetic felines.

HYPERADRENOCORTICISM

Hyperadrenocorticism (HAC) indicates a state of excess glucocorticoid activity and can be caused by excess administration of drugs with glucocorticoid activity or increased endogenous glucocorticoid activity (**Fig. 7**). Excess glucocorticoid activity can also result in diabetes and therefore represents another possible form of "other specific type of diabetes." Glucocorticoids are able to induce diabetes through a variety of mechanisms, including impairment of insulin-dependent glucose uptake in the periphery and enhanced gluconeogenesis in the liver.[32–36] In addition, glucocorticoids oppose several other actions of insulin, including its central inhibitory effect on appetite.[32] Finally, steroid-induced inhibition of insulin secretion of pancreatic beta-cells has also been shown to occur.[37,38]

PREVALENCE OF HYPERADRENOCORTICISM

Noniatrogenic or spontaneous hyperadrenocorticism, with or without subsequently induced diabetes, seems to be a rare condition in cats with approximately 100 cases reported in veterinary literature.[39–55] However, it is currently still unknown what proportion of the diabetic cat population, especially poorly controlled diabetic cats, has this form of diabetes induced by hyperadrenocorticism. Unfortunately, any screening studies are hampered by the lack of a specific and easily performed confirmatory test for this endocrinopathy, although a rough estimate of the likely *maximum* prevalence could be achieved by assessing urine cortisol:creatinine ratios (UCCRs) in morning urine samples collected at home from diabetic cats (see diagnostics). However, the true prevalence would be significantly lower than estimates using UCCRs, given the known lack of specificity of this test in animals with concurrent disease (ie, poorly controlled diabetes).

Iatrogenic feline hyperadrenocorticism is also rare and certainly less common than iatrogenic hyperadrenocorticism in dogs. Interestingly, 7.5% of diabetic cats included in a study concerning insured diabetic cats in the United Kingdom, had a confirmed history of glucocorticoid administration indirectly implicating glucocorticoids in the

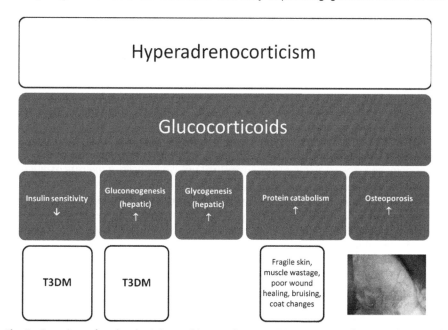

Fig. 7. Overview of pathophysiology of hyperadrenocorticism. T3DM, other specific type of diabetes/type 3 diabetes.

etiology of their diabetes (assumed type 2).[1] In another study, 4 of 12 cats on long-term steroids developed diabetes and subsequently achieved remission in a mean of 4.9 months after cessation of steroids and treatment with insulin.[56] Recent cortico-steroid administration before onset of diabetes in cats has been shown to be associated with increased probability of diabetic remission.[57] In human patients, diabetes induced by iatrogenic steroid administration generally occurs in individuals with pre-existing defects in insulin secretion, and hyperglycemia typically resolves when the hormone excess is resolved.[58] The increased probability of remission raises the question of whether cats that develop diabetes following chronic steroid use represent an "other specific type of diabetes," or the steroid use just precipitated signs of diabetes when there were preexisting defects in insulin secretion, for example associated with the pathogenesis of type 2 diabetes. The fact that many cats in remission subsequently relapse provides a more convincing argument that these cats have other underlying defects in insulin secretion and their diabetes is not solely attributable to steroids. In line with the classification system used for humans, cats developing diabetes while on steroids and achieving remission with cessation of steroids and insulin treatment, should be classed as "other specific type of diabetes — subclass endocrinopathy." They should be reclassified as "type 2 diabetes," however, if they later relapse in the absence of steroids or other identifiable disease processes associated with "other specific types of diabetes."

ETIOLOGY OF HYPERADRENOCORTICISM

Just like canine hyperadrenocorticism, spontaneous feline hyperadrenocorticism is caused by either a functional pituitary tumor (PDH) oversecreting adrenocorticotropic hormone (ACTH) or a functional tumor of the adrenal cortex oversecreting hormones with glucocorticoid activity. PDH is the most prevalent form (75%–80% of cases) and is usually caused by an adenoma of the pars intermedia or pars distalis of the pituitary gland. Rare pituitary carcinomas have been described. The remaining 20% to 25% of cases have adrenal-dependent hyperadrenocorticism (ADH). Of the latter group, a benign functional adenoma of the cortex of one of the adrenals is most likely (65%) with a malignant cortical carcinoma affecting a minority of cats with ADH.[39,41,55]

Variations of these etiologies have also been described in individual cases. These include unilateral and bilateral cortical carcinomas producing excess sex hormones with glucocorticoid effects (eg, progesterone, androstenedione, testosterone), a case of a diabetic cat with assumed ACTH-independent cortisol production caused by excess alpha-MSH production by a pituitary tumor exerting glucocorticoticotropic effects, and a double pituitary adenoma overproducing both GH and ACTH causing acromegaly and hyperadrenocorticism.[39–49] Finally, rare cases of multiple-endocrine neoplasia have been described to include hyperadrenocorticism.[43,51]

Although cats are more resistant to the effects of steroids, iatrogenic hyperadrenocorticism should be considered in any cat that becomes diabetic while receiving glucocorticoid supplementation. Such supplementation could include topical preparations for dermatologic (including ear disease) or ophthalmic disease. Nevertheless, an underlying predisposition for type 2 diabetes should be suspected in cats with onset of diabetes after exogenous steroid administration, which subsequently proves permanent despite quick withdrawal of these exogenous glucocorticoids, or in cats that achieve remission but subsequently relapse in the absence of steroids.

The excess of exogenous or endogenous glucocorticoid activity will usually result in a range of changes in the cat's body, all related to the physiologic function of glucocorticoids (see **Fig. 7**). Marked insulin resistance can therefore ensue and it is unsurprising that 80% to 90% of cases with hyperadrenocorticism are presented with signs referable to overt diabetes.[39–41,55,59]

SIGNALMENT AND PRESENTATION OF HYPERADRENOCORTICISM

A comparison of basic characteristics between hypersomatotropism and hyperadrenocorticism is shown in **Table 1**. Frequent physical examination findings are shown in **Box 1**.[39–55] Like with hypersomatotropism, most cats with hyperadrenocorticism will present with signs referable to diabetes (polyuria, polydipsia, polyphagia and peripheral neuropathy), which, as time goes on, often turns out to be insulin resistant in nature. Nevertheless, the insulin requirements tend to be less extreme than those found in some cats with hypersomatotropism and indeed not all diabetic cats with hyperadrenocorticism are in fact insulin-resistant. Interestingly, weight loss, instead of weight gain, is most common with hyperadrenocorticism. This therefore represents a significant difference compared with the dog and a useful difference in differentiating from the diabetic cat with hypersomatotropism (**Table 4**).

A minority of cats with hyperadrenocorticism will present differently and focus might lie instead on dermatologic abnormalities, such as skin fragility or polyphagia and weight gain, instead of diabetes-related clinical signs. The perceived lack of polyuria and polydipsia in the latter cases without overt diabetes illustrates the inherent resistance cats have (compared with dogs) to the glucocorticoid-induced inhibition of secretion and action of antidiuretic hormone.[39] Polyuria and polydipsia tends to ensue only once diabetes has arisen.

Specific signs that cats share with their canine counterparts include abdominal enlargement or pot-bellied appearance (**Fig. 8**), panting, muscle atrophy, unkempt hair coat (**Fig. 9**), bilateral symmetric alopecia, and predisposition for infections (urinary tract, skin, abscesses, respiratory tract, toxoplasmosis).[39,44,55] More specific to the cat is the so-called "fragile skin syndrome" (**Figs. 10** and **11**), which is thought to relate to the protein catabolism and can result in tearing of the skin under otherwise innocuous circumstances, such as self-grooming or owners grasping their cat. Also

---

Box 1
Reported physical examination findings in hyperadrenocorticism

Pot belly (see **Fig. 8**)

Unkempt coat (see **Fig. 9**)

Muscle wastage

Bilateral symmetric hair thinning, seborrhea, or alopecia

Thin skin (see **Figs. 8** and **10**)

Change in coat color (see **Fig. 11**)

Ecchymoses (see **Fig. 10**)

Inappropriate body condition score

Cutaneous lacerations or fragile skin (see **Fig. 11**)

Obesity/weight gain (less frequent)

Hepatomegaly

Signs of (recurrent) infection (including abscess)

Plantegrade stance (see **Fig. 9**)

Table 4
Clues toward the differentiation between the diabetic cat with HS and the diabetic cat with HAC

HS	HAC
Frequent weight gain	Frequent weight loss
Lack of dermatologic signs apart from possible unkempt coat	Frequent dermatologic signs
Lack of muscle wasting	Frequent muscle wasting
Ultimately severe or extreme insulin resistance	Lack of insulin resistance, or, more frequent, modest insulin resistance
Infrequent generalized poor condition	Frequent generalized poor condition
Absence of diabetes very rare	Absence of diabetes possible
IGF-1 elevated	IGF-1 usually not elevated

Abbreviations: HAC, hyperadrenocorticism; HS, hypersomatotropism; IGF-1, insulinlike growth factor 1.

in contrast to the dog, cats with hyperadrenocorticism have not been reported to develop calcinosis cutis. Cats can, however, develop hair coat color changes (see **Fig. 11**).

Finally, rare cases in which cats presented with blindness (caused by a pituitary macroadenoma or hypertension induced),[54] abnormal behavior, compulsive walking, circling, and continuous vocalization have also been reported.[44,45] Virilization has been encountered in cases with sex hormone–secreting (androstenedione and testosterone) adrenal carcinomas, which might be picked up by observing spines on the penis of a castrated male cat.

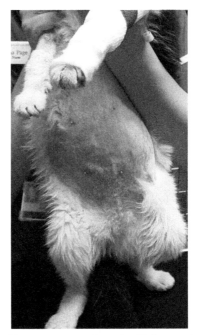

Fig. 8. Pot belly and thin skin appearance of a cat with hyperadrenocorticism.

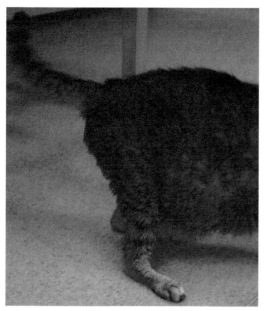

Fig. 9. Unkempt hair coat and plantegrade stance in a cat with hyperadrenocorticism.

DIAGNOSIS OF HYPERADRENOCORTICISM
Routine Clinical Pathology

In most cases, changes in hematology, biochemistry, and urine analyses are attributable to diabetes. A stress leukogram is inconsistently present, although elevation of neutrophils might also be related to a secondary infection evoked by decreased

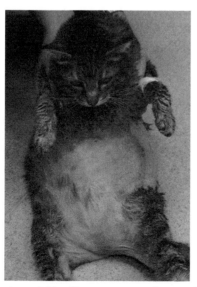

Fig. 10. Pot belly, ecchymosis, and thin skin appearance of a cat with hyperadrenocorticism.

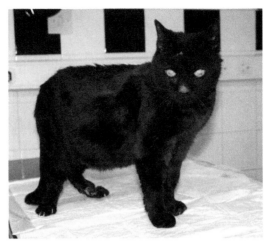

Fig. 11. Coat color changes induced by hypercortisolemia caused by PDH, as well as evidence of fragile skin syndrome on the left hind paw.

immunity or bacterial infection of skin wounds. Given the lack of a steroid-inducible ALP isoenzyme and therefore in contrast to the situation in the dog, less than one-fifth of cats with hyperadrenocorticism will show elevation of alkaline phosphatase (ALP). If found, it will be related to the unregulated diabetes. Another interesting difference with canine hyperadrenocorticism is the relative rareness of finding dilute urine in cats with hyperadrenocorticism, demonstrating the lack of effect of cortisol on feline ADH secretion and/or sensitivity. Only 1 of 43 cats reported in a hyperadrenocorticism case series had a urine specific gravity of less than 1.043,[39] although this parameter will also be partially affected by the presence of glucosuria in many cases. Proteinuria can also be encountered.

Endocrine Testing: Which Test is Best for Screening?

Endocrine tests that may be useful in substantiating a diagnosis of feline hyperadrenocorticism include the low-dose dexamethasone suppression test (LDDST), the ACTH stimulation test, and the UCCR. The latter can be combined with the administration of oral dexamethasone. The advantages and disadvantages of each screening test are discussed in the following sections. The protocols and interpretation of each test are described in **Table 5**, as well as an indication of each test's characteristics in terms of sensitivity and specificity. As is the case with almost any endocrine test, as well as any diagnostic test in general which is not 100% accurate, these diagnostics will demonstrate a superior positive predictive value only when used when the clinical picture sufficiently suggests the possible presence of hyperadrenocorticism. Conversely, also given the low prevalence of feline hyperadrenocorticism in general, routine screening in clinically unremarkable diabetic cats is therefore not advocated.

The LDDST

Many consider the LDDST the test of choice for diagnosis of feline hyperadrenocorticism. Clinicians should note that a higher dose of dexamethasone (0.1 mg/kg intravenously) is used than in the dog, because a high proportion of normal cats will not show suppression when using the traditional lower dose (0.01 mg/kg).[39,59,60] Intramuscular

Table 5
Overview and characteristics of endocrine screening tests for feline hyperadrenocorticism

Screening Test	Protocol	Interpretation	Sensitivity	Specificity
LDDST	1. Baseline serum cortisol (t = 0) 2. Intravenous 0.1 mg/kg dexamethasone (or intramuscular) 3. Serum cortisol t = 4 and 8 h	No suppression at t = 4 and/or 8 h (cortisol <35 nmol/or 1.3 µg/dL): HAC possible	★★★★★	★★
ACTH stim	1. Baseline serum cortisol (t = 0) 2. Intravenous 125 µg synthetic ACTH (or intramuscular) 3. Timings post-ACTH sample serum cortisol t = 60 min (recommendations vary according to source, please consult your local laboratory, some suggest adding time points t = 30, 90 min, or even 120 min, the latter particularly when using compounded ACTH)	Post-ACTH cortisol > upper end reference interval: HAC possible Modest, suppressed/flatline response (lack of stimulation): iatrogenic HAC possible as well as sex hormone–secreting ADH (consider requesting additional adrenal hormones)	★	★★★★
UCCR	1. Home-collected morning sample 2. Kept in fridge until analysis 3. Ideally multiple samples	$\geq 3.6 \times 10^{-5}$ suggestive of HAC $\leq 1.3 \times 10^{-5}$ unlikely cortisol producing HAC	★★★★★	★
UCCR with oral dexamethasone suppression (as screening test)	1. Two at-home collected morning samples for UCCR: calculate average 2. Owner administers 0.5 mg dexamethasone orally at 12 PM, 6 PM, and 12 midnight 3. Next morning: home-collected morning sample for UCCR	Average of 2 initial samples $\geq 3.6 \times 10^{-5}$ suggestive of HAC $\leq 50\%$ suppression UCCR 3rd sample: seen with most ADH cases and 25% of PDH cases	★★★★	★★
POMC (please note: data based on 1 small study only)	1. Basal EDTA blood sample 2. Immediate centrifugation at 4°C 3. Plasma transferred to plastic tubes and stored at -80°C until analysis/transported on dry ice	High plasma concentration of ACTH precursors in cats (>100 pmol/L) is highly suggestive of PDH	★★★★	★★★★

Abbreviations: The star rating indicates the degree of sensitivity or specificity with: ☆, indicating very poor sensitivity or specificity; ☆☆☆☆☆, indicating very good sensitivity or specificity; ACTH, adrenocorticotrophic hormone; ACTH stim, ACTH stimulation test; ADH, adrenal dependent HAC; EDTA, ethylenediaminetetraacetic acid; HAC, hyperadrenocorticism; LDDST, low-dose dexamethasone suppression test; PDH, pituitary dependent HAC; POMC, pro-opiomelanocortin; UCCR, urine cortisol:creatinine ratio.

injection could be considered in particularly fractious cats, although the risk for false-positive hyperadrenocorticism screening testing will also be increased in this patient cohort.

The protocol is outlined in **Table 5**. Suppression at the intermediate point (often 4 hours), but especially at the final point (8 hours) (usually $< \pm 40$ nmol/L but dependent on the laboratory) is suggestive of absence of hyperadrenocorticism. It should be noted that although virtually all ADH cases will not show such suppression, there might be some PDH cases that will. In the latter case, clinical judgment will have to be used to establish the need for further testing. The use of an LDDST using the canine dose of 0.01 mg/kg dexamethasone has been suggested in such cases, although seems not helpful in the authors' opinion given the lack of suppression in a proportion of normal cats.

The ACTH stimulation test

In up to two-thirds of cats with hyperadrenocorticism, cortisol concentrations during an ACTH stimulation test are within the normal reference range, which demonstrates the lack of sensitivity of this particular endocrine test for feline hyperadrenocorticism. The test remains useful in case of iatrogenic hyperadrenocorticism, where we expect a suppressed stimulation result in conjunction with a history of glucocorticoid exposure (including topical). The test might also prove useful when dealing with adrenal tumors producing other adrenal hormones, such as 17-hydroxyprogesterone, estradiol, androstenedione, progesterone, and testosterone. There is therefore still some advantage to using the ACTH stimulation test, as test results might suggest the presence of such atypical adrenal tumor through the presence of modest or even suppressed post-ACTH cortisol concentrations in a cat with clinical signs of hyperadrenocorticism. The laboratory can then be asked to use the already submitted serum sample for further assessment of these other adrenal hormones. In these cases, the basal serum samples are often already conclusive, showing extremely high concentrations of one of these cortisol precursors and in fact only little further increase in concentration is seen in the post-ACTH samples. Gray-zone elevations in these concentrations should be assessed with caution, as there is significant scope for healthy animals to show a concentration just outside the reference interval. The additional advantage of the ACTH stimulation test is its shorter duration (compared with the LDDST) and the possibility to inject the ACTH intramuscularly as well as intravenously. However, results of one study confirmed that intravenous administration of cosyntropin induced significantly greater and more prolonged adrenocortical stimulation than intramuscular administration.[61,62] Clinicians should bear in mind the timing for intravenous protocols versus intramuscular protocols in cats, and the difference in timing of post-ACTH sample collection in cats compared with dogs, because of the more variable timing of maximal stimulation of the adrenals in cats compared with dogs (see **Table 5**).

UCCR

UCCR is a useful screening test for hyperadrenocorticism.[39,63,64] Collection of a morning sample at home will help minimize the influence of stress on the test's results.[65] The test is the most sensitive screening test, and therefore a negative result makes hyperadrenocorticism unlikely. Hyperadrenocorticism, but also any concurrent illness (including hyperthyroidism) and stress could result in an elevated UCCR.[63–66] The test can be combined with the oral administration of dexamethasone to improve specificity (although when used in this fashion will lose some sensitivity), although mainly helps by concurrently attempting to differentiate PDH from ADH.

Plasma ACTH Precursors

ACTH is derived from its precursor, pro-opiomelanocortin (POMC), which is first processed to pro-ACTH and then cleaved to ACTH by the prohormone convertase 1 (PC1). Plasma ACTH precursor (POMC and pro-ACTH) concentrations have been shown to be high in large or aggressive pituitary corticotrophic tumors in both humans and dogs and recently also in 8 of 9 cats with PDH. This small study has provided the only data thus far, and therefore more rigorous assessment is required to determine the specificity and sensitivity for feline PDH.[67]

Endocrine Testing: Which Test is Best for Differentiating PDH from ADH in Cats?

As is the case with canine hyperadrenocorticism, performing discriminatory tests is a wise investment of time and money and therefore highly recommended. A cat with PDH will have a different prognosis and will face different long-term complications than a cat with ADH; additionally, the gold standard treatment is different for each subset of diseases (see later in this article). Finally, the response to medical treatment will likely be different in each patient category.

The main discriminatory tests are shown in **Table 6**, alongside the most popular protocols and main (dis)advantages. Discriminatory tests should be performed only once a diagnosis of hyperadrenocorticism has been reached on the basis of clinical signs and a positive screening test. The exception is the UCCR with oral dexamethasone suppression, which could serve both functions, although further validation of this test is desirable.

THE ROLE OF IMAGING IN HYPERADRENOCORTICISM

The role of imaging is traditionally thought most useful in the discriminatory phase of the diagnostic process (see **Table 6**). Imaging of adrenals and/or pituitary could also serve the role of substantiating a diagnosis of hyperadrenocorticism in the first instance. Nevertheless, it seems more logical to use functional (hormonal) tests for this, rather than imaging only, because the latter provides purely structural assessment and therefore can provide only indirect evidence for a diagnosis of hyperadrenocorticism. In feline hyperadrenocorticism, pituitary imaging (using CT or MRI) lacks the sensitivity that endocrine testing can offer the clinician (45% of cats with PDH had a normal CT)[39] and is usually more expensive, as well as requiring sedation/anesthesia. Additionally, a misdiagnosis could result in cases with nonfunctional pituitary tumors or nonfunctional adrenal enlargements ("incidentelomas") when endocrine testing is omitted.

Nevertheless, during the discriminatory phase, performing an abdominal ultrasound in a cat suspected of hyperadrenocorticism represents a wise investment. The adrenals in the cat have been reported to be easier to image than in dogs, although this obviously remains operator and equipment dependent.[39,68] Visualization of the adrenal glands will be informative in terms of differentiating PDH from ADH. On the premise of cats with ADH having one large adrenal/adrenal mass (**Fig. 12**) and one small one, versus cats with PDH having equal-sized to normal or enlarged adrenals (**Fig. 13**), 34 of 41 cats (83%) were correctly diagnosed in one study.[39] Abdominal ultrasound therefore seems a good discriminatory tool. Nevertheless, 10% had misleading results, suggesting a healthy dose of caution should be maintained. Ultrasound-guided biopsy of adrenal masses is possible, although not without danger (especially hemorrhage, although also risk of failure to reach a histologic diagnosis) and one could question the need for this, if adrenalectomy represents the gold-standard treatment option for ADH.

Table 6
Overview and characteristics of discriminating tests for feline hyperadrenocorticism

Differentiating Test	Protocol	Interpretation	Advantage	Disadvantage
HDDST	1. Baseline serum cortisol (t = 0) 2. Intravenous 1.0 mg/kg dexamethasone (or intramuscular) 3. Serum cortisol t = 4 and 8 h	If suppression >50% is seen, ADH unlikely	Easy to perform	In-hospital: stress 50% of PDH cats do not show suppression
UCCR with oral dexamethasone suppression (as differentiating test)	1. Two at-home collected morning samples for UCCR: calculate average 2. Owner administers 0.5 mg dexamethasone orally at 12 PM, 6 PM, and 12 midnight 3. Next morning: home collected morning sample for UCCR	75% of cats with PDH will show >50% suppression of the average UCCR	At home: less influence of stress Can serve as screening test and as discriminating test	25% of PDH cats do not show suppression
Endogenous ACTH	1. Usually collected in EDTA-collection tube 2. Put immediately on ice 3. Plasma separated and stored at −80°C 4. Transported to laboratory on dry ice 5. Exact protocol to be verified with laboratory performing the assay	If high or high normal: PDH likely If low or low normal: ADH likely	Only 1 sample needed	Unstable hormone: false low results (special sampling and transport conditions crucial, contact laboratory)

Adrenal size and morphology on abdominal ultrasound or CT	1. Measurements of adrenal width are taken 2. Structure of adrenals is assessed 3. Includes assessment for vena cava invasion	Bilaterally enlarged adrenals suggestive of PDH One large adrenal and small contralateral adrenal suggestive of ADH Vena cava invasion suggests adrenal carcinoma	Availability Vena cava invasion or evidence of metastases suggest presence of a carcinoma and informs treatment decisions Other causes of insulin resistant diabetes can be screened for (eg, pancreatitis)	Equipment and experience needed
Pituitary size and morphology on intracranial imaging (CT, MRI)	1. Imaging of the sella turcica 2. Precontrast and postcontrast enhancement	If macroadenoma present (pituitary height >3 mm) usually definitive	If no macroadenoma present, abdomen can also be imaged using the same modality Essential step for planning of hypophysectomy or radiation therapy	Limited availability Costs Need for sedation or anesthesia Micro-adenoma (50% of PDH cases) could be missed/limited sensitivity Rare immediate contrast side effects (usually only limited to waking up from sedation and vomiting) Screening for ADH and PDH
POMC (please note: data based on 1 small study only)	1. Basal EDTA blood sample 2. Immediate centrifugation at 4°C 3. Plasma transferred to plastic tubes and stored at −80°C until analysis	If high: PDH likely	Only 1 sample needed	Not validated as differentiating test Unstable hormone: false low results (special sampling and transport conditions crucial, contact laboratory)

Abbreviations: ACTH, adrenocorticotrophic hormone; ADH, adrenal dependent HAC; EDTA, ethylenediaminetetraacetic acid; HAC, hyperadrenocorticism; HDDST, high-dose dexamethasone suppression test; PDH, pituitary dependent HAC; POMC, pro-opiomelanocortin; UCCR, urine cortisol:creatinine ratio.

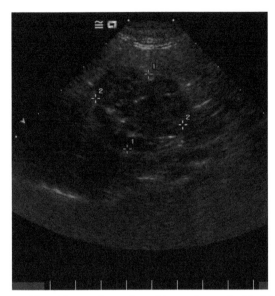

Fig. 12. Ultrasonographic evidence of an adrenal tumor in a cat with ADH.

Abdominal radiography adds little value to the diagnostic process, especially when abdominal ultrasound is available, with the exception of large adrenal tumors, which can sometimes be seen on regular radiographs. It is also important to emphasize that adrenal gland calcification can occur in cats as part of the normal aging process and does not indicate presence of an adrenal tumor as such.

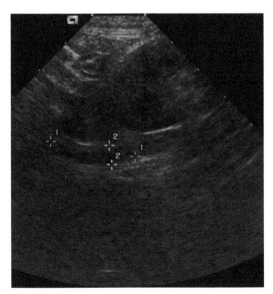

Fig. 13. Location and measurements of the adrenal gland in a cat with PDH. Both adrenals were homogeneously enlarged and a pituitary tumor was evident on a CT scan. Please note the location of the adrenal (*middle*) in relation to the kidney (*right top*).

Abdominal CT is increasingly being used for a variety of diseases affecting the abdomen and can also prove useful in the assessment of adrenal morphology, as well as assessment for vena cava invasion or metastases from an adrenal carcinoma (**Fig. 14**). In the differentiation process, both the pituitary and the adrenals could be imaged in one CT session.

Finally, a sex hormone–secreting tumor should be suspected in cats with clinical signs of hyperadrenocorticism and an adrenal mass on ultrasonography or CT, yet normal or even suppressed cortisol results.

TREATMENT OPTIONS FOR HYPERADRENOCORTICISM

Hyperadrenocorticism treatment options consist of medical treatment, surgical options, radiotherapy, and palliative treatment. As with feline hypersomatotropism, when treatment is initiated, clinicians and owners need to be vigilant for rapid changes in insulin demands. Which of the treatment options is preferred depends on the nature of the hyperadrenocorticism (ie, PDH vs ADH), hence highlighting the importance of the discrimination process.

Medical Treatment (PDH and ADH)

Medical treatment could be considered if (1) a definitive treatment option (hypophysectomy or adrenalectomy) is declined; (2) in the preoperative period to improve patient health, especially in terms of improving wound healing; (3) preradiation, periradiation, and postradiation (PDH) to assist in controlling signs; and (4) as a palliative option for cats with metastatic disease. Dosing protocols, mechanisms of action, and main (dis)advantages are shown in **Table 7**; however, currently, the authors recommend using

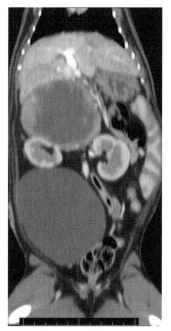

Fig. 14. CT reconstruction of the abdomen of a cat with ADH. A large adrenal tumor is apparent cranial to the right kidney.

Table 7
Overview and characteristics of medical treatment options for feline hyperadrenocorticism

Drug	Protocol	Mechanism of Action	Advantage	Disadvantage
Trilostane	1. 10 mg SID PO 2. ACTH stim after 14 d (4 h post pill) 3. Increase to 10 mg BID or 20 mg SID if necessary 4. ACTH stim after 14 d 5. Increase further as required on basis of clinical image and post-ACTH stim serum cortisol concentration (authors' target range: 50–150 nmol/L)	Steroidogenesis enzyme inhibitor (3-beta-hydroxysteroid-dehydrogenase)	Most effective of all medical options In principle, reversible action	Has no antineoplastic effect Limited experience in cats Lack of knowledge of pharmacokinetics, including impact of renal disease Extremely rare sudden death described in dogs may also occur in cats
Mitotane (not recommended)	25 mg/kg BID PO	Adrenocorticolytic	Has antineoplastic effect Widely available	Cats are much less sensitive to its effects than dogs: likely ineffective Chlorinated hydrocarbon sensitivity of cats (although rarely reported) Limited experience in cats
Ketoconazole (not recommended)	1. 5 mg/kg BID PO for 7 d, then 10 mg/kg BID 2. 14 d: ACTH stim 3. If no result: 15 mg/kg BID	Steroidogenesis enzyme inhibitor (targets imidazole ring and cytochrome P450)	Widely available In principle, reversible action	Cats are less sensitive to its effects than dogs: likely insufficient suppression Recognized ketoconazole side effects Limited experience in cats
Metyrapone (if trilostane not available)	1. 30 mg/kg BID PO 2. ACTH stim after 14 d 3. Increase dose gradually if needed 4. Recommended not to exceed 70 mg/kg BID	Steroidogenesis enzyme inhibitor (11-beta-hydroxylase)	Has shown some efficacy In principle, reversible action	Lack of efficacy in a proportion of cats Vomiting and inappetence Limited experience in cats

Abbreviations: ACTH, adrenocorticotrophic hormone; ACTH stim, ACTH stimulation test; BID, twice a day; PO, by mouth; SID, once a day.

trilostane above all other medical options, given its superior efficacy, relative lack of side effects, and ease of use. For cats that prove sensitive to trilostane, a good quality of life can be achieved long term in a significant proportion of cats (Drs Stijn Niessen, David Church, and Yaiza Forcada, personal communication, 2013).[49,69,70] When treating with trilostane, the authors aim for clinical improvement in conjunction with post-ACTH serum cortisol concentrations between 50 and 150 nmol/L.

Surgery

Hypophysectomy (PDH)

As is the case for feline hypersomatotropism, hypophysectomy is considered the treatment of choice in human, canine, and feline PDH. The largest case series to date consisted of 7 cats with PDH,[46] but likely underestimates the ultimate potential of this procedure, as experience in Dr Meij and colleagues' institution has since increased further, alongside the success rates. It still represents a major intervention; one cat in this initial series did not recover from anesthesia, and a second cat developed neurologic abnormalities 2 weeks after surgery. Nevertheless, the remaining 5 cats showed clinical and clinical pathologic resolution of their hyperadrenocorticism. Given the nature of the procedure (the pituitary is approached through an incision in the soft palate), oronasal fistulas can occur (and resulting chronic rhinitis), although increased experience will reduce the frequency of such occurrence. More information can be found in the hypersomatotropism surgery section earlier in this article.

Unilateral or bilateral adrenalectomy (ADH or PDH)

A second preferred surgical option for PDH constitutes bilateral adrenalectomy and, for ADH, unilateral adrenalectomy. The procedure requires less expertise than a hypophysectomy, although perioperative and postoperative management are equally important and (hypercortisolemia-associated) impaired wound healing can represent an added level of difficulty. In the authors' institution, a hydrocortisone infusion is started as soon as the surgeon starts working on the adrenal(s) and is continued until the patient is eating again after the procedure. At this stage, the patient is transitioned to oral glucocorticoids, either a low dose of prednisolone (0.1 mg/kg once a day) or hydrocortisone (0.5 mg/kg once a day). Whenever possible, presurgical treatment with trilostane is advocated by the authors to ensure normalization of the wound-healing processes. Vitamin A supplementation has also been used on the basis of the theoretical advantage in terms of beneficial effects on wound healing. When impaired wound healing and/or skin fragility is a great concern, a flank incision approach to the adrenal(s) is often preferred, as this might reduce the risk of wound breakdown post-operatively given the decreased tension on the wound compared with a midline incision approach. Laparoscopy can prove even more advantageous in terms of wound healing and has been shown to be feasible for the purpose of adrenalectomy in a cat with ADH.[71]

In case of bilateral adrenalectomy for PDH, the patient is then treated as an Addisonian animal. In case of unilateral adrenalectomy for ADH, glucocorticoid treatment is continued in the immediate postoperative period, and then tapered gradually over 6 weeks so the remaining adrenal gland can gradually resume glucocorticoid production. Basal cortisol checks on serum samples taken 12 hours after the administration of prednisolone or hydrocortisone can guide the assessment of the activity levels of this contralateral adrenal during the last part of this period and can inform the ultimate decision to stop medication completely. Alternatively, an ACTH stimulation test can give additional information about this adrenal, and will be less influenced by prior chronic exogenous steroid administration. If this approach fails (flatline ACTH stimulation test results are consistently seen even when the cat has been on a very low dose of steroids for a month), a final approach would be to taper the exogenous gluco-corticoids gradually and completely anyway and then perform a basal cortisol or ACTH stimulation test 4 weeks after cessation of the steroids to document adequate functioning of the remaining adrenal. In the latter case, it is advisable to ensure that the cat's owners will have steroids available at home, to be given in case of an Addisonian crisis.

Radiation Therapy (PDH)

Radiation therapy is also discussed in the feline hypersomatotropism section earlier in this article. In summary, the unreliability in terms of response to treatment is the great-est pitfall of using this modality, as is the case when treating feline hypersomatotrop-ism.[39] Hypophysectomy and bilateral adrenalectomy are therefore often preferred. When this modality is used for treatment of PDH, concurrent start of trilostane treat-ment is often indicated to reliably and immediately start controlling the ill effects of the hypercortisolemic state.

Palliative Treatment

Unlike the situation in hypersomatotropism and given the more readily available and often effective medical treatment or surgical options for hyperadrenocorticism (trilostane, adrenalectomy), treating the diabetes without addressing the underlying endocrinopathy (hyperadrenocorticism) is usually not indicated. Additionally, hypera-drenocorticism tends to result in more acute complications with seriously debilitating effects compared with feline hypersomatotropism, and intervention to reduce the endogenous cortisol levels is therefore usually more urgently needed. Meticulous wound management might be indicated in case of fragile skin syndrome–associated wounds, as well as adequate prevention and treatment and management of opportu-nistic infections and screening for hyperadrenocorticism-associated hypertension and proteinuria. A low carbohydrate canned diet recommended for diabetic felines, would be advocated to reduce demand on beta cells to produce insulin.

DIFFERENTIATING FELINE HYPERSOMATOTROPISM AND FELINE HYPERADRENOCORTICISM

Because both hypersomatotropism and hyperadrenocorticism can present with insulin-resistant diabetes and a pituitary tumor, it is of practical importance to be able to differentiate hypersomatotropism from hyperadrenocorticism. **Table 4** provides useful hints toward the differentiation process.

QUALITY OF LIFE AND PROGNOSIS IN FELINE HYPERSOMATOTROPISM AND HYPERADRENOCORTICISM

Continuous quality of life assessment is crucial to ensure the patient is managed in the most appropriate way, and if necessary, a timely decision to consider alternative treat-ment options or euthanasia is made by all parties involved. Feline hyperadrenocorti-cism tends to more acutely cause severe quality-of-life issues when left untreated or if treatment fails. In contrast, quality of life will be affected in a more chronic and slowly progressive fashion in feline hypersomatotropism when left unattended. Because both diabetic cats with hyperadrenocorticism and those with hypersomato-tropism can have suboptimal glycemic control, a diabetes-specific quality-of-life quantification tool is used in the authors' diabetic cat clinic.[31] Using such a tool regu-larly facilitates and stimulates conversations between owners and clinicians, as well as enables more objective tracking of the quality of life of these diabetic patients, especially when undergoing treatment.

Because feline hyperadrenocorticism is more debilitating in nature, traditionally a guarded to grave prognosis has been suggested. The advent of advanced surgical techniques (hypophysectomy), improved perioperative protocols for bilateral adrenalectomy, as well as trilostane treatment, justify modifying this perception, because, when the hypercortisolemia is reduced effectively, a good quality of life can be achieved for a long period. Similarly, advances in the treatment of feline hypersomatotropism, especially in terms of increased availability of hypophysectomy and identification of effective somatostatins, will likely lead to modification of expected life expectancy and life quality expectations. When effective treatment is initiated early enough, an improved quality of life and even diabetic remission can be achieved.

REFERENCES

1. McMann TM, Simpson KE, Shaw DJ, et al. Feline diabetes mellitus in the UK: the prevalence within an insured cat population and a questionnaire-based putative risk factor analysis. J Feline Med Surg 2007;9:289–99.
2. Rand JS, Fleeman LM, Farrow HA, et al. Canine and feline diabetes mellitus: nature or nurture? J Nutr 2004;134:2072S–80S.
3. Forcada Y, Holder A, Jepson R, et al. A missense mutation in the coding sequence of MC4R (MC4R: C.92 C4T) is associated with diabetes mellitus in DSH cats. J Vet Intern Med 2011;25:681.
4. Niessen SJ. Feline acromegaly: an essential differential diagnosis for the difficult diabetic. J Feline Med Surg 2010;12(1):15–23.
5. Niessen SJ, Petrie G, Gaudiano F, et al. Feline acromegaly: an underdiagnosed endocrinopathy? J Vet Intern Med 2007;21(5):899–905.
6. Elliott DA, Feldman EC, Koblik PD, et al. Prevalence of pituitary tumors among diabetic cats with insulin resistance. J Am Vet Med Assoc 2000;216(11):1765–8.
7. Niessen SJ, Forcada Y, Jensen K, et al. Routine screening of diabetic cats for acromegaly: overdue or overkill? [abstract]. J Vet Intern Med 2011;25:1489–90.
8. Berg RI, Nelson RW, Feldman EC, et al. Serum insulin-like growth factor-I concentration in cats with diabetes mellitus and acromegaly. J Vet Intern Med 2007; 21(5):892–8.
9. Niessen SJ, Khalid M, Petrie G, et al. Validation and application of an ovine radioimmunoassay for the diagnosis of feline acromegaly. Vet Rec 2007;160:902–7.
10. Niessen S. Acromegaly in cats: what do we know & what don't we know. In: ACVIM Forum Proceedings Committee, editor. Proceedings of the American College of Veterinary Medicine Annual Forum. Denver (CO): CD-ROM; 2011.
11. Feldman EC, Nelson RW. Disorders of growth hormone. In: Feldman EC, Nelson RW, editors. Canine and feline endocrinology and reproduction. 3rd edition. St Louis (MO): Saunders; 2004. p. 69–80.
12. Niessen SJ, Petrie G, Gaudiano F, et al. Routine clinical pathology findings in feline acromegaly. In: BSAVA Congress Proceedings Committee, editor. Proceedings of the British Small Animal Veterinary Association (BSAVA) congress. BSAVA, Gloucester, UK, Birmingham (United Kingdom): 2007. p. 482.
13. Peterson ME, Taylor RS, Greco DS, et al. Acromegaly in 14 cats. J Vet Intern Med 1990;4:192–201.
14. Norman EJ, Mooney CT. Diagnosis and management of diabetes mellitus in five cats with somatotrophic abnormalities. J Feline Med Surg 2000;2:183–90.

15. Niessen SJ, Forcada Y, Church DB. Serum type III procollagen propeptide: an alternative measure of growth hormone bioactivity bioactivity in cats with diabetes mellitus and hypersomatotropism. J Vet Intern Med 2012;26(6):1520 TBC.

16. Jensen K, Forcada Y, Glanemann B, et al. Physiology and diagnostic potential of serum ghrelin in cats with diabetes mellitus and hypersomatotropism. J Vet Intern Med 2012;26b(6):1519 TBC.

17. Chang-DeMoranville BM, Jackson IM. Diagnosis and endocrine testing in acromegaly. Endocrinol Metab Clin North Am 1992;21:649–68.

18. Eigenmann J, Wortman J, Haskins M. Elevated growth hormone levels and diabetes mellitus in a cat with acromegalic features. J Am Anim Hosp Assoc 1984;20:747–52.

19. Kokka N, Garcia JF, Morgan M, et al. Immunoassay of plasma growth hormone in cats following fasting and administration of insulin, arginine, 2-deoxyglucose and hypothalamic extract. Endocrinology 1971;88:359–66.

20. Posch B, Dobson J, Herrtage M. Magnetic resonance imaging findings in 15 acromegalic cats. Vet Radiol Ultrasound 2011;52(4):422–7.

21. Fischetti AJ, Gisselman K, Peterson ME. CT and MRI evaluation of skull bones and soft tissue in six cats with presumed acromegaly versus 12 unaffected cats. Vet Radiol Ultrasound 2012;53(5):535–9 online only at moment.

22. Troxel MT, Vite CH, Van Winkle TJ, et al. Feline intracranial neoplasia: retrospective review of 160 cases (1985-2001). J Vet Intern Med 2003;17(6):850–9.

23. Timian J, Lunn KF. Evaluation of a long-acting somatostatin receptor ligand for the treatment of feline acromegaly. J Vet Intern Med 2012;26:757.

24. Abraham LA, Helmond SE, Mitten RW, et al. Treatment of an acromegalic cat with the dopamine agonist L-deprenyl. Aust Vet J 2002;80:479–83.

25. Slingerland LI, Voorhout G, Rijnberk A, et al. Growth hormone excess and the effect of octreotide in cats with diabetes mellitus. Domest Anim Endocrinol 2008;35(4):352–61.

26. Meij BP, Auriemma E, Grinwis G, et al. Successful treatment of acromegaly in a diabetic cat with transsphenoidal hypophysectomy. J Feline Med Surg 2010; 12:406–10.

27. Meij BP, Galac S, Kooistra H. Surgical treatment of acromegaly in cats. In: Voorjaarsdagen Proceedings Committee, editor. Proceedings of the Voorjaarsdagen. Amsterdam (The Netherlands): 2012. p. 232–3.

28. Blois SL, Holmberg DL. Cryohypophysectomy used in the treatment of a case of feline acromegaly. J Small Anim Pract 2008;49:596–600.

29. Brearley MJ, Polton GA, Littler RM, et al. Coarse fractionated radiation therapy for pituitary tumours in cats: a retrospective study of 12 cases. Vet Comp Oncol 2006;4:209–17.

30. Dunning MD, Lowrie CS, Bexfield NH, et al. Exogenous insulin treatment after hypofractionated radiotherapy in cats with diabetes mellitus and acromegaly. J Vet Intern Med 2009;23(2):243–9.

31. Niessen SJ, Powney S, Guitian J, et al. Evaluation of a quality-of-life tool for cats with diabetes mellitus. J Vet Intern Med 2010;24(5):1098–105.

32. Andrews RC, Walker BR. Glucocorticoids and insulin resistance: old hormones, new targets. Clin Sci (Lond) 1999;96:513–23.

33. Rooney DP, Neely RD, Cullen C, et al. The effect of cortisol on glucose-6-phosphate cycle activity and insulin action. Clin Endocrinol Metab 1994;77:1180–3.

34. Rizza RA, Mandarino LJ, Gerich J. Cortisol-induced insulin resistance in man: impaired suppression of glucose production and stimulation of glucose utilization due to a postreceptor defect of insulin action. J Clin Endocrinol Metab 1982;54:131–8.

35. Chavez M, Seeley RJ, Green PK, et al. Adrenalectomy increases sensitivity to central insulin. Physiol Behav 1997;62:631–4.
36. Ling ZC, Khan A, Delaunay F, et al. Increased glucocorticoid sensitivity in islet beta-cells: effects on glucose 6-phosphatase, glucose cycling and insulin release. Diabetologia 1998;41:634–9.
37. Delaunay F, Khan A, Cintra A, et al. Pancreatic beta cells are important targets for the diabetogenic effects of glucocorticoids. J Clin Invest 1997;100:2094–8.
38. Lambillotte C, Gilon P, Henquin JC. Direct glucocorticoid inhibition of insulin secretion: an in vitro study of dexamethasone effects in mouse islets. J Clin Invest 1997;99:414–23.
39. Feldman EC, Nelson RW. Hyperadrenocorticism in cats (Cushing's syndrome). In: Feldman EC, Nelson RW, editors. Canine and feline endocrinology and reproduction. St Louis (MO): Saunders; 2004. p. 358–93.
40. Nelson RW, Feldman EC, Smith MC. Hyperadrenocorticism in cats: seven cases (1978–1987). J Am Vet Med Assoc 1988;193:245–50.
41. Watson PJ, Herrtage ME. Hyperadrenocorticism in six cats. J Small Anim Pract 1998;39:175–84.
42. Rossmeisl JH Jr, Scott-Moncrieff JC, Siems J, et al. Hyperadrenocorticism and hyperprogesteronemia in a cat with an adrenocortical adenocarcinoma. J Am Anim Hosp Assoc 2000;36:512–7.
43. Blois SL, Dickie EL, Kruth SA, et al. Multiple endocrine diseases in cats: 15 cases (1997–2008). J Feline Med Surg 2010;12:637–42.
44. Spada E, Proverbio D, Giudice C, et al. Pituitary-dependent hyperadrenocorticism and generalised toxoplasmosis in a cat with neurological signs. J Feline Med Surg 2010;12:654–8.
45. Fracassi F, Mandrioli L, Diana A, et al. Pituitary macroadenoma in a cat with diabetes mellitus, hypercortisolism and neurological signs. J Vet Med A Physiol Pathol Clin Med 2007;54:359–63.
46. Meij BP, Voorhout G, van den Ingh TS, et al. Transsphenoidal hypophysectomy for treatment of pituitary-dependent hyperadrenocorticism in 7 cats. Vet Surg 2001; 30:72–86.
47. Meij BP, van der Vlugt-Meijer RH, van den Ingh TS, et al. Somatotroph and corticotroph pituitary adenoma (double adenoma) in a cat with diabetes mellitus and hyperadrenocorticism. J Comp Pathol 2004;130:209–15.
48. Schwedes CS. Mitotane (o, p'-DDD) treatment in a cat with hyperadrenocorticism. J Small Anim Pract 1997;38:520–4.
49. Boag AK, Neiger R, Church DB. Trilostane treatment of bilateral adrenal enlargement and excessive sex steroid hormone production in a cat. J Small Anim Pract 2004;45:263–6.
50. Calsyn JD, Green RA, Davis GJ, et al. Adrenal pheochromocytoma with contralateral adrenocortical adenoma in a cat. J Am Anim Hosp Assoc 2010;46(1): 36–42.
51. Roccabianca P, Rondena M, Paltrinieri S, et al. Multiple endocrine neoplasia type-I-like syndrome in two cats. Vet Pathol 2006;43(3):345–52.
52. Briscoe K, Barrs VR, Foster DF, et al. Hyperaldosteronism and hyperprogesteronism in a cat. J Feline Med Surg 2009;11(9):758–62.
53. Quante S, Sieber-Ruckstuhl N, Wilhelm S, et al. Hyperprogesteronism due to bilateral adrenal carcinomas in a cat with diabetes mellitus. Schweiz Arch Tierheilkd 2009;151(9):437–42.
54. Brown AL, Beatty JA, Lindsay SA, et al. Severe systemic hypertension in a cat with pituitary-dependent hyperadrenocorticism. J Small Anim Pract 2012;53(2):132–5.

55. Duesberg CA, Nelson RW, Feldman EC, et al. Adrenalectomy for treatment of hyperadrenocorticism in cats: 10 cases (1988-1992). J Am Vet Med Assoc 1995;207(8):1066–70.
56. Lien YH, Huang HP, Chang PH. Iatrogenic hyperadrenocorticism in 12 cats. J Am Anim Hosp Assoc 2006;42(6):414–23.
57. Roomp K, Rand J. Intensive blood glucose control is safe and effective in diabetic cats using home monitoring and treatment with glargine. J Feline Med Surg 2009;11(4):668–82.
58. Wajngot A, Giacca A, Grill V, et al. The diabetogenic effects of glucocorticoids are more pronounced in low- than in high-insulin responders. Proc Natl Acad Sci U S A 1992;89:6035–9.
59. Peterson M. Feline hyperadrenocorticism. In: Mooney CM, Peterson ME, editors. BSAVA manual of canine and feline endocrinology. Quedgeley (Gloucester): BSAVA; 2012. p. 190–8.
60. Kley S, Alt M, Zimmer C, et al. Evaluation of the low-dose dexamethasone suppression test and ultrasonographic measurements of the adrenal glands in cats with diabetes mellitus. Schweiz Arch Tierheilkd 2007;149:493–500.
61. Peterson ME, Kemppainen RJ. Comparison of intravenous and intramuscular routes of administering cosyntropin for corticotropin stimulation testing in cats. Am J Vet Res 1992;53(8):1392–5.
62. Peterson ME, Kemppainen RJ. Dose-response relation between plasma concentrations of corticotropin and cortisol after administration of incremental doses of cosyntropin for corticotropin stimulation testing in cats. Am J Vet Res 1993;54(2):300–4.
63. Goossens MM, Meyer HP, Voorhout G, et al. Urinary excretion of glucocorticoids in the diagnosis of hyperadrenocorticism in cats. Domest Anim Endocrinol 1995;12(4):355–62.
64. Henry CJ, Clark TP, Young DW, et al. Urine cortisol:creatinine ratio in healthy and sick cats. J Vet Intern Med 1996;10(3):123–6.
65. Cauvin AL, Witt AL, Groves E, et al. The urinary corticoid:creatinine ratio (UCCR) in healthy cats undergoing hospitalisation. J Feline Med Surg 2003;5(6):329–33.
66. De Lange MS, Galac S, Trip MR, et al. High urinary corticoid/creatinine ratios in cats with hyperthyroidism. J Vet Intern Med 2004;18(2):152–5.
67. Benchekroun G, de Fornel-Thibaud P, Dubord M, et al. Plasma ACTH precursors in cats with pituitary-dependent hyperadrenocorticism. J Vet Intern Med 2012;26(3):575–81.
68. Zimmer C, Hörauf A, Reusch C. Ultrasonographic examination of the adrenal gland and evaluation of the hypophyseal-adrenal axis in 20 cats. J Small Anim Pract 2000;41(4):156–60.
69. Neiger R, Witt AL, Noble A, et al. Trilostane therapy for treatment of pituitary-dependent hyperadrenocorticism in 5 cats. J Vet Intern Med 2004;18(2):160–4.
70. Skelly BJ, Petrus D, Nicholls PK. Use of trilostane for the treatment of pituitary-dependent hyperadrenocorticism in a cat. J Small Anim Pract 2003;44(6):269–72.
71. Smith RR, Mayhew PD, Berent AC. Laparoscopic adrenalectomy for management of a functional adrenal tumor in a cat. J Am Vet Med Assoc 2012;241(3):368–72.

Diabetes and the Kidney in Human and Veterinary Medicine

Carly Anne Bloom, DVM[a],*,
Jacquie S. Rand, BVSc, DVSc, MANZVS, DACVIM[b]

KEYWORDS

- Diabetes mellitus • Diabetic nephropathy • Microalbuminuria • Hypertension

KEY POINTS

- Clinical diabetic nephropathy is neither routinely recognized nor well studied in veterinary medicine; however, various studies in the past 40 years have suggested that some of the risk factors and structural renal changes of human diabetes also exist in diabetic dogs and cats.
- Some diabetic cats and dogs do have risk factors or consequences of diabetes that are consistent with classification as diabetic nephropathy according to the American Diabetes Association, including renal azotemia, proteinuria, and hypercholesterolemia.
- In human medicine, proteinuria is predictive for development and progression of diabetic nephropathy; although not widely studied, there is recent evidence to suggest that diabetic cats may be proteinuric.
- Further study in this area is urgently needed to both confirm and understand the cause of proteinuria in feline diabetes mellitus.

INTRODUCTION TO DIABETES MELLITUS

Diabetes mellitus is classified into 4 broad types in human and veterinary medicine[1]:

- Type 1 diabetes is a result of β-cell destruction from immune-mediated mechanisms, usually leading to an absolute insulin deficiency.
- Type 2 diabetes is characterized by insulin resistance with concomitant β-cell failure, which in humans is often relative, rather than absolute, failure of insulin secretion. Insulin secretion is defective and is insufficient to compensate for the insulin resistance. At the time of diagnosis, most cats have absolute insulin deficiency, which may be reversible if the glucose toxic effects on the β cells are reversed; in other cats, there is irreversible and permanent absolute loss of

The authors have no relevant relationships to disclose.
[a] Small Animal Internal Medicine, Small Animal Clinic & Veterinary Teaching Hospital, School of Veterinary Science, Therapies Road, The University of Queensland, St Lucia, Queensland 4072, Australia; [b] Centre for Companion Animal Health, School of Veterinary Science, Slip Road, The University of Queensland, Queensland 4072, Australia
* Corresponding author.
E-mail address: c.bloom@uq.edu.au

0195-5616/13/$ – see front matter © 2013 Elsevier Inc. All rights reserved.

endogenous insulin secretion. The risk of developing this form of diabetes increases with age, obesity, and lack of physical activity.
- "Other specific types of diabetes" includes most other forms of diabetes in cats that do not fit type 2 diabetes, including exocrine pancreatic disease, endocrinopathies that antagonize insulin action, or drug-induced or chemical-induced diabetes. In humans, monogenetic defects in β-cell function or insulin action are also included.
- Gestational diabetes is not a significant cause of diabetes in cats, because most owned cats are desexed.

DIABETIC NEPHROPATHY: INTRODUCTION, DEFINITIONS, AND INCIDENCE
Human Medicine

People with type 1 or type 2 diabetes mellitus are predisposed to renal disease, commonly called diabetic nephropathy. Diabetic nephropathy is defined as structural or functional abnormalities of the kidneys as a complication of diabetes mellitus and is primarily but not exclusively a glomerular disease. Diabetic nephropathy occurs in 5 stages of increasing severity.[2] Stages 1, 2, and 3 reflect hyperfiltration and structural glomerular changes that lead to subclinical increase in renal albumin excretion, called microalbuminuria. Stage 4 diabetic nephropathy reflects functional impairment of the kidney and is defined as a clinical disease with persistent proteinuria, hypertension, and reduced glomerular filtration rate (GFR). The fifth stage reflects end-stage impairment of kidney structure and function. The incidence of diabetic nephropathy in type 1 and type 2 diabetic people is widely cited at 25% to 40%.[2] Because not all diabetic nephropathy progresses to clinical stage 4 or 5 disease, the incidence of earlier stages of diabetic renal disease is believed to be higher.[3] Diabetic nephropathy is the leading cause of end-stage renal disease in Western countries and is believed to take more than 10 to 20 years to develop, with wide variation.

Veterinary Medicine

Clinical diabetic nephropathy is not routinely recognized in veterinary medicine. However, chronic kidney disease is common in cats and the cause is often unknown; in a single study,[4] the incidence of glomerular disease of unknown cause in cats was nearly 15%. In a small postmortem study, 3 of 6 diabetic cats had glomerular changes similar to those seen in human diabetic nephropathy.[5] In addition, some diabetic cats do have risk factors or consequences of diabetes that are consistent with classification as diabetic nephropathy according to the American Diabetes Association, including renal azotemia, proteinuria, and hypercholesterolemia. Similar findings apply to diabetic dogs. Therefore, some of the histologic renal changes and some of the risk factors of human diabetic nephropathy certainly exist in diabetic cats, and these data warrant closer inspection.

HISTOPATHOLOGY OF DIABETIC NEPHROPATHY
Kidney Histopathology in Diabetic Humans

Diabetic renal disease is characterized by hallmark ultrastructural changes in the kidneys. In type 1 diabetes mellitus, morphologic changes occur throughout the kidney; however, the hallmark changes occur in the glomerulus. Two main changes occur: thickening of the glomerular basement membrane and tubular basement membrane and mesangial expansion, mainly as increased mesangial matrix.[6,7] Thickening of the glomerular basement membrane, as well as fewer podocytes (glomerular epithelial cells), are pathologic processes that lead to proteinuria by reducing the barrier to movement of proteins across the glomerular capillaries and into the ultrafiltrate.[6,7] Mesangial expansion is believed to lead to a decline in GFR by inward restriction of the lumen of the glomerular capillaries, thus restricting and reducing the total glomerular filtration surface, which directly correlates with GFR.[7,8] Ultrastructural changes in type 2 diabetes mellitus may mirror the changes seen with type 1, but overall are more heterogeneous.[9] Three main ultrastructural patterns are recognized in type 2 diabetics with normal kidney function: typical diabetic glomerulopathy, as described earlier; nearly normal renal ultrastructure; or atypical renal injury (global glomerulosclerosis, advanced glomerular arteriolar hyalinosis, and tubulointerstitial lesions). Three main ultrastructural patterns are recognized in type 2 diabetics with abnormal kidney function and proteinuria: typical diabetic glomerulopathy, as described earlier; atypical diabetic nephropathy with interstitial and vascular changes; and renal ultrastructural changes that are not typically associated with diabetes and may reflect nondiabetic renal disease.[7,9] A good review of the histopathology of type 1 and type 2 human diabetic nephropathy is available in the ninth edition of Brenner and Rector's *The Kidney*.[8]

Kidney Histopathology in Diabetic Cats

Chronic tubulointerstitial nephritis is the most common histologic lesion in cats with renal azotemia from chronic kidney disease. However, in 1 study reporting on histology of renal biopsies in azotemic cats, nearly 15% of cats had primarily glomerular lesions (this did not include amyloidosis, which was categorized separately). The glomerular lesions were noted to be comparable with human glomerulopathies, but cause was not pursued in this study.[4] A necropsy study in 6 cats with diabetes mellitus as diagnosed by persistent hyperglycemia reported predominantly glomerular changes (including mesangial proliferation and diffuse glomerular sclerosis) in 3 of 6 cats (50%), and glomerular change was more common than tubular or interstitial change in 2 of 6 cats (33%). Only 1 cat had no renal changes on histology.[5] Although this was a small study, investigators have used these data as histologic evidence suggestive of diabetic nephropathy in cats.[10,11] In veterinary medicine, advances are being made in techniques and understanding of glomerular histopathology. Using electron microscopy and a combination of staining techniques, including routine and special light microscopy staining and immunofluorescent staining, veterinary nephropathologists are now able to diagnose and understand ultrastructural changes in renal and particularly glomerular disease, at a level not achievable with routine staining and light microscopy alone.[12] It is recommended to visually assess renal biopsy samples using light microscopy (10–40x power) or an ocular loupe before submission to verify the presence of glomeruli, and to carefully process at least 2 or 3 biopsy samples using appropriate fixatives and additives. Samples should be submitted to a laboratory specializing in nephropathology and equipped to perform light microscopy with routine and special stains, electron microscopy, and immunostaining on all glomerular samples. A review of renal biopsy acquisition, and the information gained by processing glomerular samples beyond tradition light microscopy and routine staining, can be found in Lees and colleagues' *Renal Biopsy and Pathologic Evaluation of Glomerular Disease*.[12]

Glomerular disease is understudied in cats, and scant data do suggest that histologic changes similar to human diabetic nephropathy may exist in diabetic cats. Recent advances in technique and understanding of glomerular histopathology should be applied to further investigation of glomerular disease in cats, and on kidney histopathology in cats with chronic diabetes mellitus at varying levels of renal azotemia, renal proteinuria, and glycemic control.

STAGES OF DIABETIC NEPHROPATHY

In the 1980s, Dr C-E Mogensen[13] in Denmark developed a classification scheme outlining the typical stages of diabetic renal disease. The scheme was developed for type 1 diabetic patients who followed the typical albuminuric pathway toward worsening renal impairment. The stages are now considered to roughly describe progression of both type 1 and type 2 diabetic renal disease, and are as follows:

1. Glomerular hyperfiltration and hypertrophy: microvascular changes in the kidney
2. Silent phase: structural changes to the glomerulus
3. Persistent microalbuminuria: subclinical, persistent increase in renal albumin excretion (microalbuminuria)
4. Clinical diabetic nephropathy: clinical nephropathy with overt, persistent increase in renal albumin excretion (macroalbuminuria), reduced GFR, and hypertension
5. End-stage renal disease: severe structural and functional renal impairment

In the first stage (glomerular hyperfiltration and hypertrophy), hyperfiltration is defined as an abnormally increased GFR more than the range of age-matched nondiabetic people (normal GFR is >135 mL/min/1.73 m^2 in young patients, and this value decreases with age). The origin of the hyperfiltration is likely multifactorial and includes hyperglycemia and poor glycemic control, increased atrial natriuretic peptide, and other factors.[13,14] Hyperfiltration and increased GFR begin in stage 1 while the patient is nonalbuminuric, and persist through stages 2 and 3. Although hyperfiltration and increased GFR imply well-preserved renal function, data suggest that hyperfiltration predisposes patients to the development of microalbuminuria, which characterizes stage 3, and, with time, a declining GFR, which characterizes stage 4 clinical diabetic nephropathy.[7,13,15] As a result, hyperfiltration and abnormally increased GFR in stage 1 diabetic nephropathy are believed to be predictive of future structural, clinicopathologic, and functional renal disease, representing the progressive stages of diabetic nephropathy.[13,15,16]

In the second or silent phase, there are no obvious functional renal abnormalities, and patients are nonalbuminuric or only sporadically microalbuminuric. However, structural abnormalities have already occurred by this stage, including the glomerular basement membrane thickening and mesangial expansion described earlier. The silent phase may last for years, and many diabetics remain in this stage for life. Patients in stage 2 experience hyperfiltration, suggesting preserved renal function, but to a lesser extent than stage 1 patients.[15] Type 1 diabetics in stage 2 are nonhypertensive with normal renal function, although many type 2 diabetics in stage 2 are hypertensive from nonrenal causes with normal renal function in this stage.[13]

The third stage is characterized by persistent microalbuminuria, which is defined as a subclinical increase in albumin excretion, leading to albumin concentrations in the urine that are more than normal, but less than the limits of detection using routine methods for proteinuria measurement such as the protein dipstick. The American Diabetes Association defines microalbuminuria as renal albumin excretion of 30 to 299 mg per day in 24-hour urine collection, or 30 to 299 μg albumin per mg creatinine on spot collection.[2] Provided that diabetics in stage 3 remain normotensive, and their albumin excretion does not increase to become overt proteinuria, GFR seems to be preserved.[7] However, type 2 diabetics are often hypertensive by this stage, as a result of nonrenal factors such as obesity, dyslipidemia, advanced age, and metabolic syndrome.[7,15]

Stage 4 is diabetic nephropathy, which is defined as a clinical disease with persistent, overtly detectable proteinuria (macroalbuminuria) in association with increased blood pressure and a decline in GFR. Previously, the decline in GFR in stage 4 was considered unrelenting; however, newer evidence suggests that control of hypertension, hyperglycemia, and other risk factors may at least mitigate the declining GFR.[17–19] If diabetics in stage 4 are left untreated, GFR continues to decline, leading to worsening renal impairment.

Stage 5, end-stage renal disease, occurs when GFR declines even further, leading to severe, end-stage renal impairment. Many diabetics in stage 5 need renal replacement therapy, such as peritoneal dialysis, or intermittent or continuous hemodialysis. Other treatment options for stage 5 patients include renal transplant or combined renal-pancreas transplant.

Not all diabetics with ultrastructural changes consistent with diabetic nephropathy are microalbuminuric. Despite this situation, measurement of microalbuminuria and macroalbuminuria is still considered the best noninvasive test to predict and follow diabetic kidney disease.[2,7]

A recent study of feline diabetics found that 70% of diabetic cats were microalbuminuric, which was significantly higher than both age-matched healthy controls (18%) and sick, nondiabetic cats (39%).[10] This finding must be explored further. Ideally, microalbuminuria should be correlated with renal histopathology to show a relationship between renal proteinuria and glomerular changes suggestive of the early stages of diabetic nephropathy in feline diabetics.

CAUSE OF DIABETIC NEPHROPATHY

In their recent article on diabetes and the kidney,[7] MacIsaac and Watts break down the cause of diabetic renal disease into initiators of diabetic nephropathy and promoters of diabetic nephropathy. Initiators of diabetic nephropathy include hyperglycemia and genetic predisposition. Promoters of diabetic nephropathy include hyperglycemia and insulin resistance, hypertension, dyslipidemia, long duration of diabetes, anemia, procoagulant state, ethnicity, and smoking. In this article, the contributions of genetics, hyperglycemia, hypertension, and dyslipidemia on the development of diabetic renal disease in human and feline medicine are reviewed. Azotemia and proteinuria as 2 important clinical consequences of diabetic nephropathy are also discussed.

Initiators of Diabetic Nephropathy: Genetics, Hyperglycemia

Genetics
Many candidate genes have been implicated in the susceptibility to development of human diabetic nephropathy. This is an active area of research in human medicine and certainly has important implications in the early recognition, therapy, and possibly prevention of human diabetic nephropathy.

Hyperglycemia
Early in the course of diabetes mellitus, even mild hyperglycemia and poor glycemic control (glycosylated hemoglobin >1.5 times more than normal and possibly as low as >1.2 times more than the normal value of 8.2% in people) is widely recognized as a risk factor for development of diabetic nephropathy in both type 1 and type 2 diabetics.[13,16,20–22] How does hyperglycemia initiate the renal microvascular and ultrastructural changes that result in altered GFR and glomerular blood-ultrafiltrate barrier? Early in the course of diabetes mellitus, hyperglycemia leads to microvascular changes throughout the body, including increased vasoconstriction and increased vascular permeability. End organs most damaged by these microvascular changes include the glomerulus, retina, and peripheral nerves. In the glomerulus, microvascular

changes contribute to the development of thickened glomerular basement membrane, reduced podocyte number, and mesangial expansion typical of diabetic renal disease. Simplistically, these microvascular changes are mediated by cytokines, growth factors, and inflammatory mediators, the expression of which is altered by hyperglycemia. With poor glycemic control, some cells develop increased intracellular glucose, because they are not able to downregulate their cellular glucose intake in response to hyperglycemia. The intracellular hyperglycemia seems to activate signaling pathways that lead to expression of inflammatory and other mediators, which lead to end-organ damage. Some of the pathways implicated include the hexosamine pathway, polyol pathway, protein kinase C activation, and advanced glycated end-product pathway. These pathways may have a common upstream element, which could be a potential therapeutic target to reduce initiation of diabetic nephropathy.[23–25] As described earlier, hyperglycemia and other factors that contribute to the microvascular and ultrastructural changes characteristic of stage 1 and 2 diabetic nephropathy lead the way for the persistent microalbuminuria of stage 3, and eventually the reduced GFR, reduced renal function, and clinical renal disease that characterize stages 4 and 5.

Promoters of Diabetic Nephropathy: Hypertension, Dyslipidemia

Hypertension in human diabetes mellitus

How do intraglomerular and systemic hypertension develop in diabetes and how do they promote diabetic nephropathy? In type 1 diabetes mellitus, systemic hypertension is usually a consequence of renal disease and develops around the time that overt proteinuria develops, in stage 4. Contrastingly, in type 2 diabetics, systemic hypertension is usually diagnosed at the time of diabetes diagnosis, before clinical nephropathy occurs. This situation is the result of a variety of nonrenal causes of hypertension, including obesity, dyslipidemia, older or geriatric age, and metabolic syndrome.[7,15] Regardless of systemic blood pressure, people with stage 1 to 3 diabetic nephropathy uniformly develop hyperfiltration and abnormally increased GFR, which cause intraglomerular hypertension. These changes in renal hemodynamics mediate the progression of diabetic nephropathy, initially by damaging the glomerulus and contributing to structural disease of the glomerular basement membrane and mesangial matrix (stages 1 and 2). This situation leads to microalbuminuria (stage 3) and eventually macroalbuminuria and functional and clinical renal disease (stages 4 and 5).[26,27] The ultrastructural and clinicopathologic changes occur early in the course of both type 1 and type 2 diabetes mellitus, regardless of systemic blood pressure.[26,27] Furthermore, in the face of systemic hypertension, as often occurs in type 2 diabetics in the preclinical stages of diabetic nephropathy, autoregulatory renal vasoconstriction and arteriolar nephrosclerosis augment and accelerate the damage to renal structure and, eventually, function. During stage 4 and 5 clinical renal disease in type 1 and type 2 diabetics, renal disease causes upregulation of the renin-angiotensin-aldosterone system, leading to increased production of the vasoconstrictor angiotensin II, aldosterone, and activation of the sympathetic nervous system. This situation results in vasoconstriction and increased blood volume through sodium and water retention, both of which exacerbate systemic hypertension. It is suspected that aldosterone may also be prosclerotic in the glomerulus.[8] Normalization of blood pressure to less than 130 mm Hg systolic generally slows the progression of diabetic renal disease in both type 1 and type 2 diabetics.[17–19] The American Diabetes Association recommends monitoring systolic and diastolic blood pressure at each routine diabetes visit, to establish repeatability of results. American Diabetes Association guidelines recommend a balanced diet, exercise, and pharmacologic agents to keep the systolic and diastolic blood pressure less than 130/80 for most patients with diabetes.[2] These guidelines also recommend dietary modifications to minimize postprandial hyperglycemia and facilitate weight loss for type 2 diabetics, including either low-fat and energy-restricted diets, or low-carbohydrate diets.

Hypertension in feline diabetes mellitus

There has been mention of blood pressure in several articles on diabetic cats. In Littman's retrospective study on the cause of hypertension in 24 cats,[28] 1 had diabetes mellitus, which was believed to have been secondary to previous dexamethasone injection, whereas 7 had mild hyperglycemia (125–202 mg/dL, normal range 70–110 mg/dL [6.94–11.2 mmol/L, normal range 3.9–6.1 mmol/L]) but no glucosuria, which was attributed to either stress hyperglycemia or insulin resistance. Most of the hyperglycemic cats were also hypercholesterolemic, suggesting that they might have been prediabetic (blood glucose > normal but < diabetic). It was not stated whether these cats had repeated blood or urine glucose measurements, or additional testing such as fructosamine, to determine whether their hyperglycemia was transient (indicating stress hyperglycemia) or persistent (indicating the possibility of prediabetes or diabetes mellitus). It is also not mentioned if any of the 7 hyperglycemic cats overlapped with any of the 6 cats on oral glucocorticoid therapy noted in the study; glucocorticoid therapy is a known risk factor for development of feline diabetes mellitus. All cats in this hypertension study had some evidence of kidney dysfunction; however, it is not known whether this caused or was caused by the hypertension. Two hypertensive cats had glomerulosclerosis, which is a nonspecific finding, but is one of the renal structural changes noted in type 2 diabetic people with nephropathy. It was not noted whether these cats were also hyperglycemic and potentially prediabetic or diabetic. The method of renal biopsy analysis (light vs electron microscopy) was also not mentioned, and light microscopy is an insensitive method for detecting early glomerular lesions associated with diabetic nephropathy. Because hyperglycemia and hypercholesterolemia are both promoters of diabetic nephropathy, and all cats in this study had evidence of kidney dysfunction (including 2 cats with glomerular disease) and hypertension, it is worthwhile considering whether diabetic nephropathy may have caused or contributed to the hypertension in some of these cats.

In a study on ocular lesions in 69 hypertensive cats, Maggio and colleagues[29] found 2 cats with hypertensive retinopathy in which the hypertension was attributed to diabetes mellitus. One of these diabetic cats had evidence of renal dysfunction, whereas the other did not, and neither cat was hyperthyroid.

Recently, Al-Ghazlat and colleagues[10] found that mean systolic blood pressure was higher in diabetic cats than healthy control cats, although the prevalence of systolic blood pressure greater than 160 mm Hg was not different between groups. However, in a more targeted study of hypertension in 14 diabetic cats, Sennello[11] found no hypertension in diabetic cats, where hypertension was strictly defined as systolic blood pressure greater than 180 mm Hg, with at least 1 of the following: hypertensive retinopathy, left ventricular hypertrophy, or proteinuria. This article is often cited as proof that diabetic cats are not hypertensive; however, the study does have certain weaknesses worth noting. First, hypertensive retinopathy in cats can be associated with blood pressure greater than 168 mm Hg, less than the cutoff for hypertension in the Sennello study.[30] Second, although this study measured blood pressure several times within 5 to 10 minutes for each cat, repeatability of blood pressure over longer time points (eg, week to week) was not assessed, as it is in some veterinary studies on hypertension, and this could have led to some hypertensive cats being undetected; this lack of long-term repeatability was likely considered acceptable because of the otherwise strict inclusion criteria in the Sennello study.[31,32] Third, the blood pressure cutoff of systolic blood pressure greater than 180 mm Hg is high compared with some other studies. It is particularly high in light of Kobayashi's finding that a population of normal cats had a mean systolic blood pressure of just 118 ± 10.6 mm Hg, and cats with chronic kidney disease had a mean systolic blood pressure of only 146.6 ± 25.4 mm Hg, and as a group, were considered hypertensive at those pressures, with statistically higher blood pressures than normal cats.[10,31–34] The American College of Veterinary Internal Medicine consensus statement on hypertension states that cats with systolic blood pressure greater than 150 mm Hg are at mild risk of target-organ damage, cats with systolic blood pressure greater than 160 mm Hg likely need antihypertensive therapy, and cats with systolic blood pressure greater than or equal to 180 mm Hg are considered at severe risk of target-organ damage.[35] Fourth, only macroalbuminuria was measured in this study, and the cutoff used (urine protein/creatinine ratio >1) is now considered high; current research suggests less than 0.2 is normal for cats.[36–38] Although Sennello and colleagues[11] reported no difference in systolic blood pressure between diabetic and healthy cats, and concluded that hypertension does not occur, or does not occur commonly, in diabetic cats, the criteria used to define hypertension and renal disease limit the conclusions of the study. Well-designed prospective studies are urgently required to investigate if there is an association between persistent hyperglycemia, hypertension, and renal disease in cats. It is important that further studies use more sensitive cut points for renal disease, hypertension, and hyperglycemia, including lower urine protein/creatinine ratios (<0.4), microalbuminuria, lower blood pressure cutoffs (<180 mm Hg) and fasting glucose concentrations more than 6.5 mmol/L (117 mg/dL). At least 50% of diabetic humans are undiagnosed, and those people classified as prediabetic with persistent mild hyperglycemia less than the level considered diabetic outnumber diabetic patients 4 to 1.[39] Statistics for cats are currently unknown, but are likely to be similar or higher. Therefore, given the incidence of idiopathic renal disease among cats, prospective studies are urgently required to determine if there are associations between persistent hyperglycemia, hypertension, and renal disease in cats, similar to those in humans. In a recent review on endocrine hypertension, Reusch and colleagues[40] concluded that "further studies using larger cohorts of diabetic cats are needed to evaluate questions, such as the definitive prevalence of hypertension and the risk of kidney damage when blood pressure is in the upper end of normal." Human diabetics are often considered hypertensive if systolic blood pressure is greater than 130 to 140 mm Hg.[2]

Severe hypertension as currently defined in veterinary medicine is not common in cats with diabetes mellitus, but well-designed large-scale studies investigating the association between hypertension, glycemic control, duration of diabetes, and renal disease have not been reported. Further investigation is urgently warranted, considering the prevalence of both diabetes mellitus and the prevalence of idiopathic chronic kidney disease in the feline population.

Dyslipidemia in human diabetes mellitus

Dyslipidemia has also been studied as a promoter of diabetic renal disease. There is a clear association in human diabetics between dyslipidemia and microalbuminuria and macroalbuminuria, and type 2 diabetics are particularly at risk for dyslipidemias, including increased low-density lipoprotein (LDL) cholesterol, reduced high-density lipoprotein (HDL) cholesterol, and increased triglycerides.[41] Most likely, dyslipidemia contributes to microvascular dysfunction in various ways, including promotion of renal vascular atherosclerosis.[7,8] In addition to promotion of renal disease, dyslipidemia plays a significant role in diabetic cardiovascular disease. Although the use of statins to control LDL cholesterol does not conclusively alter albumin excretion rate or GFR, dietary and pharmacologic control of dyslipidemia is still routinely recommended for its benefits on cardiovascular disease.[2] The American Diabetes Association recommends a fasting lipid profile including LDL and HDL cholesterol and triglycerides every 1 to 2 years in most adult diabetic patients. American Diabetes Association guidelines recommend diet (limited saturated and trans fat, limited dietary cholesterol, and increased intake of n-3 polyunsaturated fatty acids), exercise, and pharmacologic agents to keep LDL cholesterol less than 70 to 100 mg/dL (1.8–2.6 mmol/L), HDL cholesterol greater than 40 to 50 mg/dL (1.0–1.3 mmol/L), and triglycerides less than 150 mg/dL (1.7 mmol/L) for most patients with diabetes, particularly in those patients with concurrent cardiovascular disease or risk factors.[2]

Dyslipidemia in feline diabetes mellitus

Although cholesterol is not a main focus in current studies on diabetic cats, there are some published data. Diabetic cats' median cholesterol was more than the reference range (median 343 mg/dL [8.9 mmol/L], reference range 77–250 mg/dL [2.0–6.5 mmol/L])and diabetic cats had the highest median cholesterol when compared with groups of cats with hypoproteinemia, hyperproteinemia, azotemia, hyperbilirubinemia, or healthy controls.[42] Three of 10 cats (30%) with diabetes mellitus had hypercholesterolemia at the time of diagnosis; all 3 cats went into diabetic remission after treatment, but follow-up cholesterol values were not reported.[43] In a retrospective study on predictors of clinical remission in 90 newly diagnosed diabetic cats, increased cholesterol decreased the chance of remission by almost 65%, which may be attributable to a direct toxic effect of cholesterol on β cells, or may reflect the role of dyslipidemia in microvascular disease, as recognized in diabetic humans.[44] Although increased cholesterol was associated with decreased probability of remission, it was not statistically analyzed to determine whether this was independent of the level of hyperglycemia. Hypercholesterolemia may also be a reflection of poor glycemic control, and therefore is a biomarker, not an initiator or promoter, of diabetes, nor an independent factor affecting probability of diabetic remission in cats. Although the relationship between glycemic control and triglycerides is linear in people, cholesterol and triglycerides did not correlate well with metabolic control in diabetic cats treated with porcine zinc insulin, when metabolic control was assessed via fructosamine and via 24-hour inhospital blood glucose curves measured 5 times over the first 1 year of treatment.[45] There are no published well-designed studies in diabetic cats investigating the association between dyslipidemia (including lipoprotein profiles), hyperglycemia (including degree and duration) and renal disease.

Diabetic cats are at increased risk of hypercholesterolemia, and this may play a role in the pathogenesis and progression of diabetes mellitus, and adversely affect renal structure and function. Further study is warranted.

Additional Clinical Consequences of Diabetic Nephropathy: Azotemia and Proteinuria

Azotemia in human diabetes mellitus

Azotemia is a consequence of any renal disease that affects the filtration function of the nephrons by more than 75%.[46] Therefore, azotemia is an indicator of the progression and severity of renal disease, including diabetic nephropathy. The American Diabetes Association recommends monitoring serum creatinine at least annually. They recommend using creatinine to estimate GFR and to stage the level of chronic kidney disease, if present.[2]

Azotemia in feline diabetes mellitus

Azotemia is defined as an increase of blood urea nitrogen (BUN) or creatinine more than normal limits. Azotemia is categorized as prerenal (dehydration), renal (kidney disease), and postrenal (lower urinary tract). Postrenal urinary obstruction or leakage is generally easy to exclude on history, clinical examination, and if needed, imaging and laboratory testing. In differentiating between prerenal and renal causes of azotemia, the urine specific gravity is often considered, which is high with prerenal azotemia (in the absence of other disease affecting concentrating ability) and less than normal in renal azotemia. Kidney size and shape are also relied on, which is often smaller and more irregular with chronic kidney disease. Many patients with kidney disease have concomitant prerenal and renal azotemia on admission, and diagnosis and quantification of the renal component can be achieved only once the prerenal dehydration is ameliorated, often with fluid therapy.

There are several complicating factors when categorizing azotemia in diabetic cats. (1) Glucosuria causes osmotic diuresis, thus decreasing the urine specific gravity. However, glucose molecules in urine can also slightly increase the refractive index of urine, artificially increasing the specific gravity reading on a nonautomated refractometer, which is the most common cage-side method of determining urine specific gravity.[47] This situation makes differentiation of prerenal and renal azotemia more difficult in a dehydrated diabetic cat than a dehydrated nondiabetic cat. (2) Diabetic cats and especially cats with diabetic ketosis or ketoacidosis are often clinically dehydrated. Thus, the difficulty separating prerenal and renal azotemia in diabetic cats is a common and important problem in clinical practice. (3) Both diabetes mellitus and chronic kidney disease are common diseases in older cats, and they may exist concurrently in up to 13% to 31% of diabetic cats.[23,48–51] When faced with an azotemic cat with diabetes mellitus and small or irregular kidneys, most clinicians would attribute the azotemia to chronic kidney disease of unknown cause and consider the diabetes mellitus a separate disease. The possibility is not often considered that the 2 could be related. (4) Urea and creatinine are the most widely used measurements of kidney function but are known to be highly insensitive and are believed to be increased only with 75% or greater loss of functional nephrons.[46,52] Thus, lack of azotemia in no way excludes the possibility of nephropathy concurrent with, or as a result of, diabetes mellitus in cats or dogs. (5) As a general rule, proteinuria is considered a marker of glomerular disease, whereas azotemia is a marker of tubular disease, although there is significant overlap in clinical disease. Because diabetic nephropathy in humans often begins as a glomerular disease, it may be that proteinuria is a more appropriate marker than azotemia for diagnosis or investigation of diabetic nephropathy in companion animals. (6) Creatinine may be artificially decreased in animals with loss of lean body mass, which may occur with undiagnosed or poorly controlled diabetes mellitus.

As with cholesterol, azotemia is rarely the main feature but may be reported in articles on diabetes mellitus in cats. In some studies, no diabetic cats are reported to be azotemic.[53–55] In others, diabetic or diabetic ketoacidotic cats are azotemic, likely because of prerenal dehydration.[29,50,56,57] There are also reports of diabetic cats with suspected renal azotemia.[23,44,48–51,58] Thus, it seems that some diabetic cats do have renal azotemia, which begets the question: are these necessarily separate and concurrent diseases or could they be related?

It is difficult to characterize azotemia as prerenal versus renal in diabetic glucosuric cats, and BUN and creatinine are insensitive markers of kidney function; however, up to 31% of diabetic cats have suspected renal azotemia. Further study is warranted and should focus on prospective studies that use multiple measures of kidney function, including urea, creatinine, proteinuria, GFR, and renal histopathology. Studies should focus on both newly diagnosed and chronic diabetics, as well as animals with varied glycemic control.

Proteinuria in human diabetes mellitus

As described earlier, the hemodynamic and ultrastructural changes to the glomerulus in stages 1 and 2 of diabetic nephropathy usually result in microalbuminuria, a hallmark of stage 3 diabetic nephropathy. Microalbuminuria is defined as a subclinical increase in albumin excretion, leading to albumin concentrations in the urine that are more than normal but less than the limits of detection using routine methods for proteinuria measurement, such as the protein dipstick or urine protein/creatinine ratio. The American Diabetes Association defines microalbuminuria as renal albumin excretion of 30 to 299 mg per day in 24-hour urine collection, or 30 to 299 µg albumin per mg creatinine (urine protein/creatinine ratio <0.3) on spot collection.[2] As renal function worsens, diabetics may move into stage 4 diabetic nephropathy, characterized by overt proteinuria or macroalbuminuria, which is defined by the American Diabetes Association as renal albumin excretion of 300 mg per day or higher, or at least 300 µg albumin per mg creatinine (urine protein/creatinine ratio ≥0.3) on spot collection. Macroalbuminuria is detectable on routine methods of urine protein assessment, including the protein dipstick, urine protein/creatinine ratio, and urine albumin/creatinine ratio. Because of their prognostic significance, monitoring of microalbuminuria and macroalbuminuria are considered the best noninvasive tests to predict and follow diabetic kidney disease.[2,7] The American Diabetes Association recommends annual assessment of urine albumin excretion starting 5 years after diagnosis in type 1 diabetics and at the time of diagnosis in type 2 diabetics. Recommendations for assessment of albuminuria include:

- Random spot collection testing for urinary albumin/creatinine ratio (ideal)
- Random spot collection testing for urinary albumin via immunoassay or dipstick that is specific for microalbuminuria (handy, but less sensitive and specific)
- Note that 24-hour or timed collections are considered burdensome without adding significant accuracy

Proteinuria in feline diabetes mellitus

Renal proteinuria in cats can be measured in a variety of ways, is repeatable, and should be interpreted from inactive urine sediment. For cats, microalbuminuria is defined as albuminuria greater than normal (>1.0 mg/dL), but less than the limit of detection using conventional dipstick urine protein screening methodology (≥30 mg/dL).[59] In the clinic, the most common measurement is the protein dipstick colorimetric test, a test for macroalbuminuria, which is easy to use and primarily measures albumin, but does not take urine specific gravity into account, and has many false-positive results and, less commonly, false-negative results.[37,59,60] The American College of Veterinary Internal Medicine guidelines recommend that a positive dipstick test be confirmed with a sulfasalicylic acid or similarly accurate test.[36] The urine protein/creatinine ratio compares urine protein (mainly albumin) with urine creatinine to adjust for urine concentration and is recommended for all companion animals with chronic kidney disease per International Renal Interest Society guidelines, or in any case in which renal proteinuria is suspected.[38,59] Less than 0.2 is believed to be normal in cats, whereas 0.4 or greater is considered overt proteinuria.[36–38] Even mild overt proteinuria of greater than 0.4 is a negative prognostic indicator in cats with chronic kidney disease, and increasing urine protein/creatinine ratio correlates with both increasing creatinine and increasing blood pressure.[61] In 2003, Sennello and colleagues[11] found that none of 14 diabetic cats was proteinuric; however, the cutoff for proteinuria used was urine protein/creatinine ratio of greater than 1, which is now considered high. Using a urine protein/creatinine ratio cutoff of 0.4, a recent study[10] found that the urine protein/creatinine ratio was significantly higher in diabetic than in control cats, with proteinuria in 75% of diabetics and only 20% of nondiabetic control cats. In human medicine, the urine albumin/creatinine ratio is also used to detect overt proteinuria. In cats, this test has been shown to correlate strongly with urine protein/creatinine ratio, but is uncommonly used in research or practice, has not been shown to be superior to urine protein/creatinine ratio measurement in cats, and has not been evaluated in feline diabetes to our knowledge.[45,61]

Microalbuminuria and particularly the semiquantitative E.R.D.-HealthScreen microalbuminuria test (Heska, Loveland, CO), has been validated in cats, is both sensitive and specific, and has been found to increase both with age and with a variety of disease states.[37,62] Microalbuminuria correlates with urine protein/creatinine ratio and is believed to be more sensitive, although instances of positive microalbuminuria with negative urine protein/creatinine ratio and (less understandably) positive urine protein/creatinine ratio with negative microalbuminuria have been reported.[10,37,63] Whittemore and colleagues[45] found no increase in microalbuminuria in cats with endocrine disease; it is not reported whether any diabetic cats were included in this study. Recently, Al-Ghazlat and colleagues[10] found that 70% of diabetic cats were microalbuminuric, which was significantly higher than both healthy controls (18%) and sick, nondiabetic cats (39%).

In human medicine, proteinuria is predictive for development and progression of diabetic nephropathy. Although not widely studied, there is recent evidence to suggest that diabetic cats may be proteinuric. Further study in this area is urgently needed to both confirm and understand the cause of proteinuria in feline diabetes mellitus.

SUMMARY

- The cause of chronic kidney disease is often unknown in cats
- Some diabetic cats do have risk factors or markers that have been reported to be associated with human diabetic renal disease, including proteinuria, hypercholesterolemia, and renal azotemia
- Diabetic cats may have higher blood pressure than nondiabetic cats
- Some diabetic cats do have glomerular disease, and some cats with chronic kidney disease have glomerular disease of unknown cause
- Undiagnosed persistent hyperglycemia consistent with prediabetes or early diabetes is likely common in cats, as it is in humans
- Further study is warranted to explore the risk factors, laboratory and histologic findings, and clinical consequences of renal disease in diabetic cats at varying levels of glycemic control, chronicity of disease, and diabetic remission

REFERENCES

1. American Diabetes Association. Diagnosis and classification of diabetes mellitus. Diabetes Care 2010;33:562–9.
2. American Diabetes Association. Standards of medical care in diabetes-2011. Diabetes Care 2011;34:S11–61.
3. Mogensen CE. Microalbuminuria as a predictor of clinical diabetic nephropathy. Kidney Int 1987;31:673–89.
4. Minkus G, Reusch C, Horauf A, et al. Evaluation of renal biopsies in cats and dogs-histopathology in comparison with clinical data. J Small Anim Pract 1994; 35:465–72.
5. Nakayama H, Uchida K, Ono K, et al. Pathological observation of 6 cases of feline diabetes mellitus. Nihon Juigaku Zasshi 1990;52(4):819–22.

6. Dalla Vestra M, Saller A, Bortoloso E, et al. Structural involvement in type 1 and type 2 diabetic nephropathy. Diabetes Metab 2000;26(Suppl 4):8–14.

7. MacIsaac RJ, Watts GF. Diabetes and the kidney. In: Shaw KM, Cummings MH, editors. Diabetes: chronic complications. Chichester (United Kingdom): John Wiley & Sons; 2006. p. 21–47.

8. Parving H-H, Mauer M, Fioretto P, et al. Diabetic nephropathy. In: Taal MW, Chertow GM, Marsden PA, et al, editors. Brenner and Rector's the kidney, vol. 1, 9th edition. Philadelphia: Elsevier Saunders; 2011. p. 1411–54.

9. Osterby R, Gall MA, Schmitz A, et al. Glomerular structure and function in proteinuric Type 2 (non-insulin-dependent) diabetic patients. Diabetologia 1993; 36(10):1064–70.

10. Al-Ghazlat SA, Langston CE, Greco DS, et al. The prevalence of microalbuminuria and proteinuria in cats with diabetes mellitus. Top Companion Anim Med 2011; 26(3):154–7.

11. Sennello KA, Schulman RL, Prosek R, et al. Systolic blood pressure in cats with diabetes mellitus. J Am Vet Med Assoc 2003;223(2):198–201.

12. Lees GE, Cianciolo RE, Clubb FJ Jr. Renal biopsy and pathologic evaluation of glomerular disease. Top Companion Anim Med 2011;26(3):143–53.

13. Mogensen CE. Microalbuminuria, blood pressure and diabetic renal disease: origin and development of ideas. Diabetologia 1999;42:263–85.

14. Bangstad HJ, Osterby R, Dahl-Jorgensen K, et al. Improvement of blood glucose control in IDDM patients retards the progression of morphologic changes in early diabetic nephropathy. Diabetologia 1994;37:483–90.

15. Mogensen CE. Glomerular hyperfiltration in human diabetes. Diabetes Care 1994;17:770–5.

16. Chase HP, Jackson WE, Hoops SL, et al. Glucose control and the renal and retinal complications of insulin-dependent diabetes. J Am Med Assoc 1989;261(7): 1155–60.

17. Bakris GL, Williams M, Dworkin L, et al. Preserving renal function in adults with hypertension and diabetes: a consensus approach. Am J Kidney Dis 2000;36: 646–61.

18. Parving HH, Jacobsen P, Rossing K, et al. Benefits of long-term antihypertensive treatment on prognosis in diabetic nephropathy. Kidney Int 1996;49:1778–82.

19. Tobe SW, McFarlane PA, Naimark DM. Microalbuminuria in diabetes mellitus. Can Med Assoc J 2002;167(5):499–503.

20. Parving HH. Renoprotection in diabetes: genetic and non-genetic risk factors and treatment. Diabetologia 1998;41:745–59.

21. Diabetes Control and Complications Trial Research Group. The effect of intensive treatment of diabetes on the development and progression of long-term complications in insulin-dependent diabetes mellitus. N Engl J Med 1993;329: 977–86.

22. Nyberg G, Blohme G, Norden G. Impact of metabolic control in progression of clinical diabetic nephropathy. Diabetologia 1987;30:82–6.

23. Ishii H, Jirousek MR, Koya D, et al. Amelioration of vascular dysfunctions in diabetic rats by an oral PKC β inhibitor. Science 1996;272(5262): 728–31.

24. Brownlee M. Biochemistry and molecular cell biology of diabetic complications. Nature 2001;414:813–20.

25. Cooper ME, Brownlee M. Reducing the burden of diabetic vascular complications. In: Greenbaum CJ, Harrison LC, editors. Diabetes: translating research into practice. 1st edition. New York: Informa Healthcare; 2008. p. 159–72.

26. Hostetter TH, Rennke HG, Brenner BM. The case for intrarenal hypertension in the initiation and progression of diabetic and other glomerulopathies. Am J Med 1982;72(3):375–80.
27. MacIsaac RJ, Deckert T, Feldt-Rasmussen T, et al. Albuminuria reflects widespread vascular damage. The Steno hypothesis. Diabetologia 1989;32:219–26.
28. Littman MP. Spontaneous systemic hypertension in 24 cats. J Vet Intern Med 1994;8(2):79–86.
29. Maggio F, DeFrancesco TC, Atkins CE, et al. Ocular lesions associated with systemic hypertension in cats: 69 cases (1985-1998). J Am Vet Med Assoc 2000;217(5):695–702.
30. Sansom J, Rogers K, Wood JL. Blood pressure assessment in healthy cats and cats with hypertensive retinopathy. Am J Vet Res 2004;65(2):245–52.
31. Elliott J, Barber P, Syme H, et al. Feline hypertension: clinical findings and response to hypertensive treatment in 30 cases. J Small Anim Pract 2001;42:122–9.
32. Jepson RE, Elliott J, Brodbelt D, et al. Effect of control of systolic blood pressure on survival in cats with systemic hypertension. J Vet Intern Med 2007;21:402–9.
33. Kobayashi DL, Petersen ME, Graves TK, et al. Hypertension in cats with chronic renal failure or hyperthyroidism. J Vet Intern Med 1990;4:58–62.
34. Henik RA, Stepien RL, Wenholz LJ, et al. Efficacy of atenolol as a single antihypertensive agent in hyperthyroid cats. J Feline Med Surg 2008;10(6):577–82.
35. Brown SA, Atkins C, Bagley R, et al. ACVIM consensus statement: guidelines for the identification, evaluation, and management of systemic hypertension in dogs and cats. J Am Vet Med Assoc 2007;21:542–58.
36. Lees GE, Brown SA, Elliott J, et al. Assessment and management of proteinuria in dogs and cats: 2004 ACVIM Forum Consensus Statement (small animal). J Vet Intern Med 2005;19:377–85.
37. Langston C. Microalbuminuria in cats. J Am Anim Hosp Assoc 2004;40:251–4.
38. International Renal Interest Society. Available at: http://www.iris-kidney.com/. Accessed February 24, 2013.
39. Gavin JR, Alberti K, Davidson MB. Report of the expert committee on the diagnosis and classification of diabetes mellitus. Diabetes Care 2000;23(1):S4–20.
40. Reusch CE, Schellenberg S, Wenger M. Endocrine hypertension in small animals. Vet Clin North Am Small Anim Pract 2010;40(2):335–52.
41. Watts GF, Naumova R, Slavin BM, et al. Serum lipids and lipoproteins in insulin-dependent diabetic patients with persistent microalbuminuria. Diabet Med 1989;6(1):25–30.
42. Reusch CE, Haberer B. Evaluation of fructosamine in dogs and cats with hypo- or hyperproteinaemia, azotaemia, hyperlipidaemia and hyperbilirubinaemia. Vet Rec 2001;148(12):370–6.
43. Nelson RW, Griffey SM, Feldman EC, et al. Transient diabetes mellitus in cats: 10 cases (1989-1991). J Vet Intern Med 1999;13:28–35.
44. Zini E, Hafner M, Osto M, et al. Predictors of clinical remission in cats with diabetes mellitus. J Vet Intern Med 2010;24(6):1314–21.
45. Whittemore JC, Miyoshi Z, Jensen WA, et al. Association of microalbuminuria and the urine albumin-to-creatinine ratio with systemic disease in cats. J Am Vet Med Assoc 2007;230(8):1165–9.
46. Hayman JM, Shumway NP, Dumke P, et al. Experimental hyposthenuria. J Clin Invest 1939;18(2):195–212.
47. Pradella M, Dorizzi RM, Rigolin F. Relative density of urine: methods and clinical significance. Crit Rev Clin Lab Sci 1988;26(3):195–242.

48. Goossens MM, Nelson RW, Feldman EC, et al. Response to insulin treatment and survival in 104 cats with diabetes mellitus (1985-1995). J Vet Intern Med 1998;12: 1–6.
49. Bailiff NL, Nelson RW, Feldman EC, et al. Frequency and risk factors for urinary tract infection in cats with diabetes mellitus. J Vet Intern Med 2006;20(4):850–5.
50. Koenig A, Drobatz KJ, Beale AB, et al. Hyperglycemic, hyperosmolar syndrome in feline diabetics: 17 cases (1995-2001). J Vet Emerg Crit Care (San Antonio) 2004;14(1):30–40.
51. Scott-Moncrieff JC. Insulin resistance in cats. Vet Clin North Am Small Anim Pract 2010;40(2):241–57.
52. Polzin DJ. Chronic kidney disease. In: Ettinger SJ, Feldman EC, editors. Textbook of veterinary internal medicine, vol. 2. St. Louis (MI): Saunders Elsevier; 2010. p. 1990–2020.
53. Michiels L, Reusch CE, Boari A, et al. Treatment of 46 cats with porcine lente insulin–a prospective, multicentre study. J Feline Med Surg 2008;10(5):439–51.
54. Nelson RW, Lynn RC, Wagner-Mann CC, et al. Efficacy of protamine zinc insulin for treatment of diabetes mellitus in cats. J Am Vet Med Assoc 2001;218(1): 38–42.
55. Sieber-Ruckstuhl N, Kley S, Tschuor F, et al. Remission of diabetes mellitus in cats with diabetic ketoacidosis. J Vet Intern Med 2008;22:1326–32.
56. Christopher MM, Broussard JD, Peterson ME. Heinz body formation associated with ketoacidosis in diabetic cats. J Vet Intern Med 1995;9(1):24–31.
57. Claus MA, Silverstein DC, Shofer FS, et al. Comparison of regular insulin infusion doses in critically ill diabetic cats: 29 cases (1999-2007). J Vet Emerg Crit Care (San Antonio) 2010;20(5):509–17.
58. Kraus MS, Calvert CA, Jacobs GJ, et al. Feline diabetes mellitus: a retrospective mortality study of 55 cats (1982-1994). J Am Anim Hosp Assoc 1997;33(2): 107–11.
59. Grauer GF. Proteinuria: measurement and interpretation. Top Companion Anim Med 2011;26(3):121–7.
60. Lyon SD, Sanderson MW, Vaden SL, et al. Comparison of urine dipstick, sulfosalicylic acid, urine protein-to-creatinine ratio, and species-specific ELISA methods for detection of albumin in urine samples of cats and dogs. J Am Vet Med Assoc 2010;236(7):874–9.
61. Syme HM, Markwell PJ, Pfeiffer D, et al. Survival of cats with naturally occurring chronic renal failure is related to severity of proteinuria. J Vet Intern Med 2006;20: 528–35.
62. Loveland, CO: Heska Corporation. Available at: http://www.heska.com/. Accessed February 24, 2013.
63. Mardell EJ, Sparkes AH. Evaluation of a commercial in-house test kit for the semiquantitative assessment of microalbuminuria in cats. J Feline Med Surg 2006;8: 269–78.

Diabetic Ketoacidosis and Hyperosmolar Hyperglycemic State in Cats

Jacquie S. Rand, BVSc, DVSc, MANZVS, DACVIM

KEYWORDS

- Feline • Diabetes mellitus • Ketoacidosis • Hyperosmolar state

KEY POINTS

- Diabetic ketoacidosis (DKA) and hyperosmolar hyperglycemic state are life-threatening presentations of diabetes mellitus.
- Treatment requires careful attention to restoring fluid volume, electrolyte deficits, and acid-base deficits.
- Rapid-acting insulin is used to reverse ketoacidosis and should be administered until blood or urine ketone concentrations have normalized.
- Insulin treatment itself can cause hypokalemia and hypophosphatemia; potassium and phosphate should be supplemented and their levels monitored frequently.
- Hyperosmolar hyperglycemic state is a rare form of complicated diabetes mellitus with a high mortality rate.

INTRODUCTION

Diabetes mellitus is defined as persistent hyperglycemia and is the result of insulin deficiency. Classically, high blood glucose concentrations lead to glucosuria, polyuria, polydipsia, and hyperphagia.[1] Insulin deficiency also results in ketosis, the result of breakdown of triglycerides.[2] Ketosis refers to the presence of triglyceride breakdown products such as β-hydroxybutyrate, acetoacetate, and acetone (the so-called ketone bodies). Insulin deficiency reduces intracellular glucose concentrations to a level that is insufficient for normal metabolism, resulting in some tissues using increased circulating ketones instead of glucose as their main energy source. However, these ketone bodies also lead to diabetic complications. Ketone bodies stimulate the chemoreceptor trigger zone in the medulla oblongata, leading to anorexia and vomiting. Ketosis also contributes to the osmotic diuresis that is present in clinical diabetes mellitus. These clinical signs all contribute to a propensity to dehydration, volume depletion, hypokalemia (and total body potassium deficits), and acidosis that characterizes DKA. Correcting these abnormalities is required to help the patient to survive in the

Centre for Companion Animal Health, School of Veterinary Science, The University of Queensland, Slip Road, Queensland 4072, Australia
E-mail address: j.rand@uq.edu.au

Vet Clin Small Anim 43 (2013) 367–379
http://dx.doi.org/10.1016/j.cvsm.2013.01.004
vetsmall.theclinics.com
0195-5616/13/$ – see front matter Crown Copyright © 2013 Published by Elsevier Inc. All rights reserved.

short term. Controlling ketoacidosis and the associated fluid and electrolyte abnormalities are the key components of stabilizing ketoacidotic diabetic cats and take precedence over controlling blood glucose concentrations on the first day of treatment.

The prognosis for recovery from DKA varies, and reported survival rates from tertiary referral hospitals range from 69% to 84%,[3,4] and up to 96% to 100% in hospitals accepting a mix of referral and primary accession patients.[5,6] Higher survival rates are reported in uncomplicated DKA cases. Cats with severe DKA can readily develop renal failure because severe dehydration coupled with sodium loss results in renal hypoperfusion. Dehydration and electrolyte derangements can also cause hyperviscosity, thromboembolism and severe metabolic acidosis. All these conditions can (and do) cause death in cats with severe DKA. However, cats with DKA that survive to discharge are as likely to achieve remission as diabetic cats without DKA.[7]

Hyperosmolar hyperglycemic state is another life-threatening presentation of diabetes mellitus. Like DKA, the hyperosmolar hyperglycemic state presents with depression, dehydration, hypovolemia, and hypokalemia.[8] Hyperosmolar hyperglycemic state was formerly called nonketotic hyperosmolar diabetes mellitus, but it has been recognized that up to one-third of humans with hyperosmolar hyperglycemia have some degree of ketonemia or acidosis, and hyperosmolar hyperglycemic state is now recognized as being on a continuous spectrum with DKA.

It is important to recognize the time course for development of ketosis and acidosis. Once insulin concentrations are suppressed to fasting levels (despite the presence of hyperglycemia) ketonemia and ketoacidosis can occur within approximately 12 and 16 days, respectively, if uncomplicated by precipitating conditions. Ketoacidosis can occur as early as 4 days after ketonemia is first detected.[9] Approximately 1 week before ketonuria is detectable on dipsticks, fasting visible lipemia is detectable, indicating breakdown of lipids. Once hyperglycemia occurs, the effect of glucose toxicity continues a cycle of suppression of insulin secretion and ever-increasing glucose concentrations. Even in cats with normal residual beta cell mass, marked suppression of insulin secretion occurs on average 4 days after blood glucose concentrations reach 30 mmol/L (540 mg/dL). This highlights the importance of instituting insulin therapy early in newly diagnosed diabetic cats to prevent the development of ketoacidosis. Risk factors for developing DKA include undiagnosed diabetes mellitus, inadequate insulin dose or dosing frequency, missed insulin doses, and intercurrent illnesses such as sepsis or acute necrotizing pancreatitis.

Both DKA and hyperosmolar hyperglycemic patients are more likely than well diabetic patients to have concurrent diseases, including acute pancreatitis, urinary tract infection, pneumonia, chronic kidney disease, neoplasia,[8] and acromegaly.[10] These concurrent diseases can contribute their own clinical signs in affected diabetic cats, altering both the prognosis and the treatment strategies required to manage complicated cases of diabetes. Identifying these diseases early is an important component of addressing the needs of diabetic cats with complications, but the treatment of these diseases is outside the scope of this article.

CLINICAL SIGNS, DIAGNOSIS, AND ASSESSMENT

DKA is suspected in diabetic cats if the cat is unwell (anorexic or inappetant, quiet or depressed), collapsed, moribund, or comatose. Diagnosis requires measurement of the levels of blood or urine ketones and confirmation of acidosis and hyperglycemia. Blood ketone levels can be measured using a portable meter similar to blood glucose meters (eg, Abbott Precision Xtra[11] or Precision Xceed,[12] Abbott GmbH, Wiesbaden,

Germany) or using urinary dipsticks.[13] Ketone meters can also be used as glucose meters with different test strips. Urine ketone levels are routinely measured using commercially available multitest strips (eg, Ketostix and Multistix 10 SG urine reagent strips; Bayer Corporation, Elkhart, IL, USA, and Combur 9 urinary test strips, Roche, Mannheim, Germany). A positive result in urine for ketones confirms the presence of ketosis. However urine testing can miss up to 12% of ketoacidotic cats because the predominant ketone body in cats, β-hydroxybutyrate, is not tested for by commonly available urine test strips and some portable blood ketone meters, which test for acetoacetate and acetone.[13] Portable meters for measuring β-hydroxybutyrate are available (both Abbott Precision Xtra and Xceed measure β-hydroxybutyrate), and these meters are more sensitive for detecting ketosis in cats.

Positive test results for blood or urine ketones alone are not sufficient to diagnose diabetic ketosis because ketone levels can also be elevated by other illnesses, notably hepatic lipidosis. Normal β-hydroxybutyrate concentrations are less than 0.5 mmol/L (5 mg/dL),[14] whereas 99% of sick cats with nondiabetic illness have β-hydroxybutyrate concentrations less than 0.58 mmol/L (6.0 mg/dL).[15] In contrast, cats with DKA typically have β-hydroxybutyrate more than 1 mmol/L (10.4 mg/dL) if acidosis is from ketone production.[13] Using a cutoff point of 1.5 mmol/L for urinary acetoacetate, the sensitivity and specificity of urine dipsticks for detecting DKA in cats were reported to be 82% and 95%, respectively; when used with a cutoff point of 4 mmol/L in plasma, sensitivity and specificity were 100% and 88% for detecting DKA.[11] One study of induced hyperglycemia in cats found that urine dipsticks that tested for acetoacetate produced a positive test result approximately 5 days after β-hydroxybutyrate was detectable in the urine and up to 11 days after β-hydroxybutyrate concentration exceeded the reference range in plasma (0.5 mmol/L).[9] Therefore, cats are ketonemic well before ketones can be detected in urine with a dipstick. Cats with ketonemia but without significant acidosis usually appear as "healthy" diabetic cats.[9] A rare differential diagnosis for ketonuria and glycosuria in cats is proximal tubulopathy (Fanconi-like syndrome). This syndrome has been associated with dried meat treats that are flavored with "smoke flavor." Typically cats have polyuria, polydipsia, and glycosuria. Ketonuria may be present, but persistent hyperglycemia greater than 12 mmol/L (216 mg/dL) is not present.

Hyperosmolar hyperglycemic state (formerly called nonketotic hyperosmolar diabetes but renamed because some human patients with this syndrome do exhibit ketonemia/ketonuria) is diagnosed if blood glucose concentrations are greater than 30 mmol/L (540 mg/dL), plasma osmolarity is greater than 350 mOsm/L, and the cat is moribund or comatose. Plasma osmolarity is measured by osmometry. However, because osmometers are not commonly used in veterinary clinics, estimates of plasma osmolarity are more usually calculated based on the concentrations of sodium, potassium, and glucose.[16] Osmolarity calculations are summarized in **Box 1**. From the formula, hypernatremia has a much greater effect on osmolarity than hyperglycemia; hence, many cats with DKA are protected from marked hyperosmolality by whole-body hyponatremia, despite significant elevation of plasma glucose levels. Although hyperosmolar hyperglycemia is a rare clinical presentation in cats, it is worth considering this entity in any cat that is severely depressed or moribund, because the prognosis is near-hopeless,[17] close 24-hour clinical monitoring is required, and much more care needs to be taken when restoring volume deficits and starting insulin treatment to avoid fatal cerebral edema.

The assessment of unwell diabetic cats should include a detailed history and examination to distinguish uncomplicated from complicated diabetes. The clinical examination should in all cases include urine analysis to detect urinary ketones, urine culture to

---

Box 1
Formula for calculating effective plasma osmolarity using plasma concentrations of sodium, potassium, and glucose

For concentrations reported in International System of units

Plasma osmolarity = 2 × [sodium + potassium] + [glucose]

For concentrations reported in mg/dL for glucose[a]

Plasma osmolarity = 2 × [sodium + potassium] + [glucose/18]

[a] This formula assumes that sodium and chloride concentrations are reported in mEq/L (mmol/L). Some laboratories report sodium and potassium concentrations in mg/dL, in which case the sodium concentration should be converted by dividing by 2.3 and the potassium concentration by 3.9.
    Data from Schermerhorn T, Barr SC. Relationships between glucose, sodium and effective osmolality in diabetic dogs and cats. J Vet Emerg Crit Care 2006;16(1):19–24.

---

check for infection, plasma electrolytes and acid/base status to assess fluid and electrolyte abnormalities, and feline pancreatic lipase (fPL) concentrations. Abdominal ultrasonography and plasma osmolarity (measured or calculated) are indicated in some cats, especially those presenting with severe signs. However, investigation for other diseases revealed by the history, physical examination, or other testing can usually be deferred until the cat has been stabilized.

TESTING FOR CONCURRENT DISEASES

Although ketoacidosis can occur purely as a result of marked insulin deficiency, in many cats, DKA is associated with precipitating factors such as infection and pancreatitis, especially necrotizing pancreatitis. Of cats dying with acute diabetes, necrotizing pancreatitis was the most common underlying cause.[18] Many diseases can be present as complicating factors in cats with complicated diabetes, but several are more common than others and should be tested for routinely. These include urinary tract infection and pancreatitis. Urinary tract infection is common in all diabetic patients, and should be tested for with urine culture, even if the urine sediment is unremarkable and body temperature is normal. If there are increased numbers of leukocytes on urine sediment examination, then antibiotics should be started empirically pending urine culture and sensitivity results. Although lesions of pancreatitis are present in up to half of cats with diabetes, they are also common in nondiabetic cats, and it is unknown in what proportion of diabetic cats pancreatitis is a precipitating cause for DKA or an underlying cause of their diabetes. In a study of 115 cats with a variety of disease conditions, prevalence of histologic evidence of acute and chronic pancreatitis was 16% and 67%, respectively, regardless of the cause of death; even 45% of healthy cats had evidence of chronic pancreatitis.[19] Diagnosis of pancreatitis in cats can be difficult because the clinical signs are nonspecific, and none of the available diagnostic tests have high sensitivity or specificity. fPL testing has a sensitivity of up to 80% for acute pancreatitis[20] and is now available as an in-clinic test[21] (Snap fPL, Idexx Laboratories, Westbrook, ME, USA). Abdominal ultrasonography can be used to assist the diagnosis of pancreatitis. Pancreatitis can result in the pancreas appearing hypoechoic (edema and inflammation) or hyperechoic (fibrosis), the peripancreatic tissues appearing hypoechoic (edema), and biliary sludging or dilation.[22] However, sensitivity of ultrasonography for pancreatitis in cats is generally low (<30%), and the pancreas can appear normal even in cats dying of acute necrotizing pancreatitis. Diagnostic sensitivity varies widely with operator experience and the characteristic of the ultrasound machine and probe. The combination of ultrasonography and fPL assay is currently the most effective way of assessing cats for the presence of pancreatic disease.[22] See article by Carney on Pancreatitis and Diabetes elsewhere in this issue.

TREATMENT OF DIABETIC KETOACIDOSIS
Fluid and Electrolyte Treatment

The first aims of managing cats with DKA are to restore fluid and electrolyte abnormalities and to stop the uncontrolled breakdown of triglycerides to reverse the ketoacidosis. Correction of electrolyte and fluid deficits, and thereby acidosis, is initiated first, followed by reversal of ketone formation with insulin therapy. Common abnormalities that need correction are intravascular fluid deficits,[23] hyponatremia, and hypokalemia.[16] Initial correction of intravascular hypovolemia can be achieved with sodium chloride–containing fluids. Although 0.9% sodium chloride solution is commonly used for water and sodium replacement, it is an unbuffered solution, which is acidifying, so a better choice in cats with DKA might be a buffered fluid such as lactated Ringer's solution or Normosol-R.[8] Although there are no studies reported in cats comparing the efficacy of different fluid therapies for DKA, there is evidence in humans that normal saline is associated with hyperchloremic metabolic acidosis, which prolongs recovery of acid-base abnormalities in humans with DKA.[24] Until evidence in cats is developed on this matter, we recommend balanced electrolyte solutions rather than 0.9% sodium chloride for fluid resuscitation of cats with DKA. The rate of fluid administration should be calculated to provide the combination of the following (**Table 1**):

1. Maintenance fluid needs of a nondiabetic cat (approximately 50 mL/kg/d)
2. Replacement of ongoing losses associated with polyuria (typically 25 mL/kg/d)
3. Correction of volume deficits over a period of 24 hours or so (typically 50–100 mL/kg/d)

The rate of fluid administration depends on clinical assessment of hydration status, degree of shock, and the presence of concurrent disease, which could limit the rate of infusion. Chronic renal failure[25,26] and cardiomyopathy[27,28] are reported to be common in diabetic cats, and the clinician should have an index of suspicion that these might be present. Prerenal azotemia is typically present in cats with DKA, but one study reported 31% of diabetic cats 10 to 15 years of age, and 18% aged 5 to less than 10 years had chronic kidney disease sufficient to cause persistent azotemia[26] and therefore would be expected to have compromised ability to secrete excess fluids. Fluid deficits should be corrected over 12 to 18 hours using typical flow rates of 60 to 150 mL/kg/24 h. Flow rates appropriate for shock therapy should be used for cats with severe signs of dehydration and poor perfusion. However, the flow rate should be reduced if depression worsens, because cerebral edema is a possible complication.

Cats receiving fluid resuscitation should be monitored for both adequate restoration of fluid volume and for adverse effects such as overhydration. Adequacy of fluid replacement can be monitored by weighing cats regularly and checking oral mucous membrane moistness and the capillary refill time.[29] Checking the resting respiratory rate is a practical, sensitive way of monitoring for overhydration. Other ways of checking for overhydration, such as central venous pressure monitoring, are possible for cats when the respiratory rate is unreliable, such as cats that are tachypneic due to severe metabolic acidosis.[29]

Table 1
Summary of key treatment strategies for cats with DKA

Potassium	Phosphate	Crystalline (Regular) Insulin and Glucose	Sodium Chloride, 0.9%
Supplement according to plasma potassium concentration.[23] Monitor every 2–12 h	Starting dose 0.01 mmol (mEq)/kg/h Monitor concentrations every 4–12 h and adjust dose accordingly Consider transfusing if hemolysis is detected or packed cell volume is <20%	Begin insulin 1–2 h after fluid therapy and potassium supplementation has begun. If hypokalemia is still present, continue potassium supplementation and delay starting insulin no longer than 4 h after initiation of fluids	Aim to replace deficit over first 12–36 h. Watch for signs of overhydration. Many diabetic cats have chronic kidney disease and therefore have compromised ability to secrete excess fluids.
Potassium concentration (mmol/L or mEq/L) required in intravenous fluids		Starting dose 0.01 U/kg/h as intramuscular bolus or constant rate infusion	Volume supplied should meet the following requirements.
Plasma potassium concentration (mmol/L; mEq/L)		Aim to decrease blood glucose concentrations by 2–4 mmol/L/h (36–75 mg/dL/h)	Maintenance (50 mL/kg/d) Ongoing losses (25 mL/kg/d) Replace deficit (50–60 mL/kg/d)
>3.5 20		Add 2.5% glucose to the intravenous fluids when blood glucose concentration decreases to <15 mmol/L (270 mg/dL)	Typical flow rates are 60–150 mL/kg/24 h
3–3.5 30		Add 5% when blood glucose level is <8 mmol/L (144 mg/dL) to maintain insulin infusion until ketones are negative in urine or blood	If infusion rates at the higher end are associated with worsening depression, reduce the flow rate because cerebral edema is a possible complication
2.5–3 40		**Glargine protocol**	
2–2.5 60		2 U glargine per cat subcutaneously on initiation of fluid and electrolyte replacement	
<2 80		Begin 1 U per cat glargine intramuscularly, 1–2 h later (up to 4 h if persistent hypokalemia)	
		Repeat intramuscular glargine 4 or more hours later if glucose is >14 mmol/L (252 mg/dL)	
		Continue subcutaneous glargine every 12 h Provide intravenous glucose as described earlier to maintain blood glucose levels 12–14 mmol/L (216–255 mg/dL) in the first 24 h	

See text for treatment of hyperosmolar hyperglycemic state.

Almost all cats with DKA or hyperosmolar hyperglycemia have total-body potassium depletion. However, this can be masked because acidosis causes translocation of intracellular potassium to the extracellular fluid space, so that some cats present with normal or increased plasma potassium concentrations. Diabetic cats also experience higher-than-normal losses of potassium due to diuresis. Total-body potassium is expected to be low in all diabetic cats regardless of the plasma potassium concentration, so supplementation should be started along with intravascular fluids. Therefore, potassium should be added routinely to resuscitation fluids of cats with DKA or hyperosmolar hyperglycemia, unless hyperkalemia is documented (see **Table 1**).[23] If plasma potassium concentrations are normal, then providing 40 mEq/L of potassium in resuscitation fluids is a reasonable starting point. If plasma potassium concentrations are low, then potassium should be added to the balanced electrolyte solution according to commonly used guidelines,[23] and plasma potassium concentrations should be measured at least 2 or 3 times daily in the first 24 to 48 hours to ensure that supplementation is adequate and covers ongoing losses through polyuria.

Acidosis usually improves rapidly with institution of fluid therapy and resolves once ketosis is corrected, so that bicarbonate or other specific treatment of acidosis is usually not necessary.[30] However, if there is severe acidosis (pH less than 7 and plasma bicarbonate concentrations less than 7 mmol/L; 7 mEq/L) and there are signs of symptomatic acidosis such as hyperventilation, decreased cardiac contractility, or peripheral vasodilation, then bicarbonate supplementation might be indicated. For human patients with DKA, the American Diabetes Association recommends bicarbonate supplementation only if arterial pH remains less than 7.0 mmol/L (mEq/L) after 1 hour of fluid therapy. The disadvantages of bicarbonate therapy include accelerated development of hypokalemia and hypophosphatemia, and unless acidosis is severe and not responsive to fluid therapy, the disadvantages of supplementation greatly outweigh the advantages. Bicarbonate is added at the rate of $0.3 \times$ body weight (kg) $\times (24 -$ patient bicarbonate) per day, with 25% to 50% of this dose in the first few hours of treatment.[23] Acid-base analysis and plasma potassium concentration should be monitored more frequently if bicarbonate therapy is instituted, because changes in plasma pH can cause rapid changes in plasma potassium concentration.

Insulin administration allows the translocation of glucose from the extracellular to the intracellular space in glucose-sensitive tissues (especially skeletal muscle and adipose tissue).[31] This translocation of glucose is accompanied by water, potassium, and phosphate.[8] It is important to anticipate the shifts in concentrations of potassium and phosphate and to monitor their concentrations regularly in cats with DKA, because failure to supplement potassium and phosphate adequately can result in life-threatening hypokalemia[2] and hypophosphatemia.[2,32] Hypokalemia can result in muscle weakness, arrhythmia, and poor renal function.[8]

Hypophosphatemia can be present at the time of diagnosis[2,32] but more commonly develops with insulin treatment in anorexic cats. Hypophosphatemia can result in hemolytic anemia if phosphate concentrations decrease to less than 0.3 to 0.45 mmol/L (1–1.5 mg/dL).[32] Prevention of this complication should be initiated before or at the same time as insulin treatment of DKA using a constant rate infusion of potassium phosphate or by adding potassium phosphate to intravenous fluids. Because potassium is also usually depleted in DKA, one approach is to divide potassium equally as potassium chloride and potassium phosphate. Alternatively, potassium phosphate (KPO4) can be infused at 0.01 to 0.03 mmol/kg/h (0.03–0.09 mg/kg/h) increasing to 0.12 mmol/kg/h (0.36 mg/kg/h) if necessary. Calcium-containing solutions such as Ringer's solution are incompatible with phosphate-containing additives. Some cats require a blood transfusion if packed cell volume drops substantially. This condition may occur despite supplementation with phosphate. Excessive phosphorus supplementation can cause iatrogenic hypocalcemia and its resultant signs, including neuromuscular signs, hypotension, and hypernatremia. Treatment recommendations are summarized in **Table 1**.

Treatment of hyperosmolar hyperglycemic state differs from treatment of DKA because these cats are more likely to be severely chronically dehydrated.[8] Cats with hyperosmolar hyperglycemia commonly have normal to elevated sodium concentrations, and because they have poor glomerular filtration, glucose concentrations are typically twice as high (average 41 mmol/L; 750 mg/dL) as in cats with DKA or uncomplicated diabetes (average 20 mmol/L; 350 mg/dL).[17] Therefore, cats with hyperosmolar hyperglycemia have substantially higher calculated total and effective osmolarity than cats with DKA or uncomplicated diabetes,[17] so that there is potential for large fluid shifts when intravenous fluids are administered, which means that if plasma osmolarity or glucose concentrations are lowered before intracellular glucose and osmolarities have equilibrated, a concentration gradient develops between plasma and intracellular fluid. If marked, this can cause catastrophic effects such as cerebral edema. In addition, almost all cats with hyperosmolar hyperglycemia have other serious diseases concurrently, including kidney failure or neoplasia (but are less likely to have pancreatitis).[17] Therefore, fluid resuscitation for these cats needs to be more conservative, aiming to restore fluid deficits over 36 to 48 hours. It is recommended that 60% to 80% of the deficit be replaced during 24 hours, but serum osmolarity should not be decreased by more than 0.5 to 1 mOsm/h. Insulin infusion rates can be lower because insulin is not required to treat severe ketosis, which by definition is not present in classical hyperosmolar hyperglycemic state.

Insulin Treatment to Control Ketosis

The key to controlling ketoacidosis is to administer insulin in a way that is easily adjustable depending on response to treatment and clinical circumstances. Four methods have been documented for this in cats—intravenous constant rate infusions of regular insulin,[6,33] intramuscular injections of regular insulin,[33] combined subcutaneous and intramuscular injections of glargine,[5] and subcutaneous glargine combined with a constant rate infusion of regular insulin. The aim of this treatment is to control ketoacidosis, not necessarily to control hyperglycemia, because it is the ketoacidosis that causes anorexia, depression, vomiting, and acid-base disturbances. However, because the level of blood glucose is more easily measured in most clinics than that of blood ketones, and because hypoglycemia is a potential adverse effect of using insulin to control ketoacidosis, a decrease in blood glucose level is often measured both as a surrogate marker to determine the effective rate of insulin administration and to check for the development of iatrogenic hypoglycemia.

It is important to commence fluid and electrolyte replacement before commencing insulin therapy, because insulin therapy worsens hypokalemia and hypophosphatemia, sometimes markedly, resulting in potentially fatal weakness, cardiac conduction disturbances, and hemolysis. Although the timing of insulin therapy varies with the experience of each veterinarian, in general it is best to wait 1 to 2 hours after commencement of fluid therapy. Insulin therapy can be started if potassium concentrations are within the normal range after 2 hours of fluid therapy. If the serum potassium concentration is still less than 3.5 mmol/L (3.5 mEq/L), insulin therapy can be delayed a further 1 to 2 hours. This method allows fluid therapy to correct the potassium deficit. However, insulin therapy should start within 4 hours of starting replacement fluids. The aim with insulin treatment is to gradually decrease blood glucose concentrations by approximately 2 to 4 mmol/L/h (36–75 mg/dL/h) until the glucose concentration is between 12 and 14 mmol/L (216–250 mg/dL). Because diabetic cats have been hyperglycemic typically for weeks, and in many cases glucose concentrations have been increasing over months, tissue function has accommodated to this increase in glucose concentration. Therefore, although it is satisfying for the clinician to rapidly normalize glucose concentrations, in humans, intensive glucose control in critically ill patients has been shown to not reduce mortality and does come with increased risk of hypoglycemia.[34]

For the intravenous insulin protocol, short-acting regular crystalline insulin (such as Actrapid) is used because both the time of onset of action and the duration of action are short so that doses can be titrated to effects. Arbitrary starting doses of 0.05 IU/kg/h (1.1 units/kg/d) have been recommended in leading texts[35] and review articles[8,30] and have traditionally been used. These values are 50% lower than those recommended for dogs. These dose rates are based on experience in dogs and humans and modified by expert opinion and clinical experience in cats,[6] but one study found that all cats had their insulin infusions reduced within the first 24 hours, and none were given more than 0.9 units/kg/d.[6] The actual administered doses of insulin were much lower than the prescribed doses, making it necessary to reassess the published recommended doses of insulin for treatment of DKA in cats. This study highlights the rapidly changing status of cats with DKA and the need to adjust insulin doses based on clinical response. Insulin infusion rates are adjusted based on the rate of decrease in glucose concentrations, and it is important that the glucose concentration is not decreased too quickly. Unpublished data (Marshall and Rand, 2007) show that glargine can also be administered intravenously in cats with DKA.

There are 2 main methods for intravenous insulin administration.

Method 1: Add 25 units of regular crystalline insulin (not Lente or Neutral Protamine Hagedorn) to a 500-mL bag of 0.9% saline, lactated Ringer's solution or Normosol-R to produce a concentration of 50 mU/mL. Infuse this at 1 mL/kg/h. Monitor blood glucose hourly and adjust the infusion rate up or down to achieve a decrease in blood glucose concentration of between 2 and 4 mmol/L/h (approximately 50–75 mg/dL/h).

Method 2: To a 250-mL bag of 0.9% saline, add 1.1 units of crystalline insulin (eg, Actrapid) per kilogram of body weight and start the infusion at 10 mL/h to provide approximately 0.05 U/kg/h. Adjust the rate of infusion based on subsequent blood glucose concentration.

For both intravenous methods described earlier, infuse insulin until blood glucose concentration decreases to 12 to 14 mmol/L (216–250 mg/dL), then halve the rate of flow or switch to intramuscular administration of regular insulin every 4 to 6 hours. Alternatively, if hydration status is good, switch to subcutaneous administration of regular insulin every 6 to 8 hours or standard maintenance insulin subcutaneously. Insulin adsorbs to the plastics used to make intravenous fluid lines. Account for this by running 50 to 100 mL of the insulin solution through the line and discarding this to saturate the insulin binding sites. Use an infusion or syringe pump to administer insulin via a second infusion line. This pump can be attached using a 3-way tap to the maintenance fluid line. Two separate catheters can also be used to provide insulin and fluids separately.

Once glucose concentrations decrease to less than 10 to 12 mmol/L (180–216 mg/dL), add 50% dextrose to the fluids to create a 5% dextrose solution (eg, 50 mL of 50% dextrose in 500 mL of fluids). This addition prevents blood glucose concentration decreasing too much and resulting in hypoglycemia while enabling insulin therapy to be maintained to reverse ketone production.

Intramuscular injection of regular insulin has been used in cats, adapted from protocols used in dogs.[36] For intramuscular insulin protocols, insulin is administered in small boluses every 1 to 4 hours. An initial bolus of 0.2 IU/kg is followed by boluses of 0.1 IU/kg until target glucose concentrations (see later) are attained; then switch to maintenance subcutaneous insulin injections. This method is less predictable than intravenous insulin administration, and insulin absorption might be affected by poor perfusion in dehydrated cats.[8]

Once glucose concentrations are less than 14 mmol/L (the renal threshold for glucose), the insulin administration rate or frequency is maintained and glucose is added to the intravenous infusion fluids to prevent hypoglycemia. Insulin infusion or intramuscular injection continues until blood or urine ketones are within the normal range. Once this is achieved, subcutaneous insulin administration can replace intravenous or intramuscular insulin. The type of insulin chosen should be that which is intended to be used long term, such as insulin glargine, detemir, or Protamine zinc insulin.[37]

In human patients, intravenously administered glargine has an almost identical effect on blood glucose as regular insulin, and the duration of action for both types of insulin is approximately 2 hours.[38] Work by the author's group has validated the use of insulin glargine administered intramuscularly for control of DKA in cats.[5] This study was one of the few studies in cats to examine the efficacy and adverse effects of a treatment method for DKA in cats. Glargine was administered either alone or, in most cats, together with subcutaneous glargine. Based on this study, it is recommended that insulin glargine be administered subcutaneously at 2 U per cat at the time of initiation of fluid therapy and intramuscularly at a dose of 1 IU per cat approximately 1 to 2 hours or longer after initiation of fluid therapy, depending on potassium concentrations. These doses are regardless of body weight and are not per kilogram. Blood glucose concentrations should be checked every 2 to 4 hours. The intramuscular dose (0.5–1 IU) should be repeated after 4 or more hours (in some cats it was as long as 22 hours) if the blood glucose concentration is greater than 14 to 16 mmol/L (250–290 mg/dL). Aim to attain blood glucose concentration decreases of 2 to 3 mmol/L/h (36–54 mg/dL/h). The subcutaneous dose should be repeated every 12 hours. In this study, the median time until the second intramuscular insulin dose was 4 hours (range 2–6 hours) for cats treated with intramuscular glargine alone and 14 hours (range 2–22 hours) for cats treated with intramuscular and subcutaneous glargine (most cats). Half the cats required only 1 intramuscular injection, and for most cats in this study transition to subcutaneous insulin was within 24 hours (range 18–72 hours). Most cats received a total of 1 to 3 doses of glargine before being managed with subcutaneous glargine alone. Intravenous glucose was administered if blood glucose concentration decreased less than 10 mmol/L (180 mg/dL) (standard protocol 1 g/kg of 50% intravenous glucose over 5 minutes followed by continuous infusion of 2.5% glucose solution). The blood glucose concentration should be kept between 10 to 14 mmol/L (180–252 mg/dL) while continuing to administer insulin—as a minimum, subcutaneous insulin twice daily. Where owner finances restricted overnight patient monitoring, the evening insulin dose was conservative or withheld and intravenous fluids were changed to a 2.5% glucose containing solution overnight to reduce the chance of life-threatening hypoglycemia occurring while there was limited or no monitoring. All cats survived to discharge, and no cases of clinical hypoglycemia were observed, although 2 of the 15 cats exhibited blood glucose concentrations lower than 3 mmol/L (54 mg/dL). One practical advantage of this method is that clinics that see cases of DKA infrequently and do not have regular insulin in stock can use the same type of insulin that is used for long-term maintenance for management of DKA.[5] This favorable outcome, and less-intensive and therefore less-expensive protocol, may encourage some owners who would euthanize because of cost and poor prognosis, to consider treating their cat. In this study and another study of cats with DKA,[7] many cats went on to achieve remission.

Subcutaneously administered glargine is also effective in human DKA patients.[39] The addition of subcutaneous glargine led to faster resolution of acidosis and reduced the duration of hospitalization in children with DKA treated with a constant rate infusion of regular insulin.[40] In cats with DKA, a protocol similar to that of the author using subcutaneous glargine combined with regular insulin intramuscularly resulted in faster resolution of ketoacidosis than did a continuous infusion of regular insulin.[5]

Hyperglycemic hyperosmolar syndrome requires much slower restoration of volume deficits and plasma glucose concentrations because the neuronal intracellular glucose concentrations and osmolarity are elevated. If plasma glucose concentrations and osmolarity are corrected too rapidly, neuronal osmolarity remains elevated, resulting in an osmotic gradient that causes a shift of water from plasma into the cerebral intracellular space. This shift has the potential to cause cerebral edema, which is difficult to observe clinically in an already moribund cat, and is often fatal before it is recognized. In these cats, it is recommended to slowly restore volume deficits before attempting to reduce glucose concentrations. Intravascular fluid deficits are corrected over 36 to 48 hours. This method improves perfusion and reduces hyperglycemia by permitting renal glucose losses. Once plasma volume is restored, insulin treatment is started using protocols similar to those for DKA but aiming to reduce blood glucose concentrations much more slowly.

Finally, cats with ketoacidosis or hyperosmolar hyperglycemic state need to eat as soon as possible because prolonged anorexia can result in further complications; this is especially the case in obese cats. Low-carbohydrate foods are preferred, but any foods preferred by the cat can be used initially to encourage voluntary food intake. Force feeding is occasionally necessary but can lead to food aversion.

SUMMARY

Treating ketoacidotic or hyperosmolar diabetic cats is challenging and requires careful attention to supportive care by restoring fluid and electrolyte deficits while addressing the underlying need for insulin to control ketosis and hyperglycemia. Hyperglycemic hyperosmolar state is a rare form of complicated diabetes with poor prognosis. DKA has a generally good prognosis with appropriate treatment, and many cats go on to achieve remission. Early diagnosis of diabetes mellitus and institution of appropriate insulin therapy prevents these complications.

ACKNOWLEDGMENTS

Manuscript preparation and editorial assistance was provided by Kurt Verkest of VetWrite vetwrite@gmail.com.

REFERENCES

1. Rand JS, Fleeman LM, Farrow HA, et al. Canine and feline diabetes mellitus: nature or nurture? J Nutr 2004;134(Suppl 8):2072S–80S.
2. Nichols R. Complications and concurrent disease associated with diabetes mellitus. Semin Vet Med Surg 1997;12(4):263–7.
3. Bruskiewicz K, Nelson R, Feldman E, et al. Diabetic ketosis and ketoacidosis in cats: 42 cases (1980-1995). J Am Vet Med Assoc 1997;211(2):188.

4. Kley S, Casella M, CR. Diabetic ketoacidosis in 22 cats (1997-2002) [abstract]. 12th ECVIM-C. A/ESVIM Congress. Munich (Germany): 2002. http://www.vin.com/ecvim/2002

5. Marshall R, Rand J, Gunew M, et al. Intramuscular glargine with or without concurrent subcutaneous administration for treatment of feline diabetic ketoacidosis: a preliminary study. Journal of Veterinary Emergency and Critical Care 2013. http://dx.doi.org/10.111/vec.12038.

6. Claus MA, Silverstein DC, Shofer FS, et al. Comparison of regular insulin infusion doses in critically ill diabetic cats: 29 cases (1999–2007). J Vet Emerg Crit Care 2010;20(5):509–17.

7. Sieber-Ruckstuhl N, Kley S, Tschuor F, et al. Remission of diabetes mellitus in cats with diabetic ketoacidosis. J Vet Intern Med 2008;22(6):1326–32.

8. O'Brien MA. Diabetic emergencies in small animals. Vet Clin North Am Small Anim Pract 2010;40(2):317.

9. Link KRJ, Allio I, Reinecke M, et al. The effect of experimentally induced chronic hyperglycaemia on serum and pancreatic insulin, pancreatic islet IGF-I and plasma and urinary ketones in domestic cat (Felis felis) Journal of General and Comparative Endocrinology in press March 2013.

10. Niessen SJ, Petrie G, Gaudiano F, et al. Feline acromegaly: an underdiagnosed endocrinopathy? J Vet Intern Med 2007;21(5):899–905.

11. Zeugswetter F, Rebuzzi L. Point-of-care β-hydroxybutyrate measurement for the diagnosis of feline diabetic ketoacidaemia. J Small Anim Pract 2012;53(6):328–31.

12. Weingart C, Lotz F, Kohn B. Validation of a portable hand-held whole-blood ketone meter for use in cats. Vet Clin Pathol 2012;41(1):114–8.

13. Zeugswetter F, Pagitz M. Ketone measurements using dipstick methodology in cats with diabetes mellitus. J Small Anim Pract 2009;50(1):4–8.

14. Aroch I, Shechter-Polak M, Segev G. A retrospective study of serum β-hydroxybutyric acid in 215 ill cats: clinical signs, laboratory findings and diagnoses. Vet J 2012;191(2):240–5.

15. Zeugswetter F, Handl S, Iben C, et al. Efficacy of plasma ß-hydroxybutyrate concentration as a marker for diabetes mellitus in acutely sick cats. J Feline Med Surg 2010;12(4):300–5.

16. Schermerhorn T, Barr SC. Relationships between glucose, sodium and effective osmolality in diabetic dogs and cats. J Vet Emerg Crit Care 2006;16(1):19–24.

17. Koenig A, Drobatz KJ, Beale AB, et al. Hyperglycemic, hyperosmolar syndrome in feline diabetics: 17 cases (1995–2001). J Vet Emerg Crit Care 2004;14(1):30–40.

18. Goossens MM, Nelson RW, Feldman EC, et al. Response to insulin treatment and survival in 104 cats with diabetes mellitus (1985–1995). J Vet Intern Med 1998;12(1):1–6.

19. De Cock H, Forman M, Farver T, et al. Prevalence and histopathologic characteristics of pancreatitis in cats. Vet Pathol 2007;44(1):39–49.

20. Forman M, Marks S, Cock H, et al. Evaluation of serum feline pancreatic lipase immunoreactivity and helical computed tomography versus conventional testing for the diagnosis of feline pancreatitis. J Vet Intern Med 2004;18(6):807–15.

21. Forman M, Shiroma J, Armstrong P, et al. Evaluation of feline pancreas-specific lipase (Spec fPL) for the diagnosis of feline pancreatitis [ACVIM abstract 165]. J Vet Intern Med 2009;23(3):733–4.

22. Zoran DL. Pancreatitis in cats: diagnosis and management of a challenging disease. J Am Anim Hosp Assoc 2006;42(1):1–9.

23. Panciera D. Fluid therapy in endocrine and metabolic disorders. Fluid, electrolyte and acid-base disorders in small animal practice. 3rd edition. Philadelphia: Saunders; 2006. p. 478–89.
24. Stowe ML. Plasma-Lyte vs. normal saline: preventing hyperchloremic acidosis in fluid resuscitation for diabetic ketoacidosis. MSc thesis 2012. http://commons.pacificu.edu/pa/296. 2012.
25. Kraus M, Calvert C, Jacobs G, et al. Feline diabetes mellitus: a retrospective mortality study of 55 cats (1982-1994). J Am Anim Hosp Assoc 1997;33(2):107–11.
26. Roomp K, Rand J. Intensive blood glucose control is safe and effective in diabetic cats using home monitoring and treatment with glargine. J Feline Med Surg 2009;11(8):668–82.
27. Peterson ME, Taylor RS, Greco DS, et al. Acromegaly in 14 cats. J Vet Intern Med 1990;4(4):192–201.
28. Little C, Gettinby G. Heart failure is common in diabetic cats: findings from a retrospective case-controlled study in first-opinion practice. J Small Anim Pract 2008; 49(1):17–25.
29. Monaghan K, Nolan B, Labato M. Feline acute kidney injury 2. Approach to diagnosis, treatment and prognosis. J Feline Med Surg 2012;14(11):785–93.
30. Kerl ME. Diabetic ketoacidosis: treatment recommendations. Compend Contin Educ Vet 2001;23(4):330–40.
31. Marshall RD, Rand JS, Morton JM. Glargine and protamine zinc insulin have a longer duration of action and result in lower mean daily glucose concentrations than lente insulin in healthy cats. J Vet Pharmacol Ther 2008;31:205–12.
32. Adams LG, Hardy RM, Weiss DJ, et al. Hypophosphatemia and hemolytic anemia associated with diabetes mellitus and hepatic lipidosis in cats. J Vet Intern Med 1993;7(5):266–71.
33. Macintire DK. Emergency therapy of diabetic crises: insulin overdose, diabetic ketoacidosis, and hyperosmolar coma. Vet Clin North Am Small Anim Pract 1995;25:639–50.
34. Wiener RS, Wiener DC, Larson RJ. Benefits and risks of tight glucose control in critically ill adults. JAMA 2008;300(8):933–44.
35. Feldman E, Nelson R. Diabetic ketoacidosis. Canine and feline endocrinology and reproduction. 3rd edition. St Louis (MO): WB Saunders Co; 2004. p. 580–615.
36. Chastain C, Nichols C. Low-dose intramuscular insulin therapy for diabetic ketoacidosis in dogs. J Am Vet Med Assoc 1981;178(6):561–4.
37. Rand JS, Marshall RD. Diabetes mellitus in cats. Vet Clin North Am Small Anim Pract 2005;35(1):211.
38. Scholtz H, Pretorius S, Wessels D, et al. Equipotency of insulin glargine and regular human insulin on glucose disposal in healthy subjects following intravenous infusion. Acta Diabetol 2003;40(4):156–62.
39. Umpierrez GE, Jones S, Smiley D, et al. Insulin analogs versus human insulin in the treatment of patients with diabetic ketoacidosis: a randomized controlled trial. Diabetes Care 2009;32(7):1164–9.
40. Shankar V, Haque A, Churchwell KB, et al. Insulin glargine supplementation during early management phase of diabetic ketoacidosis in children. Intensive Care Med 2007;33(7):1173–8.

Continuous Glucose Monitoring in Small Animals

Sean Surman, DVM, MS, DACVIM[a],*, Linda Fleeman, BVSc, PhD, MANZCVS[b]

KEYWORDS

- Diabetes mellitus • Continuous glucose monitoring systems
- Self-monitoring of blood glucose • Interstitial fluid • Subcutaneous • Cat • Dog

KEY POINTS

- Continuous glucose monitoring systems have proved to be accurate in small animal patients for monitoring sick/hospitalized and long-term stable diabetic patients.
- The most important advantage of continuous glucose monitoring over intermittent blood glucose measurements is that it facilitates detection of brief periods of hypoglycemia and provides information overnight. A greater number of data points are obtained over a longer time frame allowing for identification of asymptomatic hypoglycemia and Somogyi phenomena that may be missed with traditional monitoring. Monitoring overnight aids in the identification of nocturnal hypoglycemia.
- Other advantages include that it is less time consuming for staff compared with traditional monitoring; reduces patient stress and stress-related hyperglycemia; reduces the frequency of venipuncture and duration of indwelling catheterization; and affords the ability to make adjustments to treatment plans that may not be indicated based on traditional glucose monitoring methods.
- Disadvantages include the initial cost associated with purchasing a system; limited recording range of 40 to 400 mg/dL (2.2–22.2 mmol/L) for the MiniMed Gold, Guardian Real-Time, i-Pro, Seven Plus, and FreeStyle Navigator, and 20 to 600 mg/dL (1.1–33.3 mmol/L) for the GlucoDay; difficulty initializing and calibrating when glucose values are outside the recording range; limited wireless range for the Guardian Real-Time of only 1.5 m; lack of accuracy in dehydrated, hypovolemic, or shock patients; and lag time that may be seen between changes in plasma and interstitial glucose.

INTRODUCTION

Continuous glucose monitoring systems were initially developed for human use as an alternative to traditional blood glucose monitoring methods. Their primary use has been in the monitoring of hospitalized patients, both diabetic and nondiabetic, and

Disclosures: None.
[a] Small Animal Internal Medicine, Small Animal Clinic & Veterinary Teaching Hospital, School of Veterinary Science, The University of Queensland, Therapies Road, St Lucia, Queensland 4072, Australia; [b] Animal Diabetes Australia, Boronia Veterinary Clinic and Hospital, 181 Boronia Road, Boronia, Victoria 3155, Australia
* Corresponding author.
E-mail address: s.surman@uq.edu.au

Vet Clin Small Anim 43 (2013) 381–406
http://dx.doi.org/10.1016/j.cvsm.2013.01.002
0195-5616/13/$ – see front matter © 2013 Elsevier Inc. All rights reserved.

vetsmall.theclinics.com

in self-monitoring of blood glucose. The goals of their use in hospitalized patients are to identify and promptly resolve hyperglycemia and hypoglycemia, which could affect morbidity and mortality, and reduce the need for frequent blood sampling. The goals of their use in self-monitoring of blood glucose are to improve glycemic control, prevent hyperglycemia and hypoglycemia, and thus delay the onset of diabetic complications and improve quality of life. Similar benefits can be achieved in veterinary patients. The use of continuous glucose monitoring systems in veterinary medicine is fairly new, but its use has increased over the past 10 years, with improved technology and veterinarian experience.

Several systems are available for human diabetic patients and some have been used in veterinary patients. These monitors differ in the method used to measure glucose and in various other features that are reviewed later in this article.

PATIENT GROUPS THAT BENEFIT FROM CONTINUOUS GLUCOSE MONITORING
Critical Care (Sick/Hospitalized Diabetic and Nondiabetic Patients): Usefulness

Diabetic cats and dogs are often hospitalized for treatment of illness both unrelated to, and as a complication of, their diabetes. Although the incidence of diabetic ketoacidosis in veterinary patients is unknown, it is recognized as a common life-threatening endocrine disorder in both cats and dogs[1–4]; 1 study found that 62% of cats with ketoacidosis were newly diagnosed diabetics.[1] Any concurrent illness in diabetic patients that causes inappetence, anorexia, or vomiting is rapidly complicated by dehydration, depression, and ketosis. Most diabetic cats that present with diabetic ketoacidosis have at least 1 concurrent disease; liver disease and pancreatitis are the most common.[1] In cats, diabetes mellitus is more commonly a sequela of pancreatitis rather than a risk factor for its development. An evaluation of pancreatitis in cats revealed that only 3% of cats with acute pancreatitis and 15% of cats with chronic pancreatitis had concurrent diabetes mellitus.[5] This is in contrast to dogs in which diabetes is usually classified as a preexisting condition.[3,6–8] Studies report concurrent pancreatitis in 13% to 36% of diabetic dogs[6–8] and in up to 52% of dogs with diabetic ketoacidosis.[3]

Hospitalized diabetics, regardless of the reason for hospitalization, still require insulin therapy. These patients are ideally treated with either a constant rate infusion[9–11] or intermittent intramuscular injections of short-acting insulin.[12] These intensive insulin treatments require close monitoring to ensure appropriate control of hyperglycemia and ketosis, while preventing complications caused by overly rapid correction of hyperglycemia, such as cerebral edema[2,13,14] or insulin-induced hypoglycemia. Such is also the case for nondiabetic patients at risk for altered glucose homeostasis, which includes critical care patients with a variety of conditions[15] including trauma, sepsis, the systemic inflammatory response syndrome,[16–18] portosystemic shunt,[19,20] insulinoma,[21] and liver failure,[22] as well as pediatric patients.

In human intensive care units, hyperglycemia occurs in up to 90% of all critically ill patients and is associated with increased morbidity and mortality.[23–26] The prevalence of hyperglycemia in critically ill nondiabetic cats has not been reported, although in dogs it is less frequent than reported for humans; in 1 study, only 16% of 245 nondiabetic dogs were hyperglycemic.[27] Whether the development of hyperglycemia in critically ill nondiabetic cats and dogs affects survival has yet to be determined. A retrospective evaluation of cats and dogs with head trauma failed to show any correlation between severity of hyperglycemia and survival,[28] although a more recent prospective study on dogs with a variety of critical illnesses did identify a significant association between the severity of hyperglycemia and length of hospital stay and survival.[27]

Continuous glucose monitoring and intensive glycemic control in critically ill human patients

Resulting from the high incidence of hyperglycemia and its association with increased morbidity and mortality, intensive protocols to maintain euglycemia have been investigated. The target and optimal method for achieving glucose control in the critical care setting are highly debated. In critically ill humans, one of the earliest studies to evaluate intensive insulin therapy with a goal of maintaining euglycemia (mean blood glucose level between 80 and 110 mg/dL; 4.4 and 6.1 mmol/L), showed a reduction in morbidity and mortality. The overall mortality rate dropped by 42%, with a decrease during hospitalization from 8.0% in the control group to 4.6% in the intensive insulin therapy group.[29] In addition, rates of infection, acute renal failure, transfusions, polyneuropathy, and mechanical ventilation were reduced.[29] Along with attaining euglycemia, reducing fluctuations and variability in glucose levels is significantly associated with decreased morbidity and mortality in humans.[30–32] Findings in subsequent studies on humans have been variable, with many showing a similar reduction in morbidity and mortality.[23,25,26,33]

Complicating the widespread acceptance of intensive insulin therapy in humans, several large prospective studies show either no benefit or even an increase in mortality for some patient groups. The largest such clinical trial, NICE-SUGAR, evaluated intensive insulin therapy in 6104 critically ill patients, and identified an increased mortality rate when the target blood glucose level was maintained between 81 and 108 mg/dL (4.5–6.0 mmol/L) compared with a less intensive protocol with a target blood glucose level of less than 180 mg/dL (10 mmol/L).[34] A follow-up meta-analysis concluded that intensive insulin protocols confer no benefit on mortality rates, but may still be useful in certain patient subsets, and may reduce the risk of end organ damage.[35] The most serious concern with intensive insulin therapy has been an increased risk of severe hypoglycemia.[25,33,35] In support of these findings, 2 large European clinical trials required early termination because of increased rates of severe hypoglycemia.[36,37] Hypoglycemia seems to be an important contributing factor in the increased mortality rates seen in intensive care patients, primarily those treated with intensive insulin therapy.[38,39] Despite these concerns, both the American Diabetes Association and the American Association of Clinical Endocrinologists recommend the use of intensive insulin protocols in the critical care setting, although with a more conservative target of 140 to 180 mg/dL (7.8–10 mmol/L).[40,41]

Conventional glucose monitoring requires the use of a point-of-care glucose meter and either frequent repeated venipuncture, capillary blood sampling, or placement of indwelling intravenous sampling catheters.[14] An important limitation of this technique is that it only allows for spot glucose determinations at a set interval, for example, every 2 to 4 hours, which limits the amount of information available on which to base treatment decisions and increases the workload on nursing staff and clinicians. It may also be a contributing factor to the frequency of severe hypoglycemia seen in patients treated with intensive insulin therapy, and directly affect morbidity and mortality rates.

The lack of improvement in morbidity and mortality seen with intensive insulin protocols may be partially due to the use of conventional glucose monitoring, as euglycemia may not actually be achieved. Using continuous glucose monitoring, investigators found that patients treated with intensive insulin therapy based on intermittent glucose monitoring achieved target blood glucose concentrations only 22% of the time.[42]

The use of a continuous glucose monitoring system would theoretically be a valuable tool in intensive insulin treatment of diabetic and nondiabetic feline patients in a critical care setting. Numerous studies on human patients have evaluated the ability of continuous glucose monitoring systems to maintain euglycemia, limit glucose variability, and reduce the risk of severe hypoglycemia. For the most part, these studies have failed to show an improvement in glycemic control in the human intensive care setting.[26,43,44] However, the investigators of one particular study do note that treatment decisions were based on the actual blood glucose value rather than the trends; the ability to follow trends is a major advantage of continuous glucose monitoring.[44]

Despite inconsistency in reducing mortality rates, continuous glucose monitoring has proved useful in reducing the risk of severe hypoglycemia in critical care patients. Use of the Guardian Real-Time (Medtronic, Northridge, CA) continuous monitoring system with intensive insulin protocols has been shown to reduce the rate and absolute risk of severe hypoglycemia in human patients.[26,43] The MiniMed Gold (Medtronic, Northridge CA) has also proved beneficial in monitoring human patients with insulinoma, documenting frequent severe hypoglycemia, of which patients were often unaware, and documenting response to treatment with diazoxide and cure following surgical excision.[45]

Continuous glucose monitoring and intensive glycemic control in feline patients

Additional large prospective studies on feline patients are necessary to first determine whether hyperglycemia affects clinical outcome in critically ill patients, and second whether intensive insulin therapy to maintain euglycemia is beneficial. Lacking this information, intensive insulin therapy is not a consensus recommendation in critically ill cats, with the exception of diabetic ketoacidosis where maintaining euglycemia is necessary for resolution of the ketoacidotic state.

Similar to the theoretic and documented benefits in critically ill humans, continuous glucose monitoring systems are likely to have similar usefulness for sick diabetic and nondiabetic cats. Their use offers several advantages over conventional blood glucose monitoring. First, the frequency of venipuncture and associated patient stress, which can have negative consequences on glycemic status, is reduced.[46,47] The need for blood collection is not eliminated completely, as the monitoring system must be calibrated 2 to 3 times per day; however, this allows for substantially fewer blood samples than the 10 to 12 required with conventional blood glucose monitoring. In addition, blood for calibration can be collected from the ear or paw pad, eliminating the need for venipuncture.[48] A practical approach is to calibrate at the same time as other scheduled blood testing such as monitoring of serum electrolyte concentrations. Second, the need for indwelling catheters or the duration of time that they are left in place may be reduced, which in turn may reduce the risk of phlebitis/catheter site infection.[49–51] Third, glucose levels can be monitored continuously during treatment with insulin, leading to more targeted titration of insulin therapy, more rapid resolution of ketosis and clinical signs, shorter hospital stays, and a reduced risk of hypoglycemia.

To date, only the MiniMed Gold has been evaluated in sick diabetic veterinary patients. This system provides clinically accurate glucose concentrations in ketoacidotic dogs, buts its use is limited as glucose measurements are only available retrospectively.[52] In the critical care setting, a system with a real-time display is required as frequent adjustments to the insulin dose, fluid therapy, and glucose therapy are necessary. Although not clinically evaluated, in the authors' experience the Guardian Real-Time continuous glucose monitoring system is useful in sick diabetic cats (**Fig. 1**). Glucose measurements are available in real time allowing clinicians to continuously monitor glucose fluctuations in their patients at the cage side. As the device samples interstitial fluid, it is possible that it might not function as well in severely dehydrated patients. Therefore, this system should not be relied on until after initial fluid resuscitation. A practical approach is to attach the system after initial rehydration of the animal at the same time that short-acting insulin therapy is started.

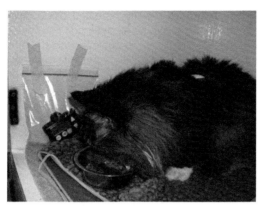

Fig. 1. The Guardian Real-Time continuous glucose monitoring system used in a sick diabetic cat (diabetic ketoacidosis). Note the monitoring device attached to the cage receiving data wirelessly from a transmitter attached to the cat's back. This reduces the amount of material that must be directly connected to the cat, which would theoretically increase patient tolerance.

The usefulness of these systems for monitoring blood glucose concentration in critically ill nondiabetic veterinary patients has not yet been evaluated. Further study is required to determine whether the use of continuous glucose monitoring systems improves glycemic control and whether the benefits observed in human critical care can be realized in critically ill veterinary patients.

Critical Care (Sick/Hospitalized Diabetic and Nondiabetic Feline Patients): Accuracy

Accuracy is critical if these systems are to replace traditional assessment methods. Accuracy has been evaluated only once in veterinary patients. The MiniMed Gold was shown to have acceptable accuracy in feline and canine patients with diabetic ketoacidosis.[52] Correlation and agreement between values obtained from the continuous glucose monitoring system and those obtained using a portable glucose meter calibrated for human use were adequate (r = 0.86); the frequency of calibration had no effect on accuracy.[52] Consensus error grid analysis revealed that greater than 98% of the paired data points were in either zone A (no effect on the clinical decision made), or zone B (altered clinical decision unlikely to affect outcome). Less than 2% of the measurements were in zone C (altered clinical decision likely to affect outcome), and there were none in zone D or E (altered clinical decision posing a significant medical risk or having dangerous consequences).[52] The median average percent difference revealed good accuracy in both dogs (9%) and cats (10%); the median percentage difference never exceeded 22.6%.[52] Glucose estimates obtained at calibration times were included in this analysis, and calibration directly influences the glucose estimate by increasing the accuracy at those times. However, the results are clinically relevant as the standard calibration protocol for the device was followed. There was no difference in average percent difference when calibrated every 8 hours versus 12 hours.[52] Significant variability between patients was noted; estimates provided by continuous glucose monitoring systems were more accurate in some patients than others. No cause for this variation was identified, because there was no association with severity of ketosis, lactate, or rectal temperature, and only a weak association with hydration status.[52]

Long-Term Monitoring in Stable Feline Diabetic Patients: Usefulness

Diabetic feline patients are not likely to wear a continuous monitor long term on a day-to-day basis; however, these systems are useful for monitoring glucose in hospitalized cats and dogs,[53–57] and may also replace repeated blood glucose concentration testing when used intermittently in the home setting.[58–60] They can be used during the initial adjustment phase of treatment to achieve stable control, and periodically thereafter to monitor that control, or to assess patients who have become uncontrolled. They are particularly useful to identify inadequate duration of insulin action, and preceding hypoglycemia as a cause for hyperglycemia.

Glycemic control is critical to abate clinical signs, maintain quality of life, and prevent complications. Effective management can decrease the amount of time patients spend with unregulated diabetes, resulting in improved health and quality of life, and reduced long-term costs. In addition, several studies have identified that improved and earlier glycemic control leads to higher rates of diabetic remission in cats.[61,62] This has been achieved with dietary therapy (low carbohydrate/high protein diet) and treatment with longer-acting insulin analogues such as protamine zinc insulin, glargine, or detemir.[61–64] Intensive protocols with either 3 consecutive days of blood glucose concentration monitoring in hospital, followed by weekly blood glucose curves in hospital or at home,[64] or daily home monitoring of blood glucose concentration have also been advocated.[61,62] These protocols have been evaluated in cats, and aim to ensure an appropriate starting dose and early glycemic control. Thus, higher rates of diabetic remission may be achieved compared with standard protocols; remission has been achieved in some cats previously treated for more than 6 months, albeit at lower rates than cats intensively treated earlier on.[61,62,64] When blood glucose concentration is closely monitored, it is expected that episodes of insulin-induced hypoglycemia can be identified earlier before clinical signs ensue, and the insulin dose adjusted appropriately.

Although intensive adjustment of insulin dose may be beneficial in achieving tight glycemic control and increasing the probability of diabetic remission in cats, it also can increase the risk of hypoglycemia, which can lead to irreversible brain damage, coma, and even death. Humans with both type 1 and 2 diabetes undergoing intensive at-home insulin therapy have a higher incidence of severe hypoglycemia compared with patients treated conventionally.[65] The prevalence of insulin-treated human patients experiencing a severe hypoglycemic event ranges from 1.5% to 7.3% annually; higher rates were seen in patients treated with intensive insulin therapy, 7.3% and 2.1%, versus 1.5% in patients with standard monitoring.[66,67] The incidence of mild asymptomatic hypoglycemia is even higher; 24% to 60% in 1 study. Some estimates indicate that many diabetics have mild hypoglycemia (<50–60 mg/dL; <2.7–3.3 mmol/L) up to 10% of the time.[68,69]

Asymptomatic nocturnal hypoglycemia is particularly common, especially in those human patients with overall good glycemic control.[70–72] A similar situation is seen in diabetic cats. In a study evaluating home monitoring of blood glucose in diabetic cats, 1/26 cats died of severe hypoglycemia.[48] Using the intensive protocols with either detemir or glargine insulin, asymptomatic hypoglycemia was common; nearly 12% and 10%, respectively, of all blood glucose concentration curves obtained had nadir values of less than 50 mg/dL (2.8 mmol/L).[61,62] Despite the high incidence of biochemical hypoglycemia, clinical hypoglycemia was seen only once for each insulin type, although episodes may have been under-reported. Both episodes were classified as mild with only restlessness and trembling seen.[61,62] Identifying hypoglycemia in insulin-treated diabetics, even when asymptomatic, is important for informing dose adjustments. If not addressed with appropriate dose adjustments, hypoglycemia may effect patient quality of life and if left untreated, could progress to fatal clinical hypoglycemia.

Insulin-induced hypoglycemic episodes can be short in duration, and easily missed with traditional in-hospital or home monitoring of serial blood glucose concentrations.

This is especially true for nocturnal hypoglycemia, as most hospitals do not have the facilities or staffing to perform overnight glucose monitoring, and most owners are unlikely to perform this task at home. In addition, hypoglycemia and the resultant Somogyi phenomenon can lead to persistent hyperglycemia during the subsequent 2 to 3 days due to counter-regulatory hormone production (**Figs. 2 and 3**).[70]

The most important advantage of continuous monitoring over intermittent blood glucose measurements is that it facilitates detection of brief periods of hypoglycemia and provides information overnight. Data can be recorded for multiple days, either in a clinic or at home. When used to monitor glycemia for a longer period, including overnight, there is evidence that a greater number of hypoglycemic events are detected.[60] When the GlucoDay (Menarini Diagnostics, Berkshire, United Kingdom) system was evaluated in the home environment in 10 diabetic dogs, investigators identified the Somogyi phenomenon, nocturnal hypoglycemia, and a brief episode of hypoglycemia in 3 of the 10 dogs.[60] In each instance, it is unlikely that traditional daytime blood glucose monitoring would have identified them, and erroneous treatment recommendations could have resulted.

The same situation occurred in diabetic cats when standard blood glucose concentration curves in the clinic were compared with curves obtained with continuous monitoring.[57] The investigators were blinded and made insulin dose recommendations based on these paired curves; this led to different dose recommendations between the 2 methodologies 30% of the time (19/63 treatment recommendations). The nadir obtained with continuous glucose monitoring was lower than that obtained with the standard curve 81% of the time. Based on these findings, the investigators concluded that the benefit was primarily in their ability to provide a more complete glucose profile and the detection of nadirs not identified with standard curves.[57]

Therefore, continuous glucose monitoring is valuable for determining the cause of hyperglycemia, and whether the most appropriate response is to increase or decrease the insulin dose or change to a longer-acting insulin.

To date, systems with or without a real-time data display have been evaluated primarily in the hospital setting to replace standard blood glucose concentration curves.[53–55,58] The readings are typically reviewed at the end of the sampling period and clinical recommendations made. Both wireless[55] and wired recording

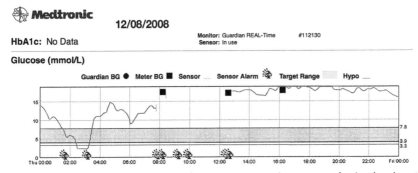

Fig. 2. Twenty-four hour continuous glucose concentration curve obtained using the Guardian Real-Time monitoring system in a diabetic dog. In this instance, use of continuous glucose monitoring identified the Somogyi phenomenon, with a blood glucose concentration less than the lower detection limit of the monitor (<40 mg/dL; 2.2 mmol/L) at 03:00 AM as shown by the flat line. This is an example of nocturnal hypoglycemia with a subsequent rapid increase in blood glucose within minutes that is sustained for the remainder of the tracing (minimum 20 hours).

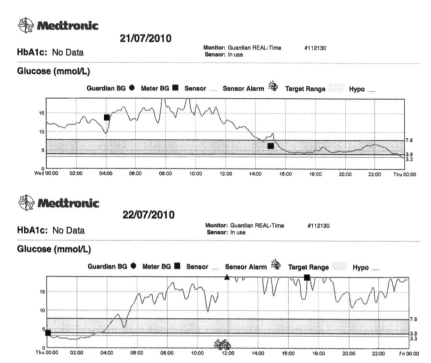

Fig. 3. Consecutive 24-hour tracings obtained using the Guardian Real-Time monitoring system in a diabetic cat. In this instance, use of continuous monitoring allowed for detection of nocturnal hypoglycemia, blood glucose <60 mg/dL (3.3 mmol/L) at around 00:00 AM and continuing until 03:00 AM.

devices[53,54,58] are reliable, but the wireless devices tend to be more convenient in the hospital setting as the monitor can be positioned outside the kennel (**Fig. 4**). In the home setting, even if a wireless device is used, it still requires attachment to the patient, because there is a maximum transmitting distance from the sensor to the monitor. The device can be attached using bandaging or garments with secured pockets, similar to those used with cardiac monitoring (Holter and event monitoring).

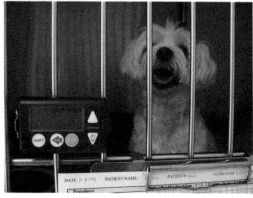

Fig. 4. Example of the Guardian Real-Time continuous glucose monitoring system monitor placed outside the patient's cage for real-time monitoring of blood glucose concentrations.

These garments are commonly used in large breed dogs for cardiovascular monitoring, and recent studies show they are well tolerated in cats.[73–75] Devices designed to record data, such as the i-Pro (Medtronic, Northridge CA), rather than transmit in real-time to a monitor would be ideal in a home setting because they are smaller and the need for extensive bandaging or garments is reduced.

Although glucose monitoring systems are a reliable alternative to conventional daytime serial blood glucose concentration monitoring[57] and are well tolerated by patients, the question arises as to whether they provide benefits over conventional monitoring that would justify the additional cost. In human diabetics receiving at home intensive insulin therapy, the introduction of long-term continuous glucose monitoring has reduced the incidence of hyperglycemia without increasing the risk of hypoglycemia,[76,77] and diabetic cats may get the same benefit.

Long-Term Monitoring in Stable Diabetic Patients: Accuracy

Continuous glucose monitoring systems rely on interstitial fluid glucose concentrations, therefore their ability to accurately predict blood glucose concentrations is critical; this was first evaluated using the MiniMed Gold on diabetic dogs with poor glycemic control.[53] Ten dogs were hospitalized for a minimum of 30 hours and received food and insulin treatment according to their usual routine. Standard blood glucose curves using a portable glucose meter calibrated for human use with samples collected every 1 to 3 hours were compared with the results of continuous monitoring, resulting in 428 hours of data and 183 paired glucose measurements. Data were similar with good correlation ($r = 0.81$); however, the blood glucose concentrations obtained with continuous glucose monitoring were statistically lower, an effect that was most pronounced during periods of hyperglycemia and 1 to 2 hours postprandially.[53] Because portable glucose meters calibrated for human use tend to give lower results than those calibrated for veterinary use or laboratory methods, it is likely that the discrepancy is greater than was reported.

For optimal accuracy, it is recommended that the correlation coefficient for compared measurements be a minimum of 0.79.[78] Subsequent studies on the accuracy of the MiniMed Gold have achieved better correlations than earlier studies, more consistent with those seen in humans using the same system.[79,80] Assessment in a population of diabetic and healthy animals gave correlations of $r = 0.997$ (dogs; $n = 7$) and 0.974 (cats; $n = 5$),[58] and evaluation in 16 diabetic cats identified similarly high correlation ($r = 0.932$) between blood and interstitial fluid measurements.[54] Excluding the blood glucose measurements used to calibrate the sensor, which are expected to be more accurate as a result of a direct effect on sensor readings, correlation was still adequate at $r = 0.862$.[54]

The MiniMed Gold has a working range of only 40 to 400 mg/dL (2.2–22.2 mmol/L). When evaluated in 14 cats, 16 blood glucose traces were obtained, with 7/16 affected by the limited recording range. Prolonged hypoglycemia and hyperglycemia were seen in 2/16 and 3/16 traces, respectively, and both hypoglycemia and hyperglycemia in 1/16, during which actual glucose concentrations were not measured. In addition, 1 cat initially had a blood glucose concentration of 282 mg/dL (15.7 mmol/L), but this increased and remained greater than 400 mg/dL (22.2 mmol/L) with the result that the device could not be calibrated and no trace was generated.[54]

Diabetic Patients Undergoing Surgery or Anesthesia: Usefulness

Anesthetized patients at risk for hypoglycemia or hyperglycemia are generally monitored using point-of-care glucose meters. As in other clinical settings, use of intermittent readings may result in failure to detect clinically significant changes in glycemic status.

Although 1 study has shown that the Guardian Real-Time provides inaccurately low glucose readings in anesthetized veterinary patients,[81] other devices may still prove useful in this situation. Even the Guardian Real-Time may be useful for monitoring impending hypoglycemia. This device tends to underestimate the blood glucose concentration, so values that are within the normal range would not require verification, reducing the frequency of venipuncture. Values in the hypoglycemic range would need to be confirmed by measuring the blood glucose concentration, but being more conservative, may provide an earlier warning of impending hypoglycemia than conventional monitoring.

Diabetic Patients Undergoing Surgery/Anesthesia: Accuracy

The accuracy of the Guardian Real-Time in anesthetized human pediatric patients is acceptable. This was shown in children undergoing cardiac surgery with 99.6% of paired values falling within zones A or B in the consensus error grid analysis, indicating no alteration in clinical action, and a mean difference of only 17.6%.[82] In addition, no negative effect was seen with hypothermia, inotrope use, or subcutaneous edema.[82] Similar results were seen in a second study on humans, with a mean difference of 13% and all paired values falling within zones A or B.[83]

To date, only 1 veterinary study has evaluated the accuracy of continuous glucose monitoring in anesthetized patients, comparing the Guardian Real-Time with the ISTAT portable chemistry analyzer (Abbott Laboratories, Abbott Park, IL).[81] In contrast to the confirmed accuracy in human patients under anesthesia, the same result was not obtained in dogs. Of 126 paired data points from 10 nondiabetic dogs under general anesthesia for routine abdominal surgery, acceptable agreement (<21% difference) was seen in only 57% of samples.[81] The Guardian Real-Time consistently recorded values lower than the blood glucose concentration for all discordant data points. In addition, hypoglycemia, blood glucose level less than 60 mg/dL (3.3 mmol/L), was recorded in 25/126 paired samples, whereas the portable chemistry analyzer recorded hypoglycemia in only 1 of these.[81]

GLUCOSE METER TECHNOLOGY
Laboratory Glucose Monitoring

Traditionally, glucose is measured as part of the routine biochemistry panel, using either in-house or reference laboratory analyzers. In the management of diabetics, serial measurements of blood glucose concentration using laboratory reference systems is impractical.

Glucose can be measured on either whole blood or on plasma/serum. Whole blood generally gives a lower glucose concentration than plasma/serum as a result of the higher water content of plasma (93% water) compared with erythrocytes (73% water). When glucose is reported based on whole blood, a multiplier of 1.1 is recommended to convert to the plasma/serum glucose concentration.[84,85]

The glucose molecule cannot be measured directly, and as a result 3 main methods have been developed to determine the concentration of glucose in a sample: reducing methods, condensation methods, and enzymatic methods. Because of problems with reducing and condensation methods, nearly all modern glucose measurements use indirect enzymatic methods.

Most reference laboratories use the enzyme hexokinase in assessing glucose concentrations. Hexokinase catalyzes the reaction between glucose and adenosine triphosphate, thereby phosphorylating glucose into glucose 6-phosphate. Subsequently, the enzyme glucose-6-phosphate dehydrogenase, in the presence of nicotinamide adenine dinucleotide (NAD), oxidizes glucose 6-phosphate to reduced NAD (NADH) and 6-phosphogluconate. NADH can then be measured spectrophotometrically.[86]

Point-of-Care Glucose Monitoring

Blood glucose concentration testing using point-of-care glucose meters is the mainstay of monitoring for human diabetics, and is becoming increasingly popular amongst the owners of diabetic dogs and cats. The greatest advance came in the late 1980s with the development of portable glucose meters that use either photometric or electrochemical methods. These meters use enzyme systems specific for glucose, called oxidoreductases, the most common being glucose oxidase and glucose dehydrogenase. In addition, they also contain coenzymes, mediator systems, and indicators. The specific oxidoreductase, mediator, coenzymes, and indicators used vary with the individual glucose meter. To quantify the concentration of glucose in the sample, 2 main technologies are used: either a photometric or an electrochemical technique. In general, oxidation of glucose via a specific oxidoreductase, in the presence of coenzymes, generates electrons that are transferred to a mediator molecule, an organic or inorganic chemical that can alternate between an oxidized and reduced state (accept or donate electrons). These mediator molecules are then capable of donating electrons to either an electrode (electrochemical method) or an indicator molecule, which forms a color (photometric method).[87] Electrochemical methods contain either glucose oxidase or glucose dehydrogenase, and most commonly rely on hexacyanoferrate III/hexacyanoferrate II as the mediator system, generating an electric current that is calibrated to measure the concentration of glucose in the specimen. Most photometric methods use glucose oxidase and rely on the generation of hydrogen peroxide (mediator), similar to the technique used in colorimetric test strips. In contrast, the light reflected off the test strip is not measured by a reflectance meter, but rather generates an electric current after contact with a photodetector.[88]

Until recently, most portable glucose meters available for use on veterinary patients were intended for human use and so their validation was based on human blood. They assume a constant and unchanging relationship between plasma and whole blood, with erythrocytes and plasma each containing 50% of glucose. This distribution is not uniform across all species. Dogs have 12.5% and 87.5% of glucose in erythrocytes and plasma, respectively, and the disparity is even greater in cats (7% and 93%, respectively).[89] Because portable glucose meters typically evaluate plasma glucose after separation of erythrocytes from plasma, use of a human glucose meter on canine or feline blood often underestimates the true glucose concentration. Veterinary-use glucose meters have now been developed that provide more accurate results for cat and dog blood. Veterinary glucose meters available at the time of writing include the AlphaTRAK meter (Abbott Laboratories, Abbot Park, IL), the g-Pet meter (Woodley Equipment Company Ltd., Horwich United Kingdom), and the i-Pet meter (UltiCare Inc., St. Paul, MN). The AlphaTRAK meter has been evaluated in dogs, cats, and horses and the results have been published.[90–92] The manufacturers of the g-Pet and i-Pet meters provide comparable results for their products, although these have not been published in the peer-reviewed literature.[93,94] In all species, there is high correlation, accuracy, and precision between the AlphaTRAK meter and the reference method. In comparison, human glucose meters typically give significantly lower results compared with the AlphaTRAK and reference method in cats and dogs.[90–92]

The AlphaTRAK meter offers several advantages over the other veterinary glucometers, most notably the small sample size required to obtain a glucose measurement. The AlphaTRAK meter requires only 0.3 µL of blood,[90–92] whereas the g-Pet and i-Pet each require 1.5 µL.[93,94] The smaller sample size means that an adequate sample volume is more reliably obtained from capillary sampling in veterinary patients, reducing or eliminating the need for venipuncture. This is especially important in individuals at risk for anemia from frequent venipuncture including feline patients in intensive care and pediatric patients. Capillary sampling is also essential for at-home continuous glucose monitoring, as owners must obtain blood samples to calibrate the system.

Interstitial and Plasma Glucose Relationships

An understanding of the relationship between interstitial and plasma glucose is essential to understanding the accuracy and limitations of devices. However, this topic is still under debate. The most commonly recognized model to explain interstitial-plasma glucose relationships is a 2-compartment model in which the capillary wall separating the plasma from the interstitial fluid acts as a barrier to the diffusion of glucose.[95,96] The interstitial glucose concentration in this model depends on the rate of diffusion across the capillary membrane, and the rate of glucose clearance from the interstitium. Glucose clearance from the interstitial space depends on insulin-mediated uptake by the surrounding cells, with a clearance rate proportional to the concentration of glucose in the interstitium and the rate of uptake by cells. If the rate of glucose uptake by surrounding cells is negligible and the diffusion rate between the plasma and interstitium is constant, a steady-state relationship will exist between interstitial and plasma glucose concentrations. Whether glucose uptake by the surrounding tissues is truly negligible is an area of debate, but, in general, there is a consensus that it is a steady-state relationship between plasma and interstitial glucose.[95,96]

Despite this steady-state relationship, diffusion of glucose from the plasma into the interstitial space is not immediate, and a corresponding lag phase exists between rapid changes in blood and interstitial glucose. Rapid changes in blood glucose concentration lead to corresponding changes in interstitial glucose, but with a delay of between 5 and 12 minutes in dogs.[79,96] Similar results have been identified in cats, with a lag time of approximately 11 minutes after an intravenous bolus of glucose.[55] Diffusion of glucose from the interstitium into the sensor may also affect the lag phase; however, available continuous glucose monitoring systems have digital filters designed to compensate for this delay.

Continuous Glucose Monitoring System Technology

Available systems use similar technology to portable blood glucose monitoring devices; glucose in the subcutaneous tissue is oxidized to gluconic acid and hydrogen peroxide. The latter is oxidized and donates electrons to the working electrode, which generates an electrochemical signal proportional to the concentration of glucose in the interstitial fluid.[55,59] Most current systems use electrochemical sensors implanted in the subcutaneous space and, to date, this remains the primary technology in the MiniMed Gold and Guardian Real-Time systems, as well as the i-Pro, Seven Plus (Dexcom, San Diego, CA), and FreeStyle Navigator (Abbott Diabetes Care, Alameda CA), all of which have been approved by the US Food and Drug Administration (FDA). More recently, a microdialysis system, GlucoDay, has been evaluated and approved for use in Europe, but is not yet FDA approved. Only the MiniMed Gold, Guardian Real-Time, and GlucoDay systems have been evaluated in veterinary patients.[52–56,58,60,81,97]

All sensor-based systems have multiple components: a glucose monitor that records data, a sterile single-use sensor, and a communication device for data download. In addition, wireless devices utilize a transmitter to distribute information from the sensor to the monitor. Each sensor is embedded in a split needle system to allow introduction into the subcutaneous space, and once in place, the needle is withdrawn;

the gauge of the needle varies with the individual system (**Table 1**). The sensor consists of an electroenzymatic 3-electrode cell that maintains a constant potential of 0.6 V between the working and reference electrodes. The sensor is enclosed in flexible tubing and contains a side window that exposes the working electrode to the subcutaneous space. A polyurethane membrane that is glucose diffusion limited, maintains a linear relationship between glucose concentration and sensor current, and covers the working electrode in the side window.[55,59] All reactions take place within the sensor and occur within the body.

In contrast, microdialysis-based systems use an implantable microdialysis fiber facilitating diffusion of interstitial fluid into the fiber, which is then carried to a central processing unit/monitoring device. The reaction that provides an estimate of blood glucose concentration is the same, but all reactions take place outside the body.[56]

SPECIFIC CONTINUOUS GLUCOSE MONITORING SYSTEMS

See **Table 1** for specific information regarding the available continuous glucose monitoring systems.

What is Available?

Currently, many systems have been approved for use throughout the world; however, only 3 systems have been clinically evaluated in dogs and cats: the MiniMed Gold; the Guardian Real-Time; and the GlucoDay. The Guardian Real-Time has effectively replaced the MiniMed Gold; however, this system is still in use and will likely continue to be in the near future. It consists of an electrochemical sensor that is inserted subcutaneously, to which a transmitting device is attached. This delivers data wirelessly to the monitor for review and storage (**Fig. 5**). Data can then be downloaded off the monitor.[55] In addition, the FDA has recently approved the i-Pro for use. The i-Pro and Guardian Real-Time use the same electrochemical sensor; however, the wireless transmitter used with the Guardian Real-Time is replaced with a recording device for data storage with the i-Pro.[98] There is no real-time display with the i-Pro, but it does allow for retrospective analysis. The Seven Plus and FreeStyle Navigator may also be applicable; however, they are yet to be evaluated in veterinary patients. These systems have similarities but there are also important differences that may affect the purchasing decision. Ultimately decisions should be based on individual needs.

Display/Recording

Continuous glucose monitoring systems can be divided based on their technology as previously discussed but also based on the display and recording type.

The MiniMed Gold and GlucoDay are wired systems, meaning the sensor or microdialysis fiber is directly connected to the recording device or processing unit.[52–54,56,58,60,81,97] The GlucoDay system is technically wireless as it can transmit wirelessly to a computer; however, the dialysis fiber is directly attached to the processing unit and thus animals must wear this even when in a hospital cage. The Guardian Real-Time, Seven Plus, and FreeStyle Navigator all function wirelessly, transmitting data to a monitor for storage and download.[55,99,100] A wireless device such as the Guardian Real-Time is more practical for hospitalized cats and dogs as the monitor can be placed outside the cage without the inconvenience of a connecting cable. In the home setting, even a wireless system requires attachment to the patient as the maximum transmitting distances are relatively short.

Table 1
Specifications of available continuous glucose monitoring systems

	MiniMed Gold[a]	Guardian Real-Time[b]	i-Pro[c]	GlucoDay[d]	FreeStyle Navigator[e]	Seven Plus[f]
Company	Medtronic	Medtronic	Medtronic	Menarini Diagnostics	Abbott	Dexcom
Availability	FDA approved, no longer manufactured	FDA approved	FDA approved	EU approved, not FDA approved	FDA approved	FDA approved
Evaluated in veterinary patients	Yes	Yes	No	Yes	No	No
Technology	Amperometric electrochemical sensor; glucose oxidase	Amperometric electrochemical sensor; glucose oxidase	Amperometric electrochemical sensor; glucose oxidase	Amperometric microdialysis fiber; glucose oxidase	Amperometric electrochemical sensor; glucose oxidase	Amperometric electrochemical sensor; glucose oxidase
Senor/transmitter weight	N/A	79 g (2.8 oz)	79 g (2.8 oz)	N/A	13.61 g (0.48 oz)	6.7 g (0.24 oz)
Transmitter/sensor size (L × W × H)	N/A	4.2 × 3.6 × 0.9 cm (1.64 × 1.4 × 0.37 in)	4.2 × 3.6 × 0.9 cm (1.64 × 1.4 × 0.37 in)	N/A	5.2 × 3.1 × 1.1 cm (2.5 × 1.23 × 0.43 in)	3.8 × 2.3 × 1.0 cm (1.5 × 0.9 × 0.4 in)
Monitor weight	113 g (4 oz)	114 g (4 oz)	N/A	245 g (8.6 oz)	100 g (3.5 oz)	100 g (3.5 oz)
Monitor size (L × W × H)	9.1 × 2.3 × 7.1 cm (3.6 × 0.9 × 2.8 in)	8.1 × 2.0 × 5.1 cm (3.2 × 0.8 × 2 in)	N/A	11 × 2.5 × 7.5 cm (4.3 × 1 × 3 in)	8.1 × 2.0 × 5.1 cm (2.5 × 3.2 × 0.9 in)	11.4 × 5.8 × 2.2 cm (4.5 × 2.3 × 0.85 in)
Recording range	40–400 mg/dL (2.2–22.2 mmol/L)	40–400 mg/dL (2.2–22.2 mmol/L)	40–400 mg/dL (2.2–22.2 mmol/L)	20–600 mg/dL (1.1–33.3 mmol/L)	40–400 mg/dL (2.2–22.2 mmol/L)	40–400 mg/dL (2.2–22.2 mmol/L)
Real-time display	No	Yes	No	Yes	Yes	Yes
Retrospective analysis	Yes	Yes	Yes	Yes	Yes	Yes

Wireless transmission	No	Yes	No	Yes	Yes	Yes[a]
Wireless transmission range	N/A	23 m (10 feet)	N/A	N/A	3 m (10 feet)	1.5 m (5 feet)
Sensor needle insertion size	24 gauge	22 gauge (Sof-sensor) 27 gauge (Enlite sensor)	24 gauge	18 gauge	21 gauge	26 gauge
Sensor life	72 h	72 h (Sof-sensor) 144 h (Enlite sensor)	72 h (Sof-sensor) 144 h (Enlite sensor)	48 h	120 h	168 h
Sensor initialization period	1 h	2 h	1 h	1 h	2 h	2 h
Calibration	2–3 times per 24 h	2 h after insertion, within the next 6 h, then every 12 h	1 and 3 h after insertion, then minimum of once every 12 h	Minimum of 1 time point per 48 h, 2 if used in real time	10 h after insertion, within the next 2–4 h, then every 12 h	2 calibrations, 2 h after insertion, then every 12 h
Recording frequency	Data collected every 10 s, mean value reported every 5 min	Data collected every 10 s, mean value reported every 5 min	Data collected every 10 s, mean value reported every 5 min	Data collected every 1 s, mean value reported every 3 min	Data collected every 10 s, mean value reported every 5 min	Data collected every 10 s, mean value reported every 5 min

a Product specifications.[108]
b Product specifications.[55,109]
c Product specifications.[98]
d Product specifications.[56]
e Product specifications.[110]
f Product specifications.[111]

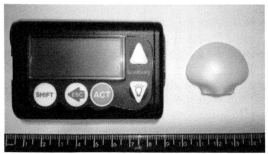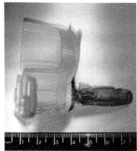

Fig. 5. The Guardian Real-Time continuous glucose monitoring system. From left to right: monitor, wireless transmitter, and electrochemical sensor.

The MiniMed Gold and i-Pro systems function retrospectively, meaning they store data that must be downloaded to a computer for analysis.[52–54,58,81,97,98] Clinical recommendations must therefore be delayed until the data can be retrospectively evaluated. Retrospective evaluation is advantageous in the home setting as owners are unable to visualize blood glucose results, reducing the likelihood they will alter treatment without consulting a veterinarian. These devices are not suitable for anesthetized or sick patients, as there is no real-time display to guide treatment. The Guardian Real-Time, Seven Plus, FreeStyle Navigator, and GlucoDay also record data but use a real-time display for immediate analysis of blood glucose data.[55,78]

Summary

- To replace or augment routine home or hospital blood glucose concentration monitoring, a continuous glucose monitoring system, with or without a real-time display, is appropriate, because the insulin dose can then be adjusted based on multiple readings.
- In anesthetized or sick patients, a real-time display is required; therefore the Guardian Real-Time or GlucoDay are the only systems applicable that have been evaluated in veterinary patients (others are available but have not been evaluated in veterinary patients).
- Wireless or wired devices are both practical options, although the wireless device is preferred in hospitalized cats and dogs.

PLACEMENT STRATEGIES AND PATIENT TOLERANCE

Placement and attachment of the various continuous glucose monitoring systems require that a site is chosen, clipped, and prepped for insertion of the sensor or dialysis fiber. Application of a small quantity of adhesive glue or suture can aid attachment of the sensor and reduce or eliminate the requirement for bandaging. Theoretically, implantation can be performed in any region that has sufficient subcutaneous space. The most commonly used sites are the flank, lateral thorax, and intrascapular region.[53,55,58,101] The most reliable site for placement of the Medtronic Guardian Real-Time sensor has been shown to be dorsal neck in cats, and the same is likely true for dogs.[102] For the GlucoDay system, a higher rate of microdialysis fiber collapse was reported in the intrascapular region than the lateral thoracic region.[56] However, collapse was attributed to the bandage technique; the use of only a protective coating rather than a firm bandage eliminated fiber collapse.[56]

The MiniMed Gold and Guardian Real-Time devices have been evaluated for in-hospital and at-home use in multiple studies, with few instances of adverse reaction.

Early studies evaluated animals in both the home and hospital setting, using the wired system. Placement of the sensor resulted in minimal discomfort, no irritation or inflammation at the site of attachment, and no abnormal behaviors, such as chewing, rolling, or biting, as reported by owners and clinical staff.[58,59] Some mild discomfort during removal of the sensor and associated redness was reported, likely related to the adhesive that was applied to attach the sensor to the skin.[58,59] A second study evaluating 16 diabetic cats in the hospital environment revealed similar results with no evidence of irritation at the site of sensor placement in any cat on any occasion. However, 1/16 patients removed the sensor after 12 hours, and 2/16 cats kinked the sensor during recording, requiring placement of a second sensor.[54]

More recently, the wireless Guardian Real-Time system has been evaluated; the patients were required to wear the sensor and a small transmitter, but not the monitor.[55] This was also the largest sample size evaluated, with 39 diseased cats and 5 healthy cats. These cats showed no signs of irritation or abnormal behavior, and no signs of skin irritation or reaction.[55] This system may be preferable as the monitor is the largest piece of equipment, and not wearing the monitor means that less material is required to secure the system, improving tolerance and compliance. This advantage only applies in the hospital setting, because the transmitting distance is only 3 m. Use of this system in the home environment would require patients to wear the monitor, as with wired systems.

The i-Pro system eliminates the need for patients to wear the monitor, because there is no wireless transmitter; the data are stored directly on the recording device. This dramatically reduces the size of the system that must be attached to the patient, even when used in the home environment.[98] This could facilitate a more simplified process for attaching the system to the patient, and improve patient tolerance. There are as yet no reports of the use of this system in veterinary medicine, but it would be ideal for at-home use.

As with standard in-hospital and at-home monitoring, critically ill patients tolerate the continuous glucose monitoring systems well.[52] The only adverse event seen was mild bleeding at the time of sensor insertion, which stopped with the application of direct pressure. No systems had to be removed because of irritation, pain, bleeding, or infection.[52] Although uncommonly reported in the literature, in our experience some cats succeed in removing the sensor despite bandaging. With small systems such as the Guardian Real-Time or i-Pro, the sensor can be taped in place to prevent removal (**Fig. 6**).

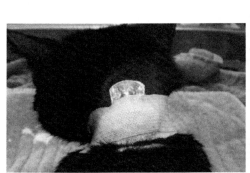
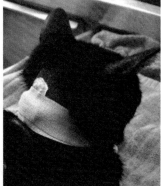

Fig. 6. Adhesive bandage tape used to secure the Guardian Real-Time sensor/transmitting device in a cat that repeatedly attempted to remove it despite standard bandaging.

Microdialysis-based systems such as the GlucoDay are also well tolerated, with limited adverse reactions. In the 2 veterinary studies evaluating this, 4/6 healthy and 3/10 diabetic dogs showed mild agitation/shaking after placement. In addition, 0/6 healthy and 4/10 diabetic dogs showed mild erythema after removal of the fiber, which soon resolved.[56,60] This system is yet to be clinically evaluated in cats, but the large processing unit may limit its use.

Summary

- The most suitable location for placement of the Medtronic Guardian Real-Time sensor is the dorsal neck, whereas the lateral thorax is preferred for the GlucoDay system.
- All systems are generally well tolerated, with no differences reported.
- Newer more compact systems like the i-Pro are likely to improve patient toler-ance and minimize adverse reactions, because they require less bandaging, leading to greater patient comfort. This has not yet been clinically evaluated in veterinary patients.

SENSOR LIFESPAN/STABILITY

All systems use the same enzymatic reaction to estimate the blood glucose concentra-tion based on interstitial glucose concentration. The MiniMed Gold, Guardian Real-Time, i-Pro, Seven Plus, and FreeStyle Navigator are sensor based, whereas the GlucoDay is microdialysis based. Although both technologies are sufficiently accurate for clinical use, some advocate the use of microdialysis fibers to harvest interstitial fluid over the use of implantable sensors.[56,60] The rationale is based on separation of the dialysis fiber from the biosensor so that all reactive substances and waste products such as hydrogen peroxide remain external to the body. As a result, they cannot diffuse into the surrounding tissues, eliminating contact with inflammatory cells and serum proteins, which can cause degradation/biofouling of the implanted material. In theory, this can interfere with the performance of the sensor.[103] Others argue that the short insertion time of only 48 to 72 hours for sensors currently available negates the effect of biofouling.[104,105]

Each sensor/dialysis fiber has a lifespan, after which time it must be replaced. The time varies with the individual sensor. The dialysis fiber used in the GlucoDay system has a lifespan of approximately 48 hours.[56] With regard to the Guardian Real-Time and i-Pro, sensor technology has recently changed. The original Sof-sensor (Medtronic, Northridge, CA) had a lifespan of 72 hours, whereas the new Enlite sensor (Medtronic, Northridge, CA) has a lifespan of 144 hours.[55,106,107] At the end of the initial 72 hour moni-toring period using the Guardian Real-Time system, the monitor will prompt the user to change the sensor. Rather than placing a new sensor, the transmitter can be reattached to the original sensor, and the system restarted to allow a further 72 hours of monitoring, although sensor accuracy subjectively may decrease after 48 hours. This would theoret-ically provide more data and contribute more information to help better guide treatment decisions.

Summary

- Microdialysis technology may prove advantageous in that performance may be less affected by inflammation/tissue reaction; however, head-to-head compari-sons have not been performed in veterinary medicine to determine clinically rele-vant superiority in short-term use.

- With the development of the Enlite sensor, the Guardian Real-Time and i-Pro now provide the option of continuous monitoring for 144 hours.

INITIALIZATION/CALIBRATION

Despite the continuous measurement of interstitial glucose, all monitors must be calibrated daily to ensure accurate results. Calibration can be performed with venous blood obtained via venipuncture or via a capillary prick. Because of the species differences in glucose homeostasis/concentrations, a veterinary glucose meter should be used for calibration if possible. There is a lag of approximately 10 to 15 minutes between blood and interstitial glucose concentrations, therefore it is important to avoid calibration whenever the glucose concentration is changing rapidly, such as during excitement or struggling. If calibration is necessary when the blood glucose concentration is changing rapidly, it is recommended that calibration be repeated once the blood glucose concentration has stabilized.

With real-time continuous glucose monitors, human patients are encouraged to calibrate before meals, at bedtime, and not within the first few hours after insulin administration to avoid periods of rapidly changing glucose concentrations. Real-time systems incorporate directional arrows on the monitor advising the user as to the direction and rate of change of the blood glucose concentration. The manufacturers advise not to calibrate if indicator arrows are showing on their device. For the Guardian Real-time, 1 arrow indicates a change of 18–36 mg/dL (1 to 2 mmol/L) in the last 20 minutes, and 2 arrows represent > 36mg/dL (2 or more mmol/L) in the last 20 minutes. With units that do not provide real-time display, such as the i-Pro, because the calibration glucose measurements are inputted into the program after the data is downloaded, having the blood glucose stable at the time of testing is not as important, because a different algorithm is used for calibration of the i-Pro compared with the real-time continuous glucose monitors.

In cats, consumption of a low carbohydrate diet is unlikely to cause rapid changes in glucose concentration. Glucose concentrations can change rapidly in some cats after insulin administration, depending on the insulin used and the individual cat, and after hypoglycemia during a Somogyi event. In most diabetic cats, the blood glucose concentration is likely to be most stable just before each insulin injection and feeding. Because the pre-insulin blood glucose concentration is also used for adjustment of dose for long-acting insulin, it would be of most benefit to measure blood glucose at this time, and use the value for calibration. For real-time units, this would provide quality control for the glucose concentrations that are important for dosing decisions; and for retrospective units being using for at-home blood glucose monitoring, it would help to prevent an inappropriately high dose of insulin being administered when the blood glucose concentration is within or less than the normal range.

For the MiniMed Gold and Guardian Real-Time systems, calibration must be performed once within the first 2 hours, with further calibration varying according to the manufacturer's recommendations.[59,97,101] For the MiniMed Gold, 3 calibrations per 24-hour period are recommended, although there are no significant differences in glucose estimates when calibrated 2 versus 3 times daily in veterinary patients. As a result, the MiniMed Gold could be used with only twice daily calibration, rather than according to the manufacturer's recommendations.[52] The manufacturer of the Guardian Real-Time recommends recalibration after 6 hours, and then 2 calibrations per 24-hour period.[55]

Manufacturer recommendations for the GlucoDay system recommend 1 or 2 calibrations per 48-hour period with the first performed 1 to 2 hours after placement. A study of varying calibration schemes in healthy dogs found that 2 calibrations, once at the beginning and again at the end of the observation period, provided the most accurate results.[56] There was no advantage to more frequent calibration.[56,60]

All these calibrations are performed prospectively during the recording period. The i-Pro manufacturer recommends calibration at 1 and 3 hours after insertion, then 2 times per 12 hours. In contrast to other available systems, the blood glucose concentration and time it was measured are entered retrospectively at the end of the recording period, which may prove advantageous, because it would simplify the process when calibration is performed by nursing staff or owners.[98,100]

As with all continuous glucose monitoring systems, more frequent calibration often provides superior accuracy. It is possible that fewer calibrations per day may be adequate for various systems, but with the exception of the MiniMed Gold and Gluco-Day systems, this has not yet been tested in veterinary patients.

In addition to the frequency of calibration needed to obtain accurate results, the ability to perform the initial calibration can sometimes be an issue. The MiniMed Gold, Guardian Real-Time, and i-Pro systems have a range of 40 to 400 mg/dL (2.2–22.2 mmol/L)[55,59,97,98,101]; values outside this range are not reported. The Gluco-Day has a wider range of 20 to 600 mg/dL (1.1–33.3 mmol/L).[56] When the initial blood glucose concentrations are outside this range, the manufacturers recommend delaying sensor insertion until the blood glucose is within range. In our experience, the Guardian Real-Time sensor can still be inserted and the system initialized even when the blood glucose concentration is outside this range. In hyperglycemic patients with blood glucose concentrations greater than 400 mg/dL (>22.2 mmol/L), calibration with a value of 400 mg/dL (22.2 mmol/L) allows for operation of the device. The specific readings will not be accurate, but trends can still be observed. For example, a patient with an initial blood glucose concentration of 580 mg/dL (32.2 mmol/L), which is outside the range for the MiniMed Gold and Guardian Real-Time systems, could be calibrated using 400 mg/dL (22.2 mmol/L) as the initial value. The system can then be used to ensure therapy is having the desired effect as represented by a gradual decrease in the glucose readings. Visualizing this decrease would eliminate the need to perform frequent blood sampling, as the trend is reliable. Because of the fairly linear relationship between plasma and interstitial glucose levels, once the display reads 184 mg/dL (10.2 mmol/L), the blood glucose concentration can be assumed to have decreased to approximately 400 mg/dL (22.2 mmol/L), and can be verified using a portable glucose meter. Once the blood glucose concentration is within range, the system can be recalibrated and subsequent values deemed accurate.

The working range of these systems is not a practical limitation in the clinical setting. For treatment decisions, it is usually sufficient to know that an animal's glucose concentration is less than 40 mg/dL (<2.2 mmol/L) or greater than 400 mg/dL (>22.2 mmol/L). Direct blood glucose measurements can be performed if a more accurate result is required.

Summary

- Calibration should be avoided when a rapid change in blood glucose concentration is anticipated, or when directional arrows are showing on the monitor.
- The GlucoDay system has a wider working range than the MiniMed Gold and Guardian Real-Time systems and so can be accurately calibrated in hyperglycemic animals (up to 600 mg/dL, 33.3 mmol/L).
- The reduced frequency of calibration (2 calibrations/48 hours), while maintaining accuracy, is a substantial advantage of the GlucoDay system compared with the

MiniMed Gold and Guardian Real-Time systems (2–3 calibrations/24 hours), primarily when calibration is inconvenient, for example at night and in the home setting.

SUMMARY

More information is needed regarding the accuracy and usefulness of continuous glucose monitoring systems for anesthetized patients; as yet, their use in monitoring nondiabetic patients with altered glucose homeostasis has not been evaluated. The Guardian Real-Time system is a versatile monitoring system because its real-time display means that it can be used in all settings. It is likely to be better tolerated due to its small size and wireless nature. The same may apply to the GlucoDay system; however, it may be less ideal for small patients or in-hospital use because patients must wear the dialysis fiber and processing unit. The i-Pro has yet to be investigated in veterinary patients, but may be the most advantageous system for at-home monitoring because of its small size, lack of a monitor, and retrospective analysis.

REFERENCES

1. Bruskiewicz KA, Nelson RW, Feldman EC, et al. Diabetic ketosis and ketoacidosis in cats: 42 cases (1980-1995). J Am Vet Med Assoc 1997;211(2):188–92.
2. Feldman E, Nelson R. Diabetic ketoacidosis. In: Feldman E, Nelson R, editors. Canine and feline endocrinology and reproduction. 3rd edition. St Louis (MO): Elsevier; 2004. p. 580–615.
3. Hume DZ, Drobatz KJ, Hess RS. Outcome of dogs with diabetic ketoacidosis: 127 dogs (1993-2003). J Vet Intern Med 2006;20(3):547–55.
4. Greco DS. Complicated diabetes mellitus. In: Bonagura JD, Twedt DC, editors. Current veterinary therapy XIV. St Louis (MO): Elsevier; 2009. p. 214–8.
5. Ferreri JA, Hardam E, Kimmel SE, et al. Clinical differentiation of acute necrotizing from chronic nonsuppurative pancreatitis in cats: 63 cases (1996-2001). J Am Vet Med Assoc 2003;223(4):469–74.
6. Cook AK, Breitschwerdt EB, Levine JF, et al. Risk factors associated with acute pancreatitis in dogs: 101 cases (1985-1990). J Am Vet Med Assoc 1993;203(5):673–9.
7. Hess RS, Kass PH, Shofer FS, et al. Evaluation of risk factors for fatal acute pancreatitis in dogs. J Am Vet Med Assoc 1999;214(1):46–51.
8. Papa K, Mathe A, Abonyi-Toth Z, et al. Occurrence, clinical features and outcome of canine pancreatitis (80 cases). Acta Vet Hung 2011;59(1):37–52.
9. Macintire DK. Treatment of diabetic ketoacidosis in dogs by continuous low-dose intravenous infusion of insulin. J Am Vet Med Assoc 1993;202(8):1266–72.
10. Claus MA, Silverstein DC, Shofer FS, et al. Comparison of regular insulin infusion doses in critically ill diabetic cats: 29 cases (1999-2007). J Vet Emerg Crit Care (San Antonio) 2010;20(5):509–17.
11. Sears KW, Drobatz KJ, Hess RS. Use of lispro insulin for treatment of diabetic ketoacidosis in dogs. J Vet Emerg Crit Care (San Antonio) 2012;22(2):211–8.
12. Chastain CB, Nichols CE. Low-dose intramuscular insulin therapy for diabetic ketoacidosis in dogs. J Am Vet Med Assoc 1981;178(6):561–4.
13. Hoorn EJ, Carlotti AP, Costa LA, et al. Preventing a drop in effective plasma osmolality to minimize the likelihood of cerebral edema during treatment of children with diabetic ketoacidosis. J Pediatr 2007;150(5):467–73.
14. O'Brien MA. Diabetic emergencies in small animals. Vet Clin North Am Small Anim Pract 2010;40(2):317–33.

15. Knieriem M, Otto CM, Macintire D. Hyperglycemia in critically ill patients. Compendium 2007;29(6):360–2, 364–72; [quiz: 372].
16. Hardie EM, Rawlings CA, George JW. Plasma-glucose concentrations in dogs and cats before and after surgery: comparison of healthy animals and animals with sepsis. Am J Vet Res 1985;46(8):1700–4.
17. Bonczynski JJ, Ludwig LL, Barton LJ, et al. Comparison of peritoneal fluid and peripheral blood pH, bicarbonate, glucose, and lactate concentration as a diagnostic tool for septic peritonitis in dogs and cats. Vet Surg 2003;32(2):161–6.
18. DeClue AE, Williams KJ, Sharp C, et al. Systemic response to low-dose endotoxin infusion in cats. Vet Immunol Immunopathol 2009;132(2–4):167–74.
19. Center SA, Magne ML. Historical, physical examination, and clinicopathologic features of portosystemic vascular anomalies in the dog and cat. Semin Vet Med Surg (Small Anim) 1990;5(2):83–93.
20. Bostwick DR, Twedt DC. Intrahepatic and extrahepatic portal venous anomalies in dogs: 52 cases (1982-1992). J Am Vet Med Assoc 1995;206(8):1181–5.
21. Greene SN, Bright RM. Insulinoma in a cat. J Small Anim Pract 2008;49(1):38–40.
22. Sherding RG. Acute hepatic failure. Vet Clin North Am Small Anim Pract 1985; 15(1):119–33.
23. Finney SJ, Zekveld C, Elia A, et al. Glucose control and mortality in critically ill patients. JAMA 2003;290(15):2041–7.
24. Krinsley JS. Association between hyperglycemia and increased hospital mortality in a heterogeneous population of critically ill patients. Mayo Clin Proc 2003;78(12):1471–8.
25. Krinsley JS. Effect of an intensive glucose management protocol on the mortality of critically ill adult patients. Mayo Clin Proc 2004;79(8):992–1000.
26. Holzinger U, Warszawska J, Kitzberger R, et al. Real-time continuous glucose monitoring in critically ill patients: a prospective randomized trial. Diabetes Care 2010;33(3):467–72.
27. Torre DM, deLaforcade AM, Chan DL. Incidence and clinical relevance of hyperglycemia in critically ill dogs. J Vet Intern Med 2007;21(5):971–5.
28. Syring RS, Otto CM, Drobatz KJ. Hyperglycemia in dogs and cats with head trauma: 122 cases (1997-1999). J Am Vet Med Assoc 2001;218(7):1124–9.
29. Van den Berghe G, Wouters P, Weekers F, et al. Intensive insulin therapy in critically ill patients. N Engl J Med 2001;345:1359–67.
30. Egi M, Bellomo R, Stachowski E, et al. Variability of blood glucose concentration and short-term mortality in critically ill patients. Anesthesiology 2006;105(2): 244–52.
31. Krinsley JS. Glycemic variability: a strong independent predictor of mortality in critically ill patients. Crit Care Med 2008;36(11):3008–13.
32. Krinsley JS, Meyfroidt G, van den Berghe G, et al. The impact of premorbid diabetic status on the relationship between the three domains of glycemic control and mortality in critically ill patients. Curr Opin Clin Nutr Metab Care 2012;15(2): 151–60.
33. Reed CC, Stewart RM, Sherman M, et al. Intensive insulin protocol improves glucose control and is associated with a reduction in intensive care unit mortality. J Am Coll Surg 2007;204(5):1048–54 [discussion: 1054–5].
34. Finfer S, Chittock DR, Su SY, et al. Intensive versus conventional glucose control in critically ill patients. N Engl J Med 2009;360(13):1283–97.
35. Griesdale DE, de Souza RJ, van Dam RM, et al. Intensive insulin therapy and mortality among critically ill patients: a meta-analysis including NICE-SUGAR study data. CMAJ 2009;180(8):821–7.

36. Brunkhorst FM, Engel C, Bloos F, et al. Intensive insulin therapy and pentastarch resuscitation in severe sepsis. N Engl J Med 2008;358(2):125–39.
37. Devos P, Presier J, Melot C. Impact of tight glucose control by intensive insulin therapy on ICU mortality and the rate of hypoglycemia: final results of the glucose control study. Intensive Care Med 2007;33:S189.
38. Krinsley JS, Grover A. Severe hypoglycemia in critically ill patients: risk factors and outcomes. Crit Care Med 2007;35(10):2262–7.
39. Krinsley J, Schultz MJ, Spronk PE, et al. Mild hypoglycemia is strongly associated with increased intensive care unit length of stay. Ann Intensive Care 2011; 1:49.
40. American Diabetes Association. Standards of medical care in diabetes–2012. Diabetes Care 2012;35(Suppl 1):S11–63.
41. Moghissi ES, Korytkowski MT, DiNardo M, et al. American Association of Clinical Endocrinologists and American Diabetes Association consensus statement on inpatient glycemic control. Endocr Pract 2009;15(4):353–69.
42. De Block C, Manuel YK, Van Gaal L, et al. Intensive insulin therapy in the intensive care unit: assessment by continuous glucose monitoring. Diabetes Care 2006;29(8):1750–6.
43. Steil GM, Langer M, Jaeger K, et al. Value of continuous glucose monitoring for minimizing severe hypoglycemia during tight glycemic control. Pediatr Crit Care Med 2011;12(6):643–8.
44. Brunner R, Adelsmayr G, Herkner H, et al. Glycemic variability and glucose complexity in critically ill patients: a retrospective analysis of continuous glucose monitoring data. Crit Care 2012;16(5):R175.
45. Munir A, Choudhary P, Harrison B, et al. Continuous glucose monitoring in patients with insulinoma. Clin Endocrinol 2008;68(6):912–8.
46. Nelson R. Stress hyperglycemia and diabetes mellitus in cats. J Vet Intern Med 2002;16(2):121–2.
47. Rand JS, Kinnaird E, Baglioni A, et al. Acute stress hyperglycemia in cats is associated with struggling and increased concentrations of lactate and norepinephrine. J Vet Intern Med 2002;16(2):123–32.
48. Kley S, Casella M, Reusch CE. Evaluation of long-term home monitoring of blood glucose concentrations in cats with diabetes mellitus: 26 cases (1999-2002). J Am Vet Med Assoc 2004;225(2):261–6.
49. Blaiset MA, Couto CG, Evans KL, et al. Complications of indwelling, silastic central venous access catheters in dogs and cats. J Am Anim Hosp Assoc 1995;31(5):379–84.
50. Mathews KA, Brooks MJ, Valliant AE. A prospective study of intravenous catheter contamination. J Vet Emerg Crit Care (San Antonio) 1996;6(1):33–43.
51. Seguela J, Pages JP. Bacterial and fungal colonisation of peripheral intravenous catheters in dogs and cats. J Small Anim Pract 2011;52(10):531–5.
52. Reineke EL, Fletcher DJ, King LG, et al. Accuracy of a continuous glucose monitoring system in dogs and cats with diabetic ketoacidosis. J Vet Emerg Crit Care (San Antonio) 2010;20(3):303–12.
53. Davison LJ, Slater LA, Herrtage ME, et al. Evaluation of a continuous glucose monitoring system in diabetic dogs. J Small Anim Pract 2003;44(10):435–42.
54. Ristic JM, Herrtage ME, Walti-Lauger SM, et al. Evaluation of a continuous glucose monitoring system in cats with diabetes mellitus. J Feline Med Surg 2005;7(3):153–62.
55. Moretti S, Tschuor F, Osto M, et al. Evaluation of a novel real-time continuous glucose-monitoring system for use in cats. J Vet Intern Med 2010;24(1):120–6.

56. Affenzeller N, Benesch T, Thalhammer JG, et al. A pilot study to evaluate a novel subcutaneous continuous glucose monitoring system in healthy Beagle dogs. Vet J 2010;184(1):105–10.

57. Dietiker-Moretti S, Muller C, Sieber-Ruckstuhl N, et al. Comparison of a continuous glucose monitoring system with a portable blood glucose meter to determine insulin dose in cats with diabetes mellitus. J Vet Intern Med 2011;25(5): 1084–8.

58. Wiedmeyer CE, Johnson PJ, Cohn LA, et al. Evaluation of a continuous glucose monitoring system for use in dogs, cats, and horses. J Am Vet Med Assoc 2003; 223(7):987–92.

59. Wiedmeyer CE, Johnson PJ, Cohn LA, et al. Evaluation of a continuous glucose monitoring system for use in veterinary medicine. Diabetes Technol Ther 2005; 7(6):885–95.

60. Affenzeller N, Thalhammer JG, Willmann M. Home-based subcutaneous continuous glucose monitoring in 10 diabetic dogs. Vet Rec 2011;169(8):206.

61. Roomp K, Rand J. Intensive blood glucose control is safe and effective in diabetic cats using home monitoring and treatment with glargine. J Feline Med Surg 2009;11(8):668–82.

62. Roomp K, Rand J. Evaluation of detemir in diabetic cats managed with a protocol for intensive blood glucose control. J Feline Med Surg 2012;14(8):566–72.

63. Marshall RD, Rand JS, Morton JM. Glargine and protamine zinc insulin have a longer duration of action and result in lower mean daily glucose concentrations than lente insulin in healthy cats. J Vet Pharmacol Ther 2008;31(3):205–12.

64. Marshall RD, Rand JS, Morton JM. Treatment of newly diagnosed diabetic cats with glargine insulin improves glycaemic control and results in higher probability of remission than protamine zinc and lente insulins. J Feline Med Surg 2009; 11(8):683–91.

65. Unger J. Uncovering undetected hypoglycemic events. Diabetes Metab Syndr Obes 2012;5:57–74.

66. Leese GP, Wang J, Broomhall J, et al. Frequency of severe hypoglycemia requiring emergency treatment in type 1 and type 2 diabetes: a population-based study of health service resource use. Diabetes Care 2003;26(4):1176–80.

67. Zoungas S, Patel A, Chalmers J, et al. Severe hypoglycemia and risks of vascular events and death. N Engl J Med 2010;363(15):1410–8.

68. Cryer PE, Davis SN, Shamoon H. Hypoglycemia in diabetes. Diabetes Care 2003;26(6):1902–12.

69. Brod M, Christensen T, Thomsen TL, et al. The impact of non-severe hypoglycemic events on work productivity and diabetes management. Value Health 2011;14(5):665–71.

70. Stephenson JM, Schernthaner G. Dawn phenomenon and Somogyi effect in IDDM. Diabetes Care 1989;12(4):245–51.

71. Wentholt IM, Maran A, Masurel N, et al. Nocturnal hypoglycaemia in Type 1 diabetic patients, assessed with continuous glucose monitoring: frequency, duration and associations. Diabet Med 2007;24(5):527–32.

72. Woodward A, Weston P, Casson IF, et al. Nocturnal hypoglycaemia in type 1 diabetes–frequency and predictive factors. QJM 2009;102(9):603–7.

73. Petrie JP. Practical application of holter monitoring in dogs and cats. Clin Tech Small Anim Pract 2005;20(3):173–81.

74. Hanas S, Tidholm A, Egenvall A, et al. Twenty-four hour Holter monitoring of unsedated healthy cats in the home environment. J Vet Cardiol 2009;11(1): 17–22.

75. Rasmussen CE, Vesterholm S, Ludvigsen TP, et al. Holter monitoring in clinically healthy Cavalier King Charles Spaniels, Wire-haired Dachshunds, and Cairn Terriers. J Vet Intern Med 2011;25(3):460–8.
76. Kovatchev B, Clarke W. Continuous glucose monitoring (CGM) reduces risks for hypo- and hyperglycaemia and glucose variability in diabetes. Diabetes 2007; 56(Suppl 1). pA23.
77. Garg S, Zisser H, Schwartz S, et al. Improvement in glycemic excursions with a transcutaneous, real-time continuous glucose sensor: a randomized controlled trial. Diabetes Care 2006;29(1):44–50.
78. Mastrototaro J. The MiniMed Continuous Glucose Monitoring System (CGMS). J Pediatr Endocrinol Metab 1999;12(Suppl 3):751–8.
79. Rebrin K, Steil GM, van Antwerp WP, et al. Subcutaneous glucose predicts plasma glucose independent of insulin: implications for continuous monitoring. Am J Phys 1999;277(3 Pt 1):E561–71.
80. Bode BW, Gross TM, Thornton KR, et al. Continuous glucose monitoring used to adjust diabetes therapy improves glycosylated hemoglobin: a pilot study. Diabetes Res Clin Pract 1999;46(3):183–90.
81. Bilicki KL, Schermerhorn T, Klocke EE, et al. Evaluation of a real-time, continuous monitor of glucose concentration in healthy dogs during anesthesia. Am J Vet Res 2010;71(1):11–6.
82. Piper HG, Alexander JL, Shukla A, et al. Real-time continuous glucose monitoring in pediatric patients during and after cardiac surgery. Pediatrics 2006; 118(3):1176–84.
83. Vriesendorp TM, DeVries JH, Holleman F, et al. The use of two continuous glucose sensors during and after surgery. Diabetes Technol Ther 2005;7(2):315–22.
84. Holtkamp HC, Verhoef NJ, Leijnse B. The difference between the glucose concentrations in plasma and whole blood. Clin Chim Acta 1975;59(1):41–9.
85. McMillin J. Blood glucose. Boston: Butterworths; 1990.
86. Henry JB. Clinical diagnosis and management by laboratory methods. Philadelphia: WB Saunders; 1979.
87. Hones J, Muller P, Surridge N. The technology behind glucose meters: test strips. Diabetes Technol Ther 2008;10(Suppl 1):s10–26.
88. Montagnana M, Caputo M, Giavarina D, et al. Overview on self-monitoring of blood glucose. Clin Chim Acta 2009;402(1–2):7–13.
89. Coldman MF, Good W. The distribution of sodium, potassium and glucose in the blood of some mammals. Comp Biochem Physiol 1967;21(1):201–6.
90. Zini E, Moretti S, Tschuor F, et al. Evaluation of a new portable glucose meter designed for the use in cats. Schweiz Arch Tierheilkd 2009;151(9):448–51.
91. Hackett ES, McCue PM. Evaluation of a veterinary glucometer for use in horses. J Vet Intern Med 2010;24(3):617–21.
92. Paul AE, Shiel RE, Juvet F, et al. Effect of hematocrit on accuracy of two point-of-care glucometers for use in dogs. Am J Vet Res 2011;72(9):1204–8.
93. Laboratory, diagnostic and critical care products direct to worldwide vet distributors. g-Pet glucose veterinary monitoring system. 2012. Available at: http://www.woodleyequipment.com/veterinary-diagnostics.html?&flag=y. Accessed November 29, 2012.
94. Ulti-Care iPet glucose monitoring system. 2012. Available at: http://www.ulti-care.com/ipet-blood-glucose-monitoring.html. Accessed November 29, 2012.
95. Sternberg F, Meyerhoff C, Mennel FJ, et al. Subcutaneous glucose concentration in humans. Real estimation and continuous monitoring. Diabetes Care 1995;18(9):1266–9.

96. Rebrin K, Steil GM. Can interstitial glucose assessment replace blood glucose measurements? Diabetes Technol Ther 2000;2(3):461–72.
97. DeClue AE, Cohn LA, Kerl ME, et al. Use of continuous blood glucose monitoring for animals with diabetes mellitus. J Am Anim Hosp Assoc 2004;40(3): 171–3.
98. i-Pro 2 Progessional continuous glucose monitoring system user guide. 2012. Available at: http://www.professional.medtronicdiabetes.com/hcp-products/ipro2. Accessed November 29, 2012.
99. Battelino T, Bolinder J. Clinical use of real-time continuous glucose monitoring. Curr Diabetes Rev 2008;4(3):218–22.
100. Hrabchak R, Taylor J. A new glucose monitoring option. J Fam Pract 2010;59(2): 81–8.
101. Wiedmeyer CE, DeClue AE. Continuous glucose monitoring in dogs and cats. J Vet Intern Med 2008;22(1):2–8.
102. Hafner M, Lutz TA, Reusch CE, et al. Evaluation of sensor sites for continuous glucose monitoring in cats with diabetes mellitus. Journal of feline medicine and surgery 2013;15(2):117–23.
103. Gerritsen M, Jansen JA, Kros A, et al. Influence of inflammatory cells and serum on the performance of implantable glucose sensors. J Biomed Mater Res 2001; 54(1):69–75.
104. Kvist PH, Iburg T, Bielecki M, et al. Biocompatibility of electrochemical glucose sensors implanted in the subcutis of pigs. Diabetes Technol Ther 2006;8(4): 463–75.
105. Kvist PH, Iburg T, Aalbaek B, et al. Biocompatibility of an enzyme-based, electrochemical glucose sensor for short-term implantation in the subcutis. Diabetes Technol Ther 2006;8(5):546–59.
106. Keenan DB, Mastrototaro JJ, Zisser H, et al. Accuracy of the Enlite 6-day glucose sensor with guardian and Veo calibration algorithms. Diabetes Technol Ther 2012;14(3):225–31.
107. Adolfsson P, Ornhagen H, Eriksson BM, et al. Continuous glucose monitoring– a study of the Enlite sensor during hypo- and hyperbaric conditions. Diabetes Technol Ther 2012;14(6):527–32.
108. Mastrototaro JJ. The MiniMed continuous glucose monitoring system. Diabetes Technol Ther 2000;2(Suppl 1):S13–8.
109. Introducing the Guardian REAL-Time continuous glucose monitoring system. 2010. Available at: http://www.medtronic-diabetes-me.com/Guardian-REAL-Time.html. Accessed November 18, 2012.
110. FreeStyle Navigator continuous glucose monitoring system. 2008. Available at: https://www.healthyoutcomes.com/pdf/freestylenavigatoruserguide.pdf. Accessed November 18, 2012.
111. Dexcom Seven continuous glucose monitoring system user's guide 2010. Available at: http://www.dexcom.com/sites/dexcom.com/files/seven/docs/SEVEN_System_Users_Guide.pdf. Accessed November 18, 2012.

Oral Hypoglycemics in Cats with Diabetes Mellitus

Carrie A. Palm, DVM[a],*, Edward C. Feldman, DVM[b]

KEYWORDS

- Hypoglycemics • Cat • Feline • Diabetes mellitus • Sulfonylurea drugs
- Meglitinides • Biguanides

KEY POINTS

- Cats with diabetes mellitus often have type 2 disease.
- When owners are unwilling to administer insulin, use of oral hypoglycemic drugs can be considered.
- Several classes of oral hypoglycemic drugs have been evaluated in cats but these drugs have not been commonly used for treatment of diabetic cats.
- The use of older oral hypoglycemics has not become common in veterinary medicine; however, the advent of newer drugs, such as DDP-4 inhibitors, which may preserve B-cell function and thereby prevent development of type 1 diabetes mellitus, necessitates the need for further studies, some of which are currently in progress.

Diabetes mellitus is relatively common in cats. Similar to diabetes mellitus in people, in whom approximately 93% are believed to have type 2 disease, most diabetic cats probably have some surviving B cells at the time of diagnosis, and have other clinical and histologic features consistent with type 2 diabetes. There are owners of diabetic cats who are fearful or who outright refuse to inject their cats with insulin, and there are cats that refuse to be injected. Because of these realities, veterinarians are often asked about alternatives to injectable insulin. Similar to type 2 diabetes in humans, hyperglycemia in cats is often largely caused by insulin resistance and dysfunctional B cells (impaired insulin secretion) but not by an absolute insulin deficiency. Some humans with type 2 diabetes mellitus benefit from exogenous insulin administration. Others do not require exogenous insulin for survival, and control of their diabetes mellitus often improves with changes in diet, exercise, and weight loss. Another subset of people with type 2 diabetes mellitus respond adequately to the use of oral hypoglycemic agents.

[a] Department of Medicine and Epidemiology, University of California-Davis School of Veterinary Medicine, University of California-Davis, 2101 Tupper Hall, One Shields Avenue, Davis, CA 95616, USA; [b] Department of Medicine and Epidemiology, University of California-Davis School of Veterinary Medicine, University of California-Davis, 2108 Tupper Hall, One Shields Avenue, Davis, CA 95616, USA
* Corresponding author.
E-mail address: cpalm@ucdavis.edu

Vet Clin Small Anim 43 (2013) 407–415
http://dx.doi.org/10.1016/j.cvsm.2012.12.002
0195-5616/13/$ – see front matter © 2013 Elsevier Inc. All rights reserved.
vetsmall.theclinics.com

Oral hypoglycemic drugs are used in patients with diabetes who have some capacity to synthesize and secrete endogenous insulin. Commonly available oral hypoglycemic drugs work through various mechanisms, including stimulation of pancreatic insulin secretion, requiring some number of functioning pancreatic B cells. Some of these drugs slow intestinal glucose absorption and others enhance tissue sensitivity to insulin.

One goal of managing diabetic cats is to prevent clinical signs, such as polyuria, polydipsia, and weight loss. Striving for perfect glucose control is often not an achievable goal and can lead to life-threatening hypoglycemia. Striving for resolution of diabetes mellitus, negating the need for oral or parenteral drugs is obvious but in some cats, illusive.

SULFONYLUREA DRUGS

Sulfonylurea derivatives have been the most commonly used oral hypoglycemic agents in cats with diabetes mellitus.[1] The primary action of sulfonylurea drugs is to bind pancreatic B-cell ATPases, which in turn stimulates insulin release. Effectiveness of drugs in this class requires the presence of functional B cells from which insulin can be secreted. Response to therapy can be variable, and is dependent in part on the number of functional B cells. For example, a patient with a large number of functional cells may have an excellent response, whereas another patient verging on becoming insulin-dependent because of loss of B cells may have little to no response. Additional explanations for variable responses to these drugs may be related to the state of B-cell health, including presence of B-cell "exhaustion," B-cell "desensitization," and B cells that are glucose "toxic."[2] Each condition can occur in response to chronic hyperglycemia. B-cell exhaustion refers to cells whose insulin stores are temporarily depleted secondary to excessive insulin secretion, whereas B-cell desensitization is temporary cell refractoriness to glucose stimulation. Both of these conditions are potentially reversible if the effected cell is "rested" by periods of glycemic control and these patients may therefore respond to oral hypoglycemics after B-cell improves. However, B cells that have experienced "glucose toxicity" are in variable states of irreversible cell damage. Affected patients will not likely respond to oral hypoglycemic drugs, unless a sufficient population of B-cells have been spared of toxicity. In addition to stimulating insulin synthesis and secretion, there is also evidence that sulfonylureas may act independent of B cells by sensitizing tissues to insulin, via limitation of hepatic glucose synthesis, and by decreasing insulin clearance by the liver.[1]

There are numerous sulfonylurea-derivative drugs available and similar to insulin, the pharmacokinetics and pharmacodynamics of the various drugs in this class can affect potency and duration of effect. In contrast to first-generation sulfonylureas, second-generation drugs have increased affinity for pancreatic B-cell receptors and are therefore more potent. This increased binding allows for less frequent dosing regimens, which is preferable in humans and cats. The second-generation sulfonylurea-derivative glipizide (Glucotrol; Pfizer, New York, NY) has been the most commonly prescribed oral hypoglycemic drug in cats and is the focus of this discussion.

It has been reported that approximately 30% of cats treated with glipizide had improvement in clinical signs of diabetes mellitus.[1] The nonresponders likely had B-cell insufficiency secondary to glucose toxicity, desensitization, or exhaustion. Other possible causes for treatment failure could include inadequate dosing by owners, discontinuation of drug administration by owners because of adverse events, or malabsorptive disorders that might prevent therapeutic drug levels from being achieved. Side effects, including vomiting immediately after administration, hypoglycemia, increases in hepatic leakage enzymes, and increased bilirubin concentrations have been reported to occur in approximately 15% of treated cats.[1] The adverse effects of glipizide can be minimized by initially using low doses. Reported dosing regimens start at 2.5 mg per os twice daily, and if no adverse effects are seen after 2 weeks and glycemic control has not been achieved, the dose can be increased to 5 mg per os twice daily. If liver enzyme abnormalities are encountered in cats, discontinuation of glipizide usually results in rapid resolution. With resolution of liver enzyme elevations, glipizide can be restarted at a lower dose. Some cats have no recurrence of hepatic enzyme abnormalities. Recurrence necessitates consideration of permanent discontinuation of the drug.[1]

Because many sulfonylurea drugs are protein-bound, their effectiveness can be altered by drugs that compete at the same binding sites. Unlike exogenously administered insulin, action of orally administered drugs requires reliable absorption from the intestinal tract. Because infiltrative bowel diseases are common in middle-aged and older cats, such problems should be considered when prescribing oral hypoglycemics. In cats, increased insulin secretion stimulated by sulfonylurea drugs may be accompanied by a concurrent increase in amylin secretion. Amylin may form toxic intracellular fibrils or amyloid deposits within the pancreatic islet, causing further B-cell dysfunction and loss, potentially resulting in permanent insulin dependency. In an experimental model of diabetes mellitus in eight cats, four neutral protamine Hagedorn (NPH) insulin-treated cats and four glipizide-treated cats were assessed for 18 months.[3] One neutral protamine Hagedorn-treated cat developed mild to moderate amyloid deposition within pancreatic B cells, whereas three of four cats in the glipizide group had these changes, suggesting that glipizide may contribute to progressive B-cell dysfunction.

Other second-generation sulfonylurea drugs include glyburide (DiaBeta, Sanofi-aventis, Bridgewater, NJ; Glynase, Pfizer; Micronase, Pfizer) and glimepiride (Amaryl; Sanofi-aventis). Glyburide has a longer duration of action compared with glipizide, and is therefore prescribed once daily. Glimepiride is a more recently marketed intermediate- to long-acting oral hypoglycemic agent. Its effectiveness was recently evaluated in a small number of healthy cats by comparing intravenous glucose tolerance testing (IVGTT) responses before and after administration.[4] Results showed that glimepiride was effective at stimulating significantly more insulin secretion with significantly lower blood glucose concentrations compared with control cats. The pattern of induced insulin secretion was prolonged with this longer-acting oral hypoglycemic, as is also the case in humans.

Given that one of the primary indications for the use of oral hypoglycemics is for cats or owners who do not tolerate insulin injections, some also may not tolerate oral administration of drugs. Given this, a study evaluating the transdermal application of glipizide in a pluronic lecithin gel was performed.[5] Results showed low and unpredictable absorption of this formulation, making it less than ideal for clinical use. Interestingly, despite lower serum glipizide levels in cats receiving transdermal glipizide (compared with equivalent oral dosing) decreases in blood glucose were similar 10 to 24 hours after administration, and were significantly different when compared with control cats. Cats administered oral glipizide did have a more significant drop in blood glucose 4 to 6 hours after administration, compared with patients given the transdermal formulation. The decreases in glucose that occurred with both formulations of glipizide were not associated with parallel increases in insulin concentration. This suggests that extrapancreatic mechanisms may be responsible for some of the glucose-lowering effects.

Although there are many potential pitfalls to the use of sulfonylurea drugs in diabetic cats, circumstances that support their use include owners unable or unwilling to give insulin injections and cats with fluctuating requirements for insulin, who may intermittently become hypoglycemic with even low doses of insulin. In a study of 20 diabetic cats treated with glipizide, 25% had resolution of clinical signs and glucosuria within 4 weeks of therapy.[6] Another 35% were nonresponders and required insulin therapy. Evidence of a clinical response is usually apparent within 4 to 6 weeks after initiation of glipizide therapy. If adequate glycemic control or control of clinical signs is not achieved in that time frame, or if ketoacidosis develops, alternate therapy should be initiated. Over time, glipizide becomes ineffective in some of the initial responders. The timeframe for this to occur can vary from weeks to years and is likely caused by progressive loss of B cells. Despite this finding, several cats were managed successfully with glipizide for years.[1]

MEGLITINIDES

Similar to the sulfonylureas, meglitinides (or glinides) bind B-cell ATPases, thereby inducing insulin secretion from functional cells. Meglinitides bind ATPase at sites independent of those that bind sulfonylureas. This would allow both drug classes to be used concurrently with potential for synergistic effects. Currently, there are two commercially available meglitinides, repaglinide (Prandin; Novo Nordisk, Princeton, NJ) and the more recently available nateglinide (Starlix, Novartis Pharma Stein AG, Stein, Switzerland).

Nateglinide was recently evaluated in healthy cats with the use of IVGTT.[4] Similar to the sulfonylurea glimepiride, oral nateglinide was found to increase insulin secretion with corresponding decreases in blood glucose concentrations compared with control cats. Compared with the effects of glimepiride, nateglinide had a more rapid onset and shorter duration of effect. Temporally, the effects of nateglinide were analogous to short-acting insulin, whereas the duration of glimepiride was similar to intermediate-acting insulin.

BIGUANIDES

Unlike the two drug classes previously discussed, biguanide drugs do not directly affect B-cell function, and therefore do not require functional B cells for efficacy. For this reason, these drugs can be used in patients with either type 1 or 2 diabetes mellitus. The exact mechanism of action for biguanides is not known, but they ultimately act to increase hepatic and peripheral tissue response to insulin. Circulating insulin must therefore be present for the biguanides to have a beneficial effect. This increase in insulin sensitivity leads to decreased hepatic gluconeogenesis, decreased glycogenolysis, and increased glucose uptake by muscle cells. Cumulatively, these actions decrease fasting blood glucose concentrations without a significant risk for development of hypoglycemia.

Gastrointestinal upset is the most common adverse effect associated with biguanides. In humans, lactic acidosis has also been uncommonly reported.[7] Currently, metformin (Glucophage; Bristol-Myers Squibb Company, Princeton, NJ) is the only commercially available oral hypoglycemic drug in this class; other previously available biguanide drugs are no longer used because of potential toxic effects. Many people with type 2 diabetes mellitus are started on metformin therapy soon after diagnosis, because it has been shown to improve long-term clinical outcomes compared with initial management with diet alone. Use of the older immediate-release of metformin has been associated with adverse gastrointestinal effects, restricting its use in some patients because of poor compliance and subsequent inadequate glycemic control.[7]

Metformin has been evaluated in cats. Serum levels similar to those needed in humans have been achieved at doses of 25 to 50 mg/cat orally twice daily, which is higher than the initially recommended dose of 2 mg/kg orally twice daily.[8,9] This dosing regimen is complicated by the commercially available 500-mg tablet size. Thus, use of metformin necessitates compounding to allow for appropriate dosing in most cats. Because compounded drugs are not consistently regulated, different formulations or batches may have different drug concentrations, which could lead to inconsistent results. After 8 weeks of metformin administration, glycemic control was evaluated in five diabetic cats.[9] Only one of the five cats responded, based on control of polyuria, polydipsia, maintenance of weight, and euglycemia. Further evaluation of these diabetic cats revealed that the responder was the only cat in the group to have measureable serum insulin levels. This supports the concept that metformin should only be used in cats known to have type 2 diabetes mellitus, and with functional B cells. It is also important to note that significant percentages of metformin are excreted by the kidneys and the drug should be used with caution in cats with abnormal glomerular filtration rates. In the study sited previously, adverse effects included vomiting, lethargy, and decreased appetite. These side effects were noted in metformin-treated cats, even with serum drug concentrations considered to be in the therapeutic range for humans. An extended-release formulation of metformin (Metformin XR; Glucophage XR; Forotmet Glucophage XR, Bristol-Myers Squibb Company) has recently become available and has shown promise in the control of diabetes mellitus in humans. This extended-release formulation has less adverse gastrointestinal effects and has been shown to achieve better glycemic control through its longer duration of action.[7]

THIAZOLIDINEDIONES

The thiazolidinediones are insulin-sensitizing agents that act to amplify hepatic, muscle, and adipose tissue responses to insulin through binding to the peroxisome proliferator-activated receptor-γ. This results in decreasing fasting blood glucose levels. Pioglitazone (Actos, Takeda Pharmaceuticals, U.S.A., Inc., Deerfield, IL) and rosiglitazone (Avandia, GlaxoSmithKline, Brentford, Middlesex, United Kingdom) are the two most commonly used thiazolidinediones in humans. Troglitazone, which has been evaluated in healthy cats, was removed from the commercial market because of the development of drug-induced hepatitis in some treated people.[10] Oral absorption of troglitazone by healthy cats was found to be poor and this drug was not evaluated in diabetic cats.[11] In a study on darglitazone, nine obese cats were treated with 2 mg/kg darglitazone orally once daily.[12] IVGTTs were performed before treatment and after 42 days of drug administration. Nine obese placebo-treated cats and four placebo-treated lean cats were also included as control populations. In all obese cats, initial IVGTT was abnormal compared with lean control cats. Darglitazone-treated cats showed significant improvement in insulin levels in response to repeat IVGTT, but secretion patterns were still not normal. Overall, treated cats showed a 40% decrease in area under the curve for insulin and a 20% decrease in the area under the curve for glucose. These findings support that darglitazone functions in large part through enhancing peripheral tissue sensitivity insulin, and not through increasing insulin secretion. This decrease in plasma insulin concentrations in treated cats may correspond with a decrease in amylin secretion, which may help to prevent or at least slow further B-cell dysfunction and loss.

CHROMIUM

Chromium picolinate is an essential trace element and a cofactor for insulin function that increases insulin binding and insulin receptor numbers, resulting in enhanced glucose transport into liver, adipose tissue, and muscle.[13] Chromium deficiency has been shown to result in insulin resistance. Older studies have demonstrated inconsistent effects among people with diabetes.[14,15] More recently, chromium has been associated with significant improvement in at least one outcome of glycemic control in people with diabetes.[13] Chromium is an inexpensive nutritional supplement that is considered to have an adjunctive role in combination diabetes therapy that may allow for dosage reduction of more expensive and potentially toxic medications.[13] Chromium picolinate supplementation was evaluated for safety and effect on IVGTT in obese and nonobese cats.[16] Results showed that supplementation of 100 μg orally for 6 weeks was safe, but had no effect on IVGTT. A more recent study used IVGTT testing to evaluate 32 healthy nonobese cats on various dosages of chromium picolinate.[17] Results showed significantly lower blood glucose levels in cats on diets supplemented with greater than 300 ppb of chromium. Further studies are needed before definitive recommendations can be made regarding the use of chromium in diabetic cats.

VANADIUM AND TUNGSTEN

Vanadium and tungsten are trace elements shown to have glucose-lowering properties and to improve pancreatic insulin secretion in rat models of experimental diabetes mellitus.[18,19] Other studies have shown that vanadium and its metabolites do not increase insulin secretion but act at a postreceptor site to increase glucose metabolism.[20,21] Administration of orthovanadate, a derivative of vanadium, to a single cat with diabetes led to resolution of clinical signs.[1] Early studies in diabetic cats suggested that vanadium might be beneficial very early in disease.[22,23] In a group of protamine zinc insulin-treated diabetic cats, those supplemented with vanadium dipicolinate had improved control.[1,23,24] Adverse effects of vanadium administration included anorexia and vomiting. Chronic administration of this trace element has been reported to lead to excessive accumulations in the liver and kidneys.[19] More recent studies in rat models of diabetes mellitus have shown vanadium derivatives to have protective effects on B cells and to improve glycemic control, without apparent toxicity.[25,26] These trace elements are not commonly administered to diabetic cats.

α-GLUCOSIDASE INHIBITORS

α-Glucosidase inhibitors, such as acarbose (Precose; Bayer Pharmaceuticals Corporation, Berkeley, CA) and miglitol (Glyset; Pfizer, New York, NY), competitively inhibit membrane-bound intestinal brush border enzymes, which normally function to hydrolyze complex carbohydrates to monosaccharides. Blockade of these brush border enzymes prevents the immediate breakdown of ingested complex carbohydrates to monosacharides. Complex carbohydrates are absorbed slower than monosacharides. Acarbose also prevents hydrolysis of complex starches by blocking pancreatic α-amylase. The combined effects help prevent postprandial blood glucose increases that can contribute to poor glycemic control. The resultant carbohydrate malassimilation can lead to diarrhea and weight loss, limiting use of these drugs. A clinical study evaluated the use of acarbose at a dose of 12.5 mg/cat orally twice daily in client-owned cats with naturally occurring diabetes mellitus.[27] At the start of the study, all cats were treated with subcutaneous insulin, in addition to acarbose and a commercially available low-carbohydrate diet. After 4 months of therapy some cats no longer needed insulin for glycemic control; however, acarbose was found to have no apparent beneficial role in controlling diabetes in these cats ingesting a low-carbohydrate diet.

This was consistent with findings from a study comparing the effects of acarbose in healthy cats fed low- and high-carbohydrate diets. Cats given acarbose and eating a high-carbohydrate diet in one daily meal had significantly reduced blood glucose concentrations for 12 hours. However, the same effect was achieved by feeding a low-carbohydrate diet (6% metabolizable energy). Acarbose is most useful in cats on a high-carbohydrate diet that are eating all their food in one or two daily meals, a typical feeding pattern seen in cats on a weight loss program. Acarbose is minimally effective when cats are eating multiple small meals or grazing throughout the day. Therefore, for the cats where acarbose is most indicated (cats with advanced renal failure eating a restricted protein, high-carbohydrate diet) their picky eating pattern tends to make acarbose ineffective. These drugs are not commonly used in diabetic cats because of the need to orally dose the medication, the associated gastrointestinal side effects, and because a low-carbohydrate diet has the same or greater effect in reducing postprandial blood glucose concentrations.[28,29]

DIPEPTIDYL-PEPTIDASE 4 INHIBITORS

Dipeptidyl-peptidase 4 (DDP-4) inhibitors, including saxagliptin (Onglyza; Bristol-Meyers Squibb, Princeton, NJ) and linagliptin (Tradjenta; Boehringer Ingelheim Pharmaceuticals, Inc., Ridgefield, CT) are the most recently available oral hypoglycemic drugs. Inhibition of DPP-4 leads to increased insulin secretion and decreased glucagon release, with a resultant lowering of blood glucose.[30] These drugs have been shown to have low risk for causing hypoglycemia and to preserve B-cell function. Given this, some clinicians recommend DPP-4 as a second agent, after metformin has failed to adequately control hyperglycemia.[31] These drugs are not yet commonly used in veterinary medicine but have been shown to be safe and to stimulate insulin secretion in healthy cats. They are currently undergoing trials in diabetic cats and are discussed elsewhere in this issue.[32]

SUMMARY

Diabetes mellitus commonly affects feline patients. Inadequate glycemic control of these patients can lead to poor patient and owner quality of life, which can ultimately lead to decisions for euthanasia. When owners are unwilling to administer insulin, use of oral hypoglycemic drugs can be considered. The use of older oral hypoglycemics has not become common in veterinary medicine; however, the advent of newer drugs, such as DDP-4 inhibitors, which may preserve B-cell function and thereby prevent development of type 1 diabetes mellitus, necessitates the need for further studies, some of which are in progress.

REFERENCES

1. Feldman EC, Nelson RW. Diabetes mellitus. In: Feldman EC, Nelson RW, editors. Canine and feline endocrinology and reproduction. 3rd edition. Philadelphia: W. B. Saunders; 2003. p. 339–91.
2. Robertson RP, Harmon J, Tran PO, et al. Glucose toxicity in beta-cells: type 2 diabetes, good radicals gone bad, and the glutathione connection. Diabetes 2003;52(3):581–7.
3. Hoenig M, Hall G, Ferguson D, et al. A feline model of experimentally induced islet amyloidosis. Am J Pathol 2000;157(6):2143–50.

4. Mori A, Lee P, Yamashita Y, et al. Effect of glimepiride and nateglinide on serum insulin and glucose concentration in healthy cats. Vet Res Commun 2009;33(8): 957–70.

5. Bennett N, Papich MG, Hoenig M, et al. Evaluation of transdermal application of glipizide in a pluronic lecithin gel to healthy cats. Am J Vet Res 2005;66(4):581–8.

6. Nelson RW, Feldman EC, Ford SL, et al. Effect of an orally administered sulfonyl-urea, glipizide, for treatment of diabetes mellitus in cats. J Am Vet Med Assoc 1993;203(6):821–7.

7. Chacra AR. Evolving metformin treatment strategies in Type-2 diabetes: from immediate-release metformin monotherapy to extended-release combination therapy. Am J Ther 2012. http://dx.doi.org/10.1097/MJT.0b013e318235f1bb.

8. Michels GM, Boudinot FD, Ferguson DC, et al. Pharmacokinetics of the anti-hyperglycemic agent metformin in cats. Am J Vet Res 1999;60(6):738–42.

9. Nelson R, Spann D, Elliott D, et al. Evaluation of the oral antihyperglycemic drug metformin in normal and diabetic cats. J Vet Intern Med 2004;18(1):18–24.

10. Ikeda T. Drug-induced idiosyncratic hepatotoxicity: prevention strategy after the troglitazone case. Drug Metab Pharmacokinet 2011;26(1):60–70.

11. Michels GM, Boudinot FD, Ferguson DC, et al. Pharmacokinetics of the insulin-sensitizing agent troglitazone in cats. Am J Vet Res 2000;61(7):775–8.

12. Hoenig M, Duncan F. Effect of darglitazone on glucose clearance and lipid metabolism in obese cats. Am J Vet Res 2003;64(11):1409–13.

13. Broadhurst CL, Domenico P. Clinical studies on chromium picolinate supplementation in diabetes mellitus: a review. Diabetes Technol Ther 2006;8(6):677–87.

14. Anderson RA, Cheng N, Bryden NA, et al. Elevated intakes of supplemental chromium improve glucose and insulin variables in individuals with type 2 diabetes. Diabetes 1997;46(11):1786–91.

15. Preuss HG, Anderson RA. Chromium update: examining recent literature 1997-98. Curr Opin Clin Nutr Metab Care 1998;1(6):509–12.

16. Cohn LA, Dodam JR, McCaw DL, et al. Effects of chromium supplementation on glucose tolerance in obese and nonobese cats. Am J Vet Res 1999;60(11):1360–3.

17. Appleton DJ, Rand JS, Sunvold GD, et al. Dietary chromium tripicolinate supplementation reduces glucose concentrations and improves glucose tolerance in normal-weight cats. J Feline Med Surg 2002;4(1):13–25.

18. Muñoz MC, Barberà A, Dominguez J, et al. Effects of tungstate, a new potential oral antidiabetic agent, in Zucker diabetic fatty rats. Diabetes 2001;50(1):131–8.

19. Domingo JL. Vanadium and tungsten derivatives as antidiabetic agents: a review of their toxic effects. Biol Trace Elem Res 2002;88(2):97–112.

20. Brichard SM, Henquin JC. The role of vanadium in the management of diabetes. Trends Pharmacol Sci 1995;16(8):265–70.

21. Goldfine AB, Simonson DC, Folli F, et al. In vivo and in vitro studies of vanadate in human and rodent diabetes mellitus. Mol Cell Biochem 1995;153(1–2):217–31.

22. Greco DS. Oral hypoglycemic agents for noninsulin-dependent diabetes mellitus in the cat. Semin Vet Med Surg (Small Anim) 1997;12(4):259–62.

23. Martin G, Rand J. Current understanding of feline diabetes. Part 2: treatment. J Feline Med Surg 2000;2(1):3–17.

24. Fondacaro JV, Greco DS, Crans DC. Treatment of feline diabetes mellitus with protamine zinc alanine insulin alone compared with PZI and oral vanadium salts [abstract]. In: Proceedings of the 17th ACVIM Forum. Chicago: p. 710.

25. Ahmadi S, Karimian SM, Sotoudeh M, et al. Pancreatic islet beta cell protective effect of oral vanadyl sulphate in streptozotocin-induced diabetic rats, an ultra-structure study. J Biol Sci 2010;13(23):1135–40.

26. Clark TA, Heyliger CE, Kopilas M, et al. A tea/vanadate decoction delivered orally over 14 months to diabetic rats induces long-term glycemic stability without organ toxicity. Metabolism 2012;61(5):742–53.
27. Mazzaferro EM, Greco DS, Turner AS, et al. Treatment of feline diabetes mellitus using an alpha-glucosidase inhibitor and a low-carbohydrate diet. J Feline Med Surg 2003;5(3):183–9.
28. Singh R, Rand JS, Morton JM. Switching to an ultra-low carbohydrate diet has a similar effect on postprandial blood glucose concentrations to administering acarbose to healthy cats fed a high carbohydrate diet [abstract]. J Vet Intern Med 2006;20(3):726.
29. Rand JS. Feline diabetes mellitus. In: Mooney CT, Peterson ME, editors. BSAVA manual of canine and feline endocrinology. 4th edition. Quedgeley, UK: British Small Animal Vet Association; 2012. p. 133–47.
30. Behme MT, Dupré J, McDonald TJ. Glucagon-like peptide 1 improved glycemic control in type 1 diabetes. BMC Endocr Disord 2003;3(1):3.
31. Derosa G, Maffioli P. Dipeptidyl peptidase-4 inhibitors: 3 years of experience. Diabetes Technol Ther 2012;14(4):350–64.
32. Padrutt I, Zini E, Kaufman J, et al. Comparison of the GLP-1 analogues exenatide (short-acting), exenatide (long-acting) and the DPP-4 inhibitor Sitagliptin to increase insulin secretion in healthy cats [abstract]. J Vet Intern Med 2012;26: 1505–38.

New Incretin Hormonal Therapies in Humans Relevant to Diabetic Cats

Claudia E. Reusch, DVM, Dr Med Vet*, Isabelle Padrutt, DVM

KEYWORDS

- Cat • Feline • Diabetes mellitus • GLP-1 receptor agonist • DPP-4 inhibitor
- Exenatide • Sitagliptin

KEY POINTS

- In humans, glucagon-like peptide 1 (GLP-1) agonists and dipeptidylpeptidase-4 (DPP-4) inhibitors are novel therapeutic options for type 2 diabetes.
- Both classes enhance glucose-dependent insulin secretion, and reduce postprandial hyperglycemia and glucagon secretion.
- GLP-1 agonists additionally decelerate gastric emptying, induce satiety and weight loss, and may have beneficial effects on blood pressure.
- In cats, GLP-1 agonists and DPP-4 inhibitors have so far only been investigated in healthy individuals, resulting in a substantial increase in insulin secretion.
- Although results of clinical studies are not yet available and costs may currently be prohibitive, it is likely that incretin-based therapy opens up an important new area in feline diabetes.

Glucagon-like peptide 1 (GLP-1) receptor agonists and dipeptidylpeptidase-4 (DPP-4) inhibitors are relatively recently developed agents for the treatment of diabetes in humans. Because of the underlying mechanism, these agents are called incretin-based therapeutics.

In general terms, incretins are hormones released from the gastrointestinal tract during food intake, which potentiate insulin secretion from the β cells of the pancreas. As early as 1906 Moore and colleagues[1] demonstrated that the oral application of an extract of porcine duodenal mucous membrane was able to reduce glucosuria in patients with diabetes mellitus, in some of whom glucosuria even disappeared.[1] Thereafter, numerous investigators tried to unravel details on the gastrointestinal factors responsible for this phenomenon. The term "incretin" (derived from the Latin word *increscere*, to increase) was used for the first time by La Barre and Still[2] in

---

Vetsuisse Faculty, Department of Small Animals, Clinic for Small Animal Internal Medicine, Winterthurerstrasse 260, CH-8057 Zurich, Switzerland
* Corresponding author.
E-mail address: creusch@vetclinics.uzh.ch

Vet Clin Small Anim 43 (2013) 417–433
http://dx.doi.org/10.1016/j.cvsm.2012.11.003
0195-5616/13/$ – see front matter © 2013 Elsevier Inc. All rights reserved.

1930, although at that time they were not able to prove that incretins definitively exist. Progress on the incretin concept was made after radioimmunoassays for the measurement of insulin became available in 1960.[3] In the following years at least 3 research groups showed that glucose given orally induces a greater insulin response than glucose given intravenously, even if the blood-glucose concentrations were higher after intravenous injection.[4–6] The first incretin, called gastric inhibitory polypeptide (GIP), was isolated and sequenced in 1971,[7] followed by the characterization of the second incretin, GLP-1, in 1985.[8] It took approximately another 20 years until incretin-based therapeutics became available for clinical use. In 2005 the first GLP-1 receptor agonist (exenatide [Byetta]; Amylin Pharmaceuticals, San Diego, CA) and in 2007 the first DDP-4 inhibitor (sitagliptin [Januvia]; MSD, Whitehouse Station, NJ) were introduced as new classes of antidiabetic agents.

BIOSYNTHESIS, SECRETION, AND METABOLISM OF GLP-1 AND GIP

GLP-1 and GIP are encoded by different genes in mammalian genomes. The proglucagon gene encodes GLP-1, as well as the nonincretin peptide hormones glucagon and GLP-2. Gene distribution includes L cells in the intestinal tract with the highest density in the ileum and colon, α cells of the endocrine pancreas, and some neurons of the hypothalamus and the brain stem.[9–12] Proglucagon processing differs in the different tissues, which is largely due to the differential expression of prohormone convertase (PC) enzymes. Whereas α cells express PC2 and generate glucagon, L cells and brain express PC1/3 and produce GLP-1 and GLP-2 (**Fig. 1**).[13] Plasma levels of GLP-1 are low in the fasted state and increase within minutes after food intake, triggered by local luminal nutrient-sensing pathways and, possibly, additional endocrine and neural factors.[13,14] Various forms of GLP-1 exist. To date, GLP-1(7–37) and GLP-1(7–36) NH_2 are known to be the biologically active forms, in humans the latter being most abundant.[15] GLP-1 acts through binding to a G-protein–coupled receptor (GLP-1-1R), which is expressed in α cells and β cells of the pancreas, kidney, lung, heart, gastrointestinal tract, and various regions of the nervous system.[16] The half-life of biologically active GLP-1 is very short (less than 2 minutes). It is degraded by the enzyme

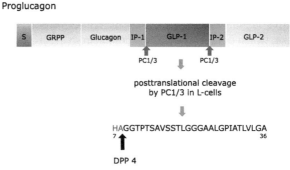

Fig. 1. Proglucagon and posttranslational cleavage of GLP-1 by prohormone convertase (PC) 1/3. GLP-1(7–36) is a major form of biologically active GLP-1 in humans. GRPP, glicentin-related pancreatic polypeptide; IP-1, IP-2, intervening peptides 1 and 2; S, signal peptide. (*Data from* Baggio LL, Drucker DJ. Islet amyloid polypeptide/GLP1/exendin. In: DeFronzo RA, Ferrannini E, Keen H, et al, editors. International textbook of diabetes mellitus. Chichester (UK): John Wiley & Sons Ltd; 2004. p. 191–223; and Kim W, Egan JM. The role of incretins in glucose homeostasis and diabetes treatment. Pharmacol Rev 2008;60:470–512.)

DPP-4, which cleaves off the 2 N-terminal residues of the GLP-1 molecule (see **Fig. 1**).[17] DPP-4 is widely expressed in many tissues as well as being present in soluble form in plasma. GIP is derived from the glucose-dependent insulinotropic polypeptide gene, the expression of which is restricted to the intestinal K cells, predominantly located in the duodenum.[11,12] As with GLP-1, food intake is the main stimulus for GIP secretion, which occurs within minutes. GIP is a 42-amino-acid peptide with a slightly longer half-life than that of GLP-1 (approximately 7 minutes in healthy humans).[9,18] GIP exerts its action through G-protein–coupled receptors distinct from the GLP-1 receptors. The GIP receptor is mainly expressed on β cells in the pancreas and, to a lesser extent, in adipose tissue and the central nervous system. Degradation is similar to degradation of GLP-1 by DPP-4.[16] Recently, the strict separation of production sites of GLP-1 and GIP in L cells and K cells has been challenged. Mortensen and colleagues[19] demonstrated that a subset of enteroendocrine cells coexpresses GIP and GLP-1 in the upper small intestine. This finding explains, at least in part, the close relationship between GIP and GLP-1 release.

BIOLOGICAL ACTIONS OF GLP-1 AND GIP

The incretin effect depends on the amount of glucose given, and accounts for 25% to 70% of the insulin secretion in healthy individuals. In functional terms GLP-1 and GIP are nearly identical in their capability to induce an insulin response, and in case of a loss they may compensate for each other.[12,20] However, on a molar basis GLP-1 is far more potent than GIP in stimulating insulin secretion.[21] The action of GLP-1 and GIP is highly glucose dependent, therefore hypoglycemia does not occur. Additional beneficial effects on β cells include stimulation of insulin biosynthesis and thereby replenishment of insulin stores, stimulation of β-cell proliferation, promotion of resistance to β-cell apoptosis, and enhanced β-cell survival.[22,23] GLP-1 but not GIP is also important for the control of fasting hyperglycemia; a lack of GLP-1 action leads to an increase in fasting blood glucose.[16]

GLP-1 also decreases blood glucose by inhibition of glucagon secretion from the α cells.[10] It is important that counterregulatory secretion of glucagon in the event of hypoglycemia is fully preserved even in the presence of a pharmacologic concentration of GLP-1.[16]

GLP-1 and GIP share the majority of effects on β cells. The main difference between the two is with regard to various extrapancreatic effects possessed by GLP-1 but not GIP (**Table 1**), the reason for which is the much wider tissue distribution of the GLP-1 receptors. Major extrapancreatic sites of GLP-1 actions are the gastrointestinal tract, the central nervous system and, possibly, the cardiovascular system. GLP-1 delays gastric emptying and decreases gastrointestinal motility; thereby the entry of nutrients into the circulation is decelerated and increase of blood glucose is attenuated. Important effects on the central nervous system are inhibition of food intake, induction of satiety, and weight loss.[10,16] Recently it has been suggested that GLP-1 has direct cardiovascular effects in addition to the well-known glucoregulatory actions. Such effects may include cardioprotection after ischemia-reperfusion injury, improvement of myocardial contractility, and vasorelaxant actions (**Fig. 2**).[24]

GLP-1 AND GIP IN HUMANS WITH TYPE 2 DIABETES MELLITUS

Type 2 diabetes mellitus is characterized by insulin resistance and β-cell dysfunction. It has been shown that the incretin effect is severely impaired in patients with type 2 diabetes and that this defect seems to play an important contributory role in the reduced secretion of insulin.[25,26]

Table 1
Comparison of GLP-1 receptor agonists and DPP-4 inhibitors

	GLP-1 Receptor Agonists	DPP-4 Inhibitors
Administration	Subcutaneous injection	Orally
Glucose-dependent insulin secretion	Enhanced	Enhanced
Glucose-dependent glucagon secretion	Reduced	Reduced
Postprandial hyperglycemia	Reduced	Reduced
Risk of hypoglycemia	Low	Low
Gastric emptying	Decelerated	No effect
Appetite	Suppressed	No effect
Satiety	Induced	No effect
Body weight	Reduced	Neutral
Main adverse effects	Nausea, vomiting	Headache, nasopharyngitis, urinary tract infection

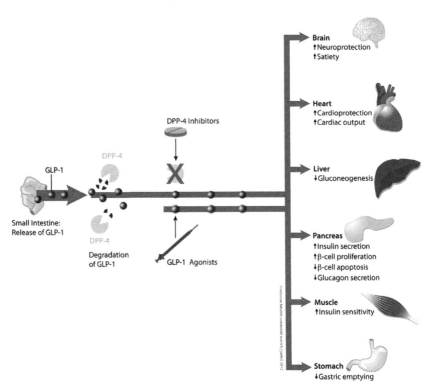

Fig. 2. Main actions of endogenous GLP-1 as well as of GLP-1 agonists in the different organs. The site and mode of action of DPP-4 and DPP-4 inhibitors are also given. (*Courtesy of* Diabetes Ratgeber; with permission. Available at: www.diabetes-ratgeber.net. Accessed June 10, 2012.)

Various studies have examined the secretion of GIP in response to oral glucose or mixed meals. Most investigators came to the conclusion that GIP concentrations are higher in patients with type 2 diabetes than in healthy controls. The overall difference was small, and in some studies not present at all.[27–30] The insulinotropic effect, however, seems to have been lost to a large extent. Insulin secretory response after application of exogenous GIP was greatly reduced, even if very high doses were given.[31] The exact mechanism is currently unknown; a GIP-receptor defect, however, seems unlikely.[32]

By contrast, the insulinotropic effect of GLP-1 is preserved in patients with type 2 diabetes. In comparison with healthy humans, however, impairment still seems to exist. At physiologic concentrations GLP-1 has little activity, and pharmacologic doses have to be used to achieve an insulinotropic effect.[25,30,32,33] As with GIP, secretion of GLP-1 has also been investigated following oral glucose loads or mixed meals. Although increased GLP-1 and normal GLP-1 concentrations have been found, most studies demonstrated small reductions in GLP-1 secretion. Impairment seems to be more pronounced in patients with poor metabolic control and long-standing diabetes.[30] The differences between the studies (ie, normal, decreased, increased GLP-1 concentrations) have been attributed to the influence of various factors, some of which (eg, higher body mass index) are associated with lower GLP-1 response, whereas others (eg, old age) are determinants of increased GLP-1 secretion.[34,35]

It has recently been shown that near-normalization of blood glucose improves the insulin response to GIP and GLP-1 by a factor of 3 to 4 in humans with type 2 diabetes. This finding suggests that the loss of the incretin effect may not be a primary defect but develops as a secondary phenomenon, possibly as a result of glucotoxicity.[36]

INCRETIN-BASED THERAPIES IN HUMANS

The discovery that GIP is ineffective, regardless of the dose, in individuals with type 2 diabetes has limited its use as a treatment modality. On the other hand, GLP-1 retains its stimulatory effect on insulin secretion and it also has beneficial effects on glucagon, gastric emptying, and satiety, which GIP lacks. Native GLP-1, however, is quickly degraded by the ubiquitous enzyme DPP-4. These findings have led to the development of GLP-1 agonists with resistance to degradation by DPP-4 and inhibitors of DPP-4 activity as therapeutic agents.[35] GLP-1 agonists are also called incretin mimetics, and DPP-4 inhibitors are known as incretin enhancers. Although both classes improve glycemic control, various differences exist between them (see **Table 1**). From a practical standpoint a major difference is the route of application: GLP-1 agonists have to be injected subcutaneously, whereas DPP-4 inhibitors are oral agents (see **Fig. 2**).

GLP-1 Receptor Agonists

Exenatide was the first GLP-1 receptor agonist to be used for the treatment of humans with type 2 diabetes. It was approved by the Food and Drug Administration in 2005, and released in Europe in 2007 under the name Byetta (Amylin Pharmaceuticals). Exenatide is the synthetic form of exendin-4, a peptide discovered in the saliva of the gila monster in 1992. It consists of 39 amino acids, with a 53% homology with human GLP-1.[37] Owing to an increased resistance to degradation by DPP-4, exenatide has a half-life of approximately 2.5 hours after subcutaneous injection. It is administered twice daily before morning and evening meals.

Exenatide has been investigated extensively under various circumstances in groups of patients with type 2 diabetes. Substantial improvement in glycemic control (reduced fasting and postprandial glucose concentration, reduced hemoglobin A1c [HbA1c] levels) and improved β-cell function (as evaluated by Homeostatic Model Assessment B) was demonstrated when exenatide was added to existing therapy (metformin, sulfonylurea, or thiazolidinedione) or used as monotherapy. Patients also experienced progressive and dose-dependent weight loss and a decrease in blood pressure.[38–42] When exenatide was compared with insulin glargine in patients who had not achieved glycemic control with metformin or sulfonylurea monotherapy, similar improvement in HbA1c was demonstrated. Exenatide therapy was associated with significant reductions in body weight and postprandial glucose excursions compared with insulin glargine, whereas insulin glargine led to a greater reduction in fasting blood glucose.[43] However, the question of whether switching from insulin to exenatide generally leads to equivalent glycemic control needs further study.[44] It has been shown that patients with longer diabetes duration and less endogenous β-cell function may experience deterioration in glycemic control if exenatide is substituted for insulin therapy.[45] Exenatide maintains its efficacy if treatment is continued long term. However, there are currently no clinical studies to confirm that exenatide therapy leads to protection and restoration of β-cell mass and function in humans. After cessation of exenatide given to type 2 diabetes patients for 52 weeks, β-cell function and glycemic control returned to pretreatment values, suggesting that continuous treatment is necessary to maintain the beneficial effects.[46]

Exenatide is not recommended for patients with severe kidney failure because it is mainly eliminated by glomerular filtration. In general, exenatide is well tolerated, and treatment discontinuation owing to adverse events is rare.[47] However, mild to moderate gastrointestinal symptoms such as nausea, vomiting, and diarrhea are common; for example, nausea has been reported in up to 50% of patients. Such events are usually transient and improve during the first 4 to 8 weeks of treatment.[47,48] Nausea and vomiting are dose dependent, and side effects may be ameliorated by gradual dose escalation.[49] There is some concern as to whether exenatide increases the risk of pancreatitis, although a causal relationship has not been established.[47,50] According to the prescribing information the drug should be discontinued immediately if pancreatitis is suspected, and should not be restarted if pancreatitis is confirmed. Other antidiabetic therapies should be considered in patients with a history of pancreatitis (www.byetta.com). There is also concern as to whether exenatide increases the risk of thyroid cancer.[51] Antibody development against exenatide is common, but except for some patients with very high titers there does not seem to be an effect on efficacy.[52] If exenatide is used as monotherapy or in combination with metformin, hypoglycemia is rare, which is consistent with the fact that its insulinotropic effect is glucose dependent.[44]

A few years after exenatide another GLP-1 agonist, liraglutide (Victoza; Novo Nordisk, Bagsvaerd, Denmark) was approved in Europe in 2009, and in the United States and Japan in 2010.[53] Liraglutide is the first human GLP-1 analogue and has 97% homology to the native GLP-1. To increase biological stability, a fatty acid side chain was added, which promotes binding to albumin, thereby increasing the half-life to 11 to 13 hours.[50] In clinical studies liraglutide was shown to be efficacious and safe, and provided improved glycemic control, improved β-cell function and weight loss, and decreased blood pressure and triglycerides with minimal risk of hypoglycemia when used as monotherapy or with other antidiabetic agents.[54,55] In a head-to-head study, liraglutide was superior to exenatide with regard to glycemic control; in addition, nausea and vomiting were less frequent with liraglutide and persisted for a shorter period of time.[56] Exenatide extended-release formulation is a new drug for once-weekly application (Bydureon; Amylin Pharmaceuticals), which was approved in Europe in summer 2011 and in the United States in January 2012. The formulation uses biodegradable microsphere technology to encapsulate the drug, enabling slow release into the circulation after subcutaneous injection.[57] The therapeutic range may be reached after 2 weeks, and after 6 to 7 weeks of treatment a steady state is achieved.[58] When exenatide extended-release was compared with exenatide twice-daily (Byetta), the once-weekly formulation resulted in significantly greater improvement in glycemic control and similar reductions in body weight, with no increased risk of hypoglycemia. Nausea and vomiting occurred less frequently with the extended-release formulation, whereas injection-site reactions were more common.[53,59,60] In comparative trials exenatide extended-release improved HbA1c to a greater extent than sitagliptin and insulin glargine; an additional difference in comparison with insulin-treated patients was weight gain in the latter and weight loss with exenatide extended-release.[61–63]

Various GLP-1 agonists are currently under investigation in the different phases of clinical trials, for example, lixisensatide (once daily), albiglutide (once weekly), dulaglutide (once weekly), and taspoglutide (once weekly, although clinical studies were stopped because of the high incidence of hypersensitivity reactions) (**Fig. 3**).

DPP-4 Inhibitors

Sitagliptin (Januvia; MSD) was the first DPP-4 inhibitor to become available for the treatment of human type 2 diabetes in the United States in 2007, followed soon by approval in other countries. Another DPP-4 inhibitor, vildagliptin (Galvus; Novartis, Basel, Switzerland) was released in Europe in 2008 and subsequently in many other

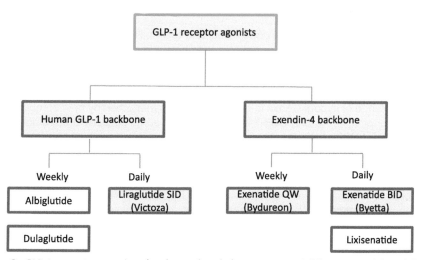

Fig. 3. GLP-1 receptor agonists that have already been approved (*blue rectangle*) and that are under investigation (*white rectangle*). The drugs are divided with regard to backbone (human or exendin-4) and frequency of application (daily or weekly). BID, twice a day; QW, once a week; SID, once a day. (*Adapted from* Madsbad S, Kielgast U, Asmar M, et al. An overview of once-weekly glucagon-like peptide-1 receptor agonists—available efficacy and safety data and perspectives for the future. Diabetes Obes Metab 2011;13:394–407; with permission.)

countries; however, it has not gained approval in the United States. More recently, additional DPP-4 inhibitors were marketed, such as saxagliptin (Onglyza; Bristol-Myers Squibb, New York, NY) and linagliptin (Tradjenta in the United States and Trajent in Europe; Boehringer Ingelheim, Ingelheim, Germany). Several DPP-4 inhibitors are currently in various phases of clinical development.[64]

DPP-4 inhibitors are given orally, either once or twice daily depending on the particular drug. These agents were shown to inhibit DPP-4 effectively and to lead to a 2- to 3-fold increase in postprandial GLP-1 concentrations compared with physiologic levels after food intake.[26,65] In patients with type 2 diabetes, it is noteworthy that infusion of GLP-1 in amounts equivalent to concentrations achieved by DPP-4 inhibition does not significantly increase insulin secretion. It has been suggested that the reason for the DPP-4 effectiveness despite only a modest increase in GLP-1 concentration lies in the restoration of the enteroinsular gradient of GLP-1; for example, stimulation of GLP-1 receptors in the enteric parasympathetic nervous system and activation of the hepatoportal glucose sensors.[50,66,67]

Comparisons between the various DPP-4 inhibitors showed that they are similar in efficacy and with regard to their adverse effects.[50] When given together with other antidiabetic drugs such as metformin, sulfonylureas, glitazones, and insulin, they effect further improvement in glycemic control, and they are also effective as monotherapy.[25,44] However, compared with metformin or sulfonylurea monotherapy, DPP-4 inhibitors are less efficient. DPP-4 inhibitors are also inferior to GLP-1 agonists with regard to glycemic control (ie, reducing HbA1c concentrations), which is most likely associated with GLP-1 concentrations being much lower with DPP-4 inhibitors than with GLP-1 agonists.[26,68] DPP-4 inhibitors (as well as GLP-1 agonists) reduce postprandial glucose to a greater extent than fasting glucose.[44]

DPP-4 inhibitors do not cause weight reduction but seem to be weight neutral. The different effect on body weight is one of the major differences between incretin mimetics and incretin enhancers. There appears to be no beneficial effect on blood pressure.[26]

DPP-4 inhibitors have shown good safety and tolerability profiles in clinical studies comprising several thousands of patients with type 2 diabetes.[26,69] Compared with the GLP-1 receptor agonists, the incidence of nausea and other gastrointestinal adverse effects is much lower. Treatment with DPP-4 inhibitors is associated with a slightly increased risk of nasopharyngitis, urinary tract infection, and headache.[70] The prevalence of hypoglycemia is low when used as monotherapy or in combination with metformin.[69,70] As with GLP-1 agonists, there is some concern about a potential association of DPP-4 inhibitors and pancreatitis; however, currently available studies did not identify an increased risk.[50]

There is also uncertainty with regard to other, nonincretin-related effects. DPP-4 is expressed on many cell types including T cells, where it was first described as a CD-26 receptor. It is involved in T-cell activation and possibly in macrophage-mediated inflammatory response.[71] Furthermore, DPP-4 has multiple substrates such as numerous neuropeptides, hormones, and chemokines.[64,72] Thus far there are no data to support that DPP-4 therapy is associated with adverse immune reactions or a negative impact of prolongation of other substrates.[64,65] There is agreement, however, that careful postmarketing surveillance and reassurance of safety in long-term clinical trials is required.[70,73]

DPP-4 inhibitors are approved either as monotherapy or in combination with other medications prescribed for type 2 diabetes (eg, metformin, sulfonylurea, glitazones). Recent developments are fixed combinations of a DPP-4 inhibitor and metformin; for example, sitagliptin and metformin is marketed as Janumet (MSD).

DIABETES MELLITUS IN CATS

Diabetes mellitus is one of the most common endocrinopathies in cats. Insulin is currently considered to be the mainstay of treatment and should be initiated as soon as possible after diagnosis. Although clinical remission can thereby be achieved in many cases,[74,75] insulin therapy harbors potential negative health effects such as hypoglycemia and weight gain.

Most cats are assumed to spontaneously develop a form of diabetes similar to human type 2 diabetes, therefore the same classes of hypoglycemic drugs can theoretically be administered (**Table 2**).

With the exception of sulfonylureas, however, these drugs have either not been investigated in diabetic cats (meglitinide, thiazolidinediones) or have been found to be unsuitable for use as a sole agent (biguanide and α-glucosidase inhibitors). Glipizide, a sulfonylurea, has been the most often used drug in this class in cats, but has shown to be successful in only 30% to 40% of affected cats.[76]

Based on the high similarity of feline diabetes to human type 2 diabetes, introducing incretins to the treatment of diabetic cats may have potential for a more efficient management of the disease. Information on its use in cats is scarce at present, and studies on their effects in diabetic cats are not available at this time.

INCRETIN SYSTEM IN THE CAT

In 1986, antigenic determinants of pancreatic proglucagon (GLP-1, glucagon, NH_2 terminus of glicentin) were immunohistochemically detected in canine and feline pancreas and gastrointestinal tracts. Proglucagons were identified in pancreatic tissue

Table 2 Drugs used for human type 2 diabetes		
Class	**Main Mode of Action**	**Main Site of Action**
Biguanides (metformin)	Reduce hepatic gluconeogenesis, increase insulin sensitivity	Liver, muscle, adipose tissue
Sulfonylureas	Enhance insulin secretion	β Cells
Nonsulfonylurea secretagogues (meglitinide)	Enhance insulin secretion	β Cells
Thiazolidinediones (glitazones)	Increase insulin sensitivity	Muscle, adipose tissue
α-Glucosidase inhibitors	Slow digestion of carbohydrates	Small intestine
GLP-1 receptor agonists	Enhance glucose-dependent insulin secretion, reduce glucagon secretion and postprandial hyperglycemia, decrease appetite and body weight, delay gastric emptying, induce satiety	β Cells, brain, heart, liver, muscle, stomach
DPP-4 inhibitors	Enhance glucose-dependent insulin secretion, reduce glucagon secretion and postprandial hyperglycemia	DPP-4 enzyme in tissue and plasma
Amylin analogues (pramlintide)	Suppress glucagon secretion, decrease appetite, delay gastric emptying	β Cells, brain, stomach

as well as in intestinal L cells and canine gastric A cells, and closely resembled those found in other mammals.[77] The GLP-1 hormone and its receptor are highly preserved across investigated species such as humans, rats, and mice (www.uniprot.org). To the authors' knowledge, the amino acid sequence of GLP-1 in cats has not been documented as yet.

As obligate carnivores, the natural diet of domestic cats consists mostly of protein and fat. Because carbohydrates only account for a minimal fraction of a feline natural meal, sugar sensing is redundant, a fact that is supported by the missing TiR2 sweet-taste receptor in cats.[78] This sweet-taste receptor in enteroendocrine K calls and L cells is one of the important factors in glucose sensing and incretin secretion in rodents and humans.[79]

The response of feline enteroendocrine cells to stimulus by different oral nutrients and the possible presence of an incretin effect have recently been investigated in healthy cats.[80] Results of this study showed that a larger amount of oral glucose administration was tolerated without development of hyperglycemia in comparison to intravenously infused glucose, thereby implying the existence of an incretin effect. Nonetheless, the glucose-dependent insulinotropic effect was shown to be much lower in cats than in other species, and GIP secretion was not stimulated by glucose. Ingestion of amino acids and lipids led to a rapid increase in GIP concentrations that exceeded the increase observed in other species. The influence of amino acids and lipids on GLP-1 secretion was similar to that in other species.

Further support of the theory of a functional incretin system in cats was provided by another study on the effects of oral glucose on GLP-1, insulin, and glucose in obese and lean cats. Insulin and GLP-1 concentrations rapidly increased after administration of oral glucose (2 g/kg) via a gastric tube in 9 healthy lean cats and 10 healthy obese cats. Areas under the curve (AUC) were significantly greater for glucose and insulin and significantly lower for GLP-1 in obese cats in comparison with lean cats.[81] These results are similar to the findings in human medicine whereby a suppressive effect of obesity on GLP-1 concentrations has been demonstrated. Although these insights show interesting aspects of the mode of action of incretins in cats, investigations are still in the early stages.

GLP-1 Receptor Agonists

The effects of the GLP-1 receptor agonist exenatide (Byetta) on insulin secretion have recently been evaluated in 2 studies on healthy cats.

Gilor and colleagues[82] studied the effect of exenatide during normoglycemia as well as during hyperglycemia in 9 healthy cats. Before the main experiment, blood-glucose levels were determined during an oral glucose tolerance test (oGTT). Thereafter, 2 iso-glycemic clamps were fixed in each cat on separate days (mimicking the glucose levels determined in the oGTT), one without prior treatment with exenatide and the other with exenatide (1 μg/kg subcutaneously).

To assess the effect of exenatide during normoglycemia, the glucose infusion was only started 2 hours after injection of exenatide. Insulin increased significantly within 15 minutes after exenatide injection, followed by a mild decrease in blood glucose and a return of insulin levels to baseline despite a continuous increase in exenatide concentrations. Hypoglycemia (54 mg/dL, 2.9 mmol/L) was seen in only 1 of the 9 cats. Subsequent glucose infusion during the clamp phase led to a significantly higher insulin AUC in cats with prior exenatide than in those without the drug. None of the cats showed any adverse reactions. The investigators concluded that exenatide has a glucose-dependent stimulatory effect on insulin secretion as well as a pronounced effect on insulin secretion during normoglycemia in cats.[82]

The authors previously compared the effects of exenatide with exenatide extended-release.[83] Because no data on dosages in cats were available, both formulations were used in a dose-escalation protocol and their influence on insulin secretion during a meal response test (MRT) was investigated. Exenatide extended-release was given to 3 cats at 40, 100, 200, and 400 μg/kg subcutaneously, with single injections each. Exenatide (Byetta) was administered to another 3 cats at dosages of 0.2, 0.5, 1, and 2 μg/kg subcutaneously for 5 consecutive days each. A washout period of 2 weeks between doses was allowed in both treatment groups. On day 5 of each treatment block, an MRT was performed with subsequent blood sampling over a period of 300 minutes. Insulin AUC of the MRT showed an increase of 127%, 169%, 178%, and 95% for exenatide extended-release and increases of 320%, 364%, 547%, and 198% for exenatide, compared with insulin AUC during MRT without administration of the drugs. Two cats of each treatment group showed gastrointestinal side effects (vomiting and diarrhea) for 1 to 3 days, irrespective of the administered drug and dose. General well-being and appetite were unaffected. The DPP-4 inhibitor sitagliptin was investigated during the same study. Comparing the 3 drugs with each other, exenatide (Byetta) most efficiently increased insulin secretion in healthy cats. Further investigations on the potential benefits of long-term administration of exenatide extended-release in cats are currently in progress.[83]

DPP-4 Inhibitors

The use of DPP-4 inhibitors in cats has been investigated in 2 studies to date. The DPP-4 inhibitor NVP-DPP728[84] was used in 12 healthy cats. In each cat, intravenous glucose tolerance tests (ivGTT) after injecting saline or NVP-DPP728 intravenously (0.5 mg/kg) or subcutaneously (1 mg/kg), and an MRT after injection of saline or

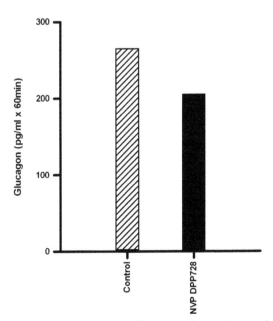

Fig. 4. The DPP-4 inhibitor NVP-DPP728 significantly reduced plasma glucagon in healthy cats, as assessed by the area under the curve 1 hour after the end of a meal. (*Adapted from* Furrer D, Kaufmann K, Tschuor F, et al. The dipeptidyl peptidase IV inhibitor NVP-DPP728 reduces plasma glucagon concentration in cats. Vet J 2010;183:355–7; with permission.)

NVP-DPP728 subcutaneously (2.5 mg/kg) were performed. The results showed a significant lowering effect of NVP-DPP728 on plasma glucagon concentrations during both ivGGT and MRT, and a significant increase of insulin secretion during ivGGT (**Fig. 4**).[85]

To further investigate the positive effects on glucagon and insulin secretion observed after the administration of the experimental NVP-DPP728 formulation, the authors recently used the DPP-4 inhibitor sitagliptin which, in contrast to NVP-DPP728, is administered orally. This route might be advantageous in facilitating therapy for some feline patients. Sitagliptin was applied in a dose-escalation study in 3 healthy cats at dosages of 1, 3, 5 and 10 mg/kg orally for 5 consecutive days each. Between all doses, a washout period of 2 weeks was instated. Insulin AUC during the MRT after each dose increased by 43%, 101%, 70%, and 56%, respectively, compared with insulin AUC during MRT without drug administration. Two cats showed gastrointestinal side effects (vomiting and diarrhea) of 1 to 3 days' duration, irrespective of the administered dose. General well-being and appetite were unaffected.[83]

To date no clinical trials in diabetic cats have been published, although work is in progress. Nonetheless, one clinical case recently showed a promising response. Sitagliptin monotherapy was given to a newly diagnosed diabetic cat in which insulin therapy was not an option for the owner. Soon after initiating therapy, clinical improvement as well as a reduction in fasting blood glucose and fructosamine concentrations was seen.

SUMMARY

In humans, GLP-1 agonists and DPP-4 inhibitors are novel therapeutic options for type 2 diabetes. Both classes enhance glucose-dependent insulin secretion, and reduce postprandial hyperglycemia and glucagon secretion. GLP-1 agonists additionally decelerate gastric emptying, induce satiety and weight loss, and may have beneficial effects on blood pressure. GLP-1 agonists are administered subcutaneously, mostly once or twice per day; however, extended-release formulations for once-weekly use recently became available. DPP-4 inhibitors are oral agents, given once or twice daily.

In cats, GLP-1 agonists and DPP-4 inhibitors have thus far only been investigated in healthy individuals, resulting in a substantial increase in insulin secretion. Although results of clinical studies are not yet available and costs may currently be prohibitive, it is likely that incretin-based therapy opens up an important new area in feline diabetes.

REFERENCES

1. Moore B, Edie ES, Abram JH. On the treatment of the diabetes mellitus by acid extract of duodenal mucous membrane. Biochem J 1906;1:28–38.
2. La Barre J, Still EU. Studies on the physiology of secretin. III. Further studies on the effects of secretin on the blood sugar. Am J Physiol 1930;91:649–53.
3. Yalow RS, Berson SA. Immunoassay of endogenous plasma insulin in man. J Clin Invest 1960 Jul;39:1157–75.
4. Elrick H, Stimmler L, Hlad CJ, et al. Plasma insulin response to oral and intravenous glucose administration. J Clin Endocrinol Metab 1964;24:1076–82.
5. McIntyre N, Holdsworth CD, Turner DS. New interpretation of oral glucose tolerance. Lancet 1964;2(7349):20–1.
6. Perley MJ, Kipnis DM. Plasma insulin responses to oral and intravenous glucose: studies in normal and diabetic subjects. J Clin Invest 1967;46(12):1954–62.

7. Brown JC, Dryburgh JR. A gastric inhibitory polypeptide. II. The complete amino acid sequence. Can J Biochem 1971;49(8):867–72.
8. Uttenthal LO, Ghiglione M, George SK, et al. Molecular forms of glucagon-like peptide-1 in human pancreas and glucagonomas. J Clin Endocrinol Metab 1985;61(3):472–9.
9. Baggio LL, Drucker DJ. Islet amyloid polypeptide/GLP1/exendin. In: DeFronzo RA, Ferrannini E, Keen H, et al, editors. International textbook of diabetes mellitus. Chichester (United Kingdom): John Wiley & Sons Ltd.; 2004. p. 191–223.
10. Drucker DJ. The biology of incretin hormones. Cell Metab 2006;3:153–65.
11. Irwin DM. Molecular evolution of mammalian incretin hormone genes. Regul Pept 2009;155(1–3):121–30.
12. Irwin DM, Prentice KJ. Incretin hormones and the expanding families of glucagon-like sequences and their receptors. Diabetes Obes Metab 2011; 13(Suppl 1):69–81.
13. Parker HE, Reimann F, Gribble FM. Molecular mechanisms underlying nutrient-stimulated incretin secretion. Expert Rev Mol Med 2010;12:1–17.
14. Nauck MA, Siemsglüss J, Orskov C, et al. Release of glucagon-like peptide 1 (GLP-1 (7-36 amide)), gastric inhibitory polypeptide (GIP) and insulin in response to oral glucose after upper and lower intestinal resections. Z Gastroenterol 1996; 34(3):159–66.
15. Orskov C, Rabenhoj L, Wettergren A, et al. Tissue and plasma concentrations of amidated and glycine-extended glucagon-like peptide I in humans. Diabetes 1994;43(4):535–9.
16. Drucker DJ, Nauck MA. The incretin system: glucagon-like peptide-1 receptor agonists and dipeptidyl peptidase-4 inhibitors in type 2 diabetes. Lancet 2006; 368:1696–705.
17. Koliaki C, Doupis J. Incretin-based therapy: a powerful and promising weapon in the treatment of type 2 diabetes mellitus. Diabetes Ther 2011;2(2):101–21.
18. Deacon CF, Nauck MA, Meier J, et al. Degradation of endogenous and exogenous gastric inhibitory polypeptide in healthy and in type 2 diabetic subjects as revealed using a new assay for the intact peptide. J Clin Endocrinol Metab 2000;85:3575–81.
19. Mortensen K, Petersen LL, Ørskov C. Colocalization of GLP-1 and GIP in human and porcine intestine. Ann N Y Acad Sci 2000;921:469–72.
20. Hansotia T, Baggio LL, Delmeire D, et al. Double incretin receptor knockout (DIRKO) mice reveal an essential role for the enteroinsular axis in transducing the glucoregulatory actions of DPP-IV inhibitors. Diabetes 2004;53(5):1326–35.
21. Kim W, Egan JM. The role of incretins in glucose homeostasis and diabetes treatment. Pharmacol Rev 2008;60:470–512.
22. Li Y, Hansotia T, Yusta B, et al. Glucagon-like peptide-1 receptor signaling modulates beta cell apoptosis. J Biol Chem 2003;278(1):471–8.
23. Farilla L, Bulotta A, Hirsberg B, et al. Glucagon-like peptide 1 inhibits cell apoptosis and improves glucose responsiveness of freshly isolated human islets. Endocrinology 2003;144(12):5149–58.
24. Treiman M, Elvekjær M, Engstrøm T, et al. Glucagon-like peptide 1—a cardiologic dimension. Trends Cardiovasc Med 2010;20(1):8–12.
25. Holst JJ, Vilsbøll T, Deacon CF. The incretin system and its role in type 2 diabetes mellitus. Mol Cell Endocrinol 2009;297:127–36.
26. Nauck MA. Incretin-based therapies for type 2 diabetes mellitus: properties, functions, and clinical implications. Am J Med 2011;124:3.

27. Ross SA, Brown JC, Dupré J. Hypersecretion of gastric inhibitory polypeptide following oral glucose in diabetes mellitus. Diabetes 1977;26(6):525–9.
28. Jones IR, Owens DR, Luzio S, et al. The glucose dependent insulinotropic poly-peptide response to oral glucose and mixed meals is increased in patients with type 2 (non-insulin-dependent) diabetes mellitus. Diabetologia 1989;32(9): 668–77.
29. Vilsbøll T, Krarup T, Deacon CF, et al. Reduced postprandial concentrations of intact biologically active glucagon-like peptide 1 in type 2 diabetic patients. Dia-betes 2001;50(3):609–13.
30. Meier JJ, Nauck MA. Is secretion of glucagon-like peptide-1 reduced in type 2 diabetes mellitus? Nat Clin Pract Endocrinol Metab 2008;4(11):606–7.
31. Nauck MA, Heimesaat MM, Orskow C, et al. Preserved incretin activity of glucagon-like peptide 1 [7-36 amide] but not of synthetic human gastric inhibitory polypeptide in patients with type-2 diabetes mellitus. J Clin Invest 1993;91(1): 301–7.
32. Nauck MA, Baller B, Meier JJ. Gastric inhibitory polypeptide and glucagon-like peptide-1 in the pathogenesis of type 2 diabetes. Diabetes 2004;53(Suppl 3): 190–6.
33. Nauck MA, Weber I, Bach I, et al. Normalization of fasting glycaemia by intrave-nous GLP-1 ([7-36 amide] or [7-37]) in type 2 diabetic patients. Diabet Med 1998; 15(11):937–45.
34. Nauck MA, Vardarli I, Deacon CF, et al. Secretion of glucagon-like peptide-1 (GLP-1) in type 2 diabetes: what is up, what is down? Diabetologia 2011;54:10–8.
35. Mudaliar S, Henry RR. The incretin hormones: from scientific discovery to prac-tical therapeutics. Diabetologia 2012;55:1865–8.
36. Højberg PV, Vilsbøll T, Rabøl R, et al. Four weeks of near-normalisation of blood glucose improves the insulin response to glucagon-like peptide-1 and glucose-dependent insulinotropic polypeptide in patients with type 2 diabetes. Diabetolo-gia 2009;52:199–207.
37. Eng J, Kleinman WA, Singh L, et al. Isolation and characterization of exendin-4, an exendin-3 analogue, from *Heloderma suspectum* venom. Further evidence for an exendin receptor on dispersed acini from guinea pig pancreas. J Biol Chem 1992;267:7402–5.
38. Buse JB, Henry RR, Han J, et al. Effects of exenatide (exendin-4) on glycemic control over 30 weeks in sulfonylurea-treated patients with type 2 diabetes. Dia-betes Care 2004;27(11):2628–35.
39. DeFronzo RA, Ratner RE, Han J, et al. Effects of exenatide (exendin-4) on glyce-mic control and weight over 30 weeks in metformin-treated patients with type 2 diabetes. Diabetes Care 2005;28(5):1092–100.
40. Kendall DM, Riddle MC, Rosenstock J, et al. Effects of exenatide (exendin-4) on glycemic control over 30 weeks in patients with type 2 diabetes treated with metformin and a sulfonylurea. Diabetes Care 2005;28(5):1083–91.
41. Zinman B, Hoogwerf BJ, Durán Garcia S, et al. The effect of adding exenatide to a thiazolidinedione in suboptimally controlled type 2 diabetes: a randomized trial. Ann Intern Med 2007;146(7):477–85.
42. Moretto TJ, Milton DR, Ridge TD, et al. Efficacy and tolerability of exenatide monotherapy over 24 weeks in antidiabetic drug-naive patients with type 2 dia-betes: a randomized, double-blind, placebo-controlled, parallel-group study. Clin Ther 2008;30(8):1448–60.
43. Barnett AH, Burger J, Johns D, et al. Tolerability and efficacy of exenatide and ti-trated insulin glargine in adult patients with type 2 diabetes previously uncontrolled

with metformin or a sulfonylurea: a multinational, randomized, open-label, two-period, crossover noninferiority trial. Clin Ther 2007;29(11):2333–48.

44. Mikhail N. Incretin mimetics and dipeptidyl peptidase 4 inhibitors in clinical trials for the treatment of type 2 diabetes. Expert Opin Investig Drugs 2008;17(6): 845–53.

45. Davis SN, Johns D, Maggs D, et al. Exploring the substitution of exenatide for insulin in patients with type 2 diabetes treated with insulin in combination with oral antidiabetes agents. Diabetes Care 2007;30(11):2767–72.

46. Bunck MC, Diamant M, Cornér A, et al. One-year treatment with exenatide improves beta-cell function, compared with insulin glargine, in metformin-treated type 2 diabetic patients: a randomized, controlled trial. Diabetes Care 2009;32(5):762–8.

47. Holst JJ, Madsbad S, Schmitz O. Non-insulin parental therapies. In: Holt RIG, Cockram CS, Flyvbjerg A, et al, editors. Textbook of diabetes. Chichester (United Kingdom): John Wiley & Sons Ltd.; 2010. p. 478–91.

48. Campbell RK. Clarifying the role of incretin-based therapies in the treatment of type 2 diabetes mellitus. Clin Ther 2011;33(5):511–27.

49. Fineman MS, Shen LZ, Taylor K, et al. Effectiveness of progressive dose-escalation of exenatide (exendin-4) in reducing dose-limiting side effects in subjects with type 2 diabetes. Diabetes Metab Res Rev 2004;20:411–7.

50. Phillips LK, Prins JB. Update on incretin hormones. Ann N Y Acad Sci 2012;00: 1–20.

51. Chiu WY, Shih SR, Tseng CH. A review on the association between glucagon-like peptide-1 receptor agonists and thyroid cancer. Exp Diabetes Res 2012;2012: 924168.

52. Fineman MS, Mace KF, Diamant M, et al. Clinical relevance of anti-exenatide anti-bodies: safety, efficacy and cross-reactivity with long-term treatment. Diabetes Obes Metab 2012;14(6):546–54.

53. Madsbad S, Kielgast U, Asmar M, et al. An overview of once-weekly glucagon-like peptide-1 receptor agonists—available efficacy and safety data and perspectives for the future. Diabetes Obes Metab 2011;13:394–407.

54. McGill JB. Insights from the liraglutide clinical development program—the liraglutide effect and action in diabetes (LEAD) studies. Postgrad Med 2009;121(3): 16–25.

55. Gallwitz B. Glucagon-like peptide-1 analogues for type 2 diabetes mellitus. Drugs 2011;71(13):1675–88.

56. Buse JB, Rosenstock J, Sesti G, et al. Liraglutide once a day versus exenatide twice a day for type 2 diabetes: a 26-week randomised, parallel-group, multinational open-label trial (LEAD-6). Lancet 2009;374(9683):39–47.

57. Murphy CE. Review of the safety and efficacy of exenatide once weekly for the treatment of type 2 diabetes mellitus. Ann Pharmacother 2012;46(6):812–21.

58. Kim D, MacConell L, Zhuang D, et al. Effects of once-weekly dosing of a long-acting release formulation of exenatide on glucose control and body weight in subjects with type 2 diabetes. Diabetes Care 2007;30(6):1487–93.

59. Drucker DJ, Buse JB, Taylor K, et al. Exenatide once weekly versus twice daily for the treatment of type 2 diabetes: a randomised, open-label, non-inferiority study. Lancet 2008;372:1240–50.

60. Blevins T, Pullman J, Malloy J, et al. DURATION-5: exenatide once weekly resulted in greater improvements in glycemic control compared with exenatide twice daily in patients with type 2 diabetes. J Clin Endocrinol Metab 2011; 96(5):1301–10.

61. Bergenstal RM, Wysham C, Macconell L, et al. Efficacy and safety of exenatide once weekly versus sitagliptin or pioglitazone as an adjunct to metformin for treatment of type 2 diabetes (DURATION-2): a randomised trial. Lancet 2010; 376(9739):431–9.

62. DeYoung MB, MacConell L, Sarin V, et al. Encapsulation of exenatide in poly-(D, L-lactide-co-glycolide) microspheres produced an investigational long-acting once-weekly formulation for type 2 diabetes. Diabetes Technol Ther 2011; 13(11):1145–54.

63. Diamant M, Van Gaal L, Stranks S, et al. Safety and efficacy of once-weekly exenatide compared with insulin glargine titrated to target in patients with type 2 diabetes over 84 weeks. Diabetes Care 2012;35(4):683–9.

64. Kirby M, Yu DM, O'Connor SP, et al. Inhibitor selectivity in the clinical application of dipeptidyl peptidase-4 inhibition. Clin Sci 2010;118:31–41.

65. Gallwitz B. GLP-1 agonists and dipeptidyl-peptidase IV inhibitors. In: Gallwitz B, editor. Diabetes—perspectives in drug therapy, handbook of experimental pharmacology 203. Berlin: Springer Verlag; 2011. p. 53–74.

66. Burcelin R, Da Costa A, Drucker D, et al. Glucose competence of the hepatoportal vein sensor requires the presence of an activated glucagon-like peptide-1 receptor. Diabetes 2001;50(8):1720–8.

67. Hiøllund KR, Deacon CF, Holst JJ. Dipeptidyl peptidase-4 inhibition increases portal concentrations of intact glucagon-like peptide-1 (GLP-1) to a greater extent than peripheral concentrations in anaesthetised pigs. Diabetologia 2011; 54(8):2206–8.

68. Karagiannis T, Paschos P, Paletas K, et al. Dipetidyl peptidase-4 inhibitors for treatment of type 2 diabetes mellitus in the clinical setting: systematic review and meta-analysis. BMJ 2012;344:e1369, 1–15.

69. Reid T. Choosing GLP-1 receptor agonists or DPP-4 inhibitors: weighing the clinical trial evidence. Clin Diabetes 2012;30(1):3–12.

70. Amori RE, Lau J, Pittas AG. Efficacy and safety of incretin therapy in type 2 diabetes. J Am Med Assoc 2007;298(2):194–206.

71. TA NN, Li Y, Schuyler CA, et al. DPP-4 (CD26) inhibitor alogliptin inhibits TLR4-mediated ERK activation and ERK-dependent MMP-1 expression by U937 histiocytes. Atherosclerosis 2010;213(2):429–35.

72. Mentlein R. Dipeptidyl-peptidase IV (CD26)—role in the inactivation of regulatory peptides. Regul Pept 1999;85(1):9–24.

73. Mikhail N. Safety of dipeptidyl peptidase 4 inhibitors for treatment of type 2 diabetes. In: Dodd S, editor. Current drug safety. 2011 Nov 1;6(5):304–9. Oak Park (IL): Bentham Science Publishers.

74. Roomp K, Rand J. Intensive blood glucose control is safe and effective in diabetic cats using home monitoring and treatment with glargine. J Feline Med Surg 2009; 11(8):668–82.

75. Zini E, Hafner M, Osto M, et al. Predictors of clinical remission in cats with diabetes mellitus. J Vet Intern Med 2010;24(6):1314–21.

76. Reusch CE, Robben JH, Kooistra HS. Endocrine pancreas. In: Rijnberk A, Kooistra HS, editors. Clinical endocrinology of dogs and cats. An illustrated text. Second, revised and extended edition. Hannover (Germany): Schlütersche; 2010. p. 155–74.

77. Vaillant CR, Lund PK. Distribution of glucagon-like peptide I in canine and feline pancreas and gastrointestinal tract. J Histochem Cytochem 1986;34(9):1117–21.

78. Li X, Li W, Wang H, et al. Cats lack a sweet taste receptor. J Nutr 2006;136(Suppl 7): 1932–4.

79. Reimann F, Habib AM, Tolhurst G, et al. Glucose sensing in L cells: a primary cell study. Cell Metab 2008;8(6):532–9.
80. Gilor C, Graves TK, Gilor S, et al. The incretin effect in cats: comparison between oral glucose, lipids, and amino acids. Domest Anim Endocrinol 2011;40:205–12.
81. Hoenig M, Jordan ET, Ferguson DC, et al. Oral glucose leads to a differential response in glucose, insulin, and GLP-1 in lean versus obese cats. Domest Anim Endocrinol 2010;38:95–102.
82. Gilor C, Graves TK, Gilor S, et al. The GLP-1 mimetic exenatide potentiates insulin secretion in healthy cats. Domest Anim Endocrinol 2011;41:42–9.
83. Padrutt I, Zini E, Kaufmann K, et al. Comparison of the GLP-1 analogues exenatide short-acting, exenatide long-acting and the DPP-4 inhibitor sitagliptin to increase insulin secretion in healthy cats. J Vet Intern Med 2012;26:1505–38. Abstract at ECVIM-CA Congress 2012.
84. Hughes TE, Mone MD, Russell ME, et al. NVP-DPP728 (1-[[[2-[(5-cyanopyridin-2-yl)amino]ethyl]amino]acetyl]-2cyano-(S)-pyrrolidine), a slow-binding inhibitor of dipeptidyl peptidase IV. Biochemistry 1999;38(36):11597–603.
85. Furrer D, Kaufmann K, Tschuor F, et al. The dipeptidyl peptidase IV inhibitor NVP-DPP728 reduces plasma glucagon concentration in cats. Vet J 2010;183:355–7.

Index

Note: Page numbers of article titles are in **boldface** type.

A

Abdominal pain
  pancreatitis in feline diabetics and
    management of, 311–312
Acromegaly
  feline
    pathogenesis of, 227
  hypersomatotropism and, 320
  long-acting insulins in feline diabetes management and, 262
ACTH stimulation test
  in hyperadrenocorticism diagnosis, 338
Adrenalectomy
  unilateral or bilateral
    in hyperadrenocorticism management, 345–346
Antibiotic(s)
  in pancreatitis management in feline diabetics, 312
Azotemia
  in diabetes mellitus
    diabetic nephropathy due to
      in cats, 359–360
      in humans, 359

B

Biguanides
  in feline diabetics, 410–411
Blood glucose monitoring
  in feline diabetics
    home-based, **283–301**. *See also* Home blood glucose monitoring, in feline diabetics

C

Cat(s)
  acromegaly in
    pathogenesis of, 227
  continuous glucose monitoring in, **381–406**
  diabetes in. *See* Diabetes mellitus, feline
  diabetic nephropathy in, **351–365**. *See also* Diabetic nephropathy, feline
  diabetic remission in, **245–249**. *See also* Diabetic remission, feline
  hyperadrenocorticism in, **330–346**. *See also* Hyperadrenocorticism, feline
  hypersomatotropism in, **319–330**. *See also* Hypersomatotropism, feline
  incretin system in, 425–426

Vet Clin Small Anim 43 (2013) 435–445
http://dx.doi.org/10.1016/S0195-5616(13)00038-7
0195-5616/13/$ – see front matter © 2013 Elsevier Inc. All rights reserved.

Moving?

Make sure your subscription moves with you!

To notify us of your new address, find your **Clinics Account Number** (located on your mailing label above your name), and contact customer service at:

Email: journalscustomerservice-usa@elsevier.com

800-654-2452 (subscribers in the U.S. & Canada)
314-447-8871 (subscribers outside of the U.S. & Canada)

Fax number: 314-447-8029

**Elsevier Health Sciences Division
Subscription Customer Service
3251 Riverport Lane
Maryland Heights, MO 63043**

*To ensure uninterrupted delivery of your subscription, please notify us at least 4 weeks in advance of move.

Printed and bound by CPI Group (UK) Ltd, Croydon, CR0 4YY

03/10/2024

01040443-0003